MW00460914

METHODS IN SOCIAL NEUROSCIENCE

Methods in Social Neuroscience

edited by
Eddie Harmon-Jones
Jennifer S. Beer

THE GUILFORD PRESS
New York   London

© 2009 The Guilford Press
A Division of Guilford Publications, Inc.
72 Spring Street, New York, NY 10012
www.guilford.com

Printed in the United States of America

This book is printed on acid-free paper.

Last digit is print number: 9   8   7   6   5   4   3   2   1

Library of Congress Cataloging-in-Publication Data

Methods in social neuroscience / edited by Eddie Harmon-Jones, Jennifer S.
Beer.
     p. ; cm.
   Includes bibliographical references and index.
   ISBN 978-1-60623-040-4 (hardcover: alk. paper)
   1. Neuropsychology.   2. Social psychology.   3. Personality and
cognition.   I. Harmon-Jones, Eddie.   II. Beer, Jennifer S., 1974–
   [DNLM: 1. Neuropsychology. 2. Social Behavior. 3. Nervous System
Physiology. WL 103.5 M5928 2009]
   QP360.M383 2009
   612.8′2—dc22

                                                                2008036611

To Cindy, Sylvia, and Leon—
Words cannot adequately express my gratitude
for all you have done and continue to do for me.
—EDDIE HARMON-JONES

To Mom and Dad—Thanks for tolerating
all of those "science experiments."
—JENNIFER S. BEER

About the Editors

Eddie Harmon-Jones, PhD, is Professor of Psychology at Texas A&M University. His research focuses on emotions and motivations, their implications for social processes and behaviors, and their underlying neural circuits. His research has been supported by the National Institute of Mental Health, the National Science Foundation, and the Fetzer Institute. Dr. Harmon-Jones coedited, with Judson Mills, *Cognitive Dissonance: Progress on a Pivotal Theory in Social Psychology* (1999, American Psychological Association) and, with Piotr Winkielman, *Social Neuroscience: Integrating Biological and Psychological Explanations of Social Behavior* (2007, Guilford Press). In 2002 he received the Award for Distinguished Early Career Contribution to Psychophysiology from the Society for Psychophysiological Research. He has also served as an associate editor of the *Journal of Personality and Social Psychology* and is on the editorial boards of five other journals.

Jennifer S. Beer, PhD, is Assistant Professor of Psychology and a faculty member in the Institute for Neuroscience at the University of Texas at Austin. Her research adopts lesion and functional magnetic resonance imaging methodologies to examine self-regulation of social behavior. Dr. Beer serves on the editorial boards of the *Journal of Personality and Social Psychology, Frontiers in Neuroscience, Social Cognition, Emotion,* and *Social, Cognitive, and Affective Neuroscience.* Additionally, she has provided service to the field of social neuroscience as a reviewer for the National Science Foundation (United States), the Economic and Social Research Council (United Kingdom), and the VENI Innovational Research Incentive Scheme (The Netherlands), and as a course instructor for training institutes in the United States and Europe.

Contributors

David M. Amodio, PhD, Department of Psychology, New York University, New York, New York

Bruce D. Bartholow, PhD, Department of Psychological Sciences, University of Missouri, Columbia, Missouri

Jennifer S. Beer, PhD, Department of Psychology, University of Texas at Austin, Austin, Texas

Terry D. Blumenthal, PhD, Department of Psychology, Wake Forest University, Winston-Salem, North Carolina

Turhan Canli, PhD, Graduate Program in Genetics and Department of Psychology, Stony Brook University, Stony Brook, New York

Joseph C. Franklin, BA, Clinical Psychology Program, Department of Psychology, University of North Carolina, Chapel Hill, North Carolina

Cindy Harmon-Jones, BS, Department of Psychology, Texas A&M University, College Station, Texas

Eddie Harmon-Jones, PhD, Department of Psychology, Texas A&M University, College Station, Texas

Ursula Hess, PhD, Department of Psychology, University of Quebec, Montreal, Quebec, Canada

Tom Johnstone, PhD, School of Psychology, University of Reading, Reading, United Kingdom

M. Justin Kim, MA, Department of Psychological and Brain Sciences, Dartmouth College, Hanover, New Hampshire

Wendy Berry Mendes, PhD, Department of Psychology, Harvard University, Cambridge, Massachusetts

Brian M. Monroe, PhD, Department of Psychology, University of Southern California, Los Angeles, California

Carly K. Peterson, BA, Department of Psychology, Texas A&M University, College Station, Texas

Stephen J. Read, PhD, Department of Psychology, University of Southern California, Los Angeles, California

Oliver C. Schultheiss, DrPhil, Department of Psychology and Sport Sciences, Friedrich-Alexander University, Erlangen, Germany

Dennis J. L. G. Schutter, PhD, Department of Experimental Psychology, Utrecht University, Utrecht, The Netherlands

Steven J. Stanton, PhD, Center for Cognitive Neuroscience, Duke University, Durham, North Carolina

Jack van Honk, PhD, Department of Experimental Psychology, Utrecht University, Utrecht, The Netherlands

Paul J. Whalen, PhD, Department of Psychological and Brain Sciences, Dartmouth College, Hanover, New Hampshire

Contents

1

Introduction to Social and Personality Neuroscience Methods

Eddie Harmon-Jones
Jennifer S. Beer

We are in the midst of an exciting time for the study of social and personality neuroscience. The explosion of interest in this area is reflected in new graduate programs, as well as books summarizing research programs (e.g., Cacioppo, Visser, & Pickett, 2006; Frith & Wolpert, 2004; Harmon-Jones & Winkielman, 2007). It is also reflected in special issues of different journals: *Biological Psychiatry* (Insel, 2002), *Journal of Personality and Social Psychology* (Harmon-Jones & Devine, 2003), *Neuropsychologia* (Adolphs, 2003), *Political Psychology* (Cacioppo & Visser, 2003), *Journal of Cognitive Neuroscience* (Heatherton, 2004), *NeuroImage* (Lieberman, 2005), and *Brain Research* (Beer, Mitchell, & Ochsner, 2006). However, no previous book has provided coverage of the wide array of methods used in neurobiological approaches to social and personality psychology. We believe that a book providing information on how to use the various methods will assist in the growth of this important field. We also hope that this book will serve as a primer to social and personality neuroscience methods, and consequently that it will be used in upper-level undergraduate and graduate courses.

1

In assembling the authors for this edited volume, we invited individuals who have published much research using their particular methodologies, and who have been very "hands-on" users of their methodologies. We feel fortunate to have assembled such a distinguished group of authors. In each chapter, the author or authors introduce their method, provide social and/or personality examples of their method, include concrete experimental design considerations, and provide a discussion of the method's advantages and disadvantages for studying social and personality questions. Consequently, we believe that the chapters will serve as useful tools for individuals planning to use one or more of the methods, or for individuals who simply want to know more about the proper techniques for collecting or manipulating the various neuroscience variables.

What Is Social and Personality Neuroscience?

"Social psychology" is often defined as the scientific study of how the thoughts, feelings, and behaviors of an individual are influenced by the actual, imagined, or implied presence of others. Traditionally, social psychologists have been interested in examining such topics as interpersonal attraction, close relationships, attitudes, prejudice and stereotyping, aggression, helping behavior, person perception, and so on. "Personality psychology" is the scientific study of how dispositional aspects of the individual influence his or her thoughts, feelings, and behavior. Personality psychologists often study the same topics as social psychologists, but from the starting point of the individual rather than the situation.

Historically, these two fields of scientific endeavor have shared much overlap, as recognized by such prominent journals as the *Journal of Personality and Social Psychology* and *Personality and Social Psychology Bulletin*. Moreover, many investigators utilize both approaches in their attempts to understand human behavior, leading to the familiar expression "trait [personality] × state [social] interactions." That is, many studies examine how individuals with differing personality characteristics respond in different ways to specific social situations.

In the last decade or so, there has been a veritable explosion of interest in understanding the neurobiological substrates and correlates of social and personality processes and behaviors. This new approach, "social and personality neuroscience," emphasizes the relationships among different levels of organization—from the molecule to the cell to the organ, system, person, interpersonal, social group, and societal levels. This multilevel analytical approach, it is hoped, will lead to an increased understanding of the human mind and behavior.

To our knowledge, however, no previous volume has given detailed descriptions of the methods used. The current book fills this important gap. By providing specific details regarding data collection and experimental design, this book presents information that is not covered in journal articles or previously published chapters. Moreover, the current volume integrates discussions of many different neuroscience methods into one convenient source.

Advantages of Social and Personality Neuroscience Methods

The appeal of neuroscience methods for social and personality psychology is clear (Harmon-Jones & Winkielman, 2007): Humans can be noninvasively monitored in various situations. This monitoring of neurobiological responses as a function of social and personality variables can inform basic neuroscientific research and theory, by pointing to the importance of self-representations and social situations (from context to culture) in altering neural, hormonal, and immunological processes. On the other hand, neuroscientific research and theory can inform social and personality psychology. The integration of neuroscience into social and personality psychology allows researchers to use what is known about neuroscience to test predicted processes underlying social phenomena. These tests may provide information that would be impossible to gather with other techniques. By applying knowledge of brain and body gained from neuroscience, researchers may develop new theories of how basic mechanisms interact to produce social and personality phenomena.

In a nutshell, neuroscience methods are invaluable for social and personality psychology, because an appreciation of the underlying biological and chemical processes will lead to a more complete understanding of psychological and behavioral processes. Being a well-trained psychological neuroscientist is much like being a well-trained automobile mechanic. The automobile can be understood at one level by observing its behaviors: It accelerates, decelerates, stops, turns to the left or the right, and so on. It can also be understood at another level by reading its gauges: The speedometer provides an index of how fast the auto is moving; the water temperature gauge indicates the temperature of the coolant circulating through the radiator; the fuel gauge indicates how much fuel is in the fuel tank; and so forth. Or the automobile can be understood through knowledge of the underlying processes that drive the outward behaviors and gauge reports. That is, the automobile's movement can be seen as the result of an internal combustion engine that uses the combustion of fuel and air in a confined space to create gases at high temperature and pressure, which are permitted to expand. The expanding hot gases cause movement of solid parts of the engine, by acting on pistons, rotors, and so on. The engine's action turns the driveshaft, which sets the automobile in motion. Of course, the details of the automobile process are much more complicated and also involve electricity, spark plugs, timing belts, coolants, oil, grease, and other materials and mechanisms. The point of this analogy is that to fully understand behavior and psychology, researchers need to "get under the hood." But knowing the outward behaviors and gauge reports will assist them in knowing where to look under the hood. For example, knowing that an automobile's overheating is probably due to problems with the radiator, thermostat, or hoses will make repairs go more quickly and cost less. Similarly, fuel efficiency and speed are behaviors of the automobile, and improving either of these will require knowledge of the operations under the hood. In other words, for a more complete understanding of human behavior, psychology needs neuroscience, and neuroscience needs psychology.

Considerations for Using Neuroscience Methods

Just as social and personality psychologists must sometimes measure their phenomena in roundabout methodologies, social and personality neuroscientists must measure neurobiological processes through skin and skull. Of course, direct recordings from human brain cells are occasionally used, but these are invasive and limited to testing of individuals undergoing brain surgery for significant medical matters. Also, some social and personality neuroscience research is conducted on nonhuman animals, and more invasive methods are permitted in animal research. However, most social and personality neuroscience studies involve intact humans and are thus noninvasive.

In addition, no single technique can measure all biological activities with excellent spatial and temporal resolution. That is, no one measure of brain function captures neuronal activity as it unfolds on the order of milliseconds or nanoseconds (temporal resolution), or can specify exactly which neurons are activated on the order of millimeters or nanometers (spatial resolution). Among the noninvasive measures typically used in research with humans, event-related potentials (ERPs) are often lauded for their excellent temporal resolution (milliseconds) but damned for their poor spatial resolution (centimeters). Functional magnetic resonance imaging (fMRI), on the other hand, is praised for its excellent spatial resolution (millimeters) but condemned for its poor temporal resolution (seconds).

Concerns with the drawing of causal inferences also appear in discussions of social and personality neuroscience methods. Measures of brain activations obtained from ERPs or fMRI are essentially correlational, in that a psychological state is manipulated and the brain activation is measured. From this type of experimental design, it is impossible to determine whether the brain activation was necessarily or sufficiently responsible for the psychological or behavioral effect. Thus other neuroscience methods are needed to establish causality more firmly. Patient methods can assist in this endeavor, as the psychological task performance of individuals who have suffered damage to one brain region can be compared to that of individuals who have suffered damage to another brain region on psychological tasks. If the groups differ in their performance, then the difference is probably due to processes supported by that specific brain region.

Likewise, repetitive transcranial magnetic stimulation (rTMS) can be used to increase or decrease neuronal activity temporarily and noninvasively over particular cortical areas. This approach permits causal statements about the role of particular cortical regions in particular psychological or behavioral outcomes. However, both patient and rTMS methods are limited. With patients, the lesions often involve a number of brain regions. With rTMS, the "virtual lesions" cannot penetrate too deeply into the brain, and the spatial resolution of the method is not very precise.

The same holds true for examinations of hormones. Many studies have manipulated or measured psychological variables and then related these variables to hormone responses. Greater causal certainty can be obtained, however, with manipulations of hormones. The chapters contained within this book illustrate the benefits of both types of approaches.

Overview of Chapters

In Chapter 2, Cindy Harmon-Jones joins us in providing practical advice about how to form collaborations across the fields of social–personality psychology and neuroscience. Because of the increased use of multiple neuroscience methods in social and personality neuroscience, this chapter is not only relevant to the behavioral scientist who plans to collaborate with a neuroscientist; it is also relevant for the neuroscientist with one set of tools who plans to collaborate with another neuroscientist with another set of tools. Because of their interdisciplinary nature, psychology–neuroscience collaborations contain the potential for great research, but also for great misunderstanding. The chapter provides insight into a number of questions that are likely to come up in initial discussions, and also frames reasonable expectations for how cross-discipline collaborations are likely to be implemented in a practical sense.

In Chapter 3, Oliver C. Schultheiss and Steven J. Stanton provide an excellent discussion of the details involved in the assessment of salivary hormones. Hormones exert lasting influences on the organism during development or during periods of hormonal flux, such as puberty. They also exert psychological and behavioral effects temporarily, without effecting lasting changes, as when peaking estradiol levels cause women to become more sensitive to sexual stimuli. In addition to reviewing research findings relevant to social and personality psychology, Schultheiss and Stanton provide a guided tour of collecting saliva samples from participants, and then assaying the samples to provide specific, sensitive, accurate, and reliable measurements of hormones. They also address important issues that arise in data analyses of hormones. They finish the chapter by discussing important guidelines for reporting hormone results, and the advantages and disadvantages of salivary hormone measures.

Jack van Honk, in Chapter 4, reviews the research literature and methodology of hormone manipulation. His review covers the manipulation of four sex hormones—estradiol, testosterone, vasopressin, and oxytocin—and these hormones' interactions with each other. Moreover, he discusses how these various hormones influence brain systems involved in social and personality psychological processes related to aggression, anxiety, love, and theory of mind. Throughout the chapter, he notes that the relationships between hormones and human behavior are intricate and implicit, and thus have properties that may be difficult to assess with self-reports.

In Chapter 5, Ursula Hess describes the methods underlying recording of electromyography (EMG), which is a measure of the electrical activity generated during muscle contraction. Often used in social and personality psychological studies to measure facial muscle activity, EMG is typically recorded noninvasively from the surface of the skin and can provide measurement of fleeting and subtle movements that often escape the naked eye. Hess reviews details regarding the recording of the signal, such as placing electrodes properly and handling ambient electrical noise. She then discusses several important methodological considerations (baselines, communication from subject to experimenter, artifact removal); reviews ways of analyzing the EMG data; and finally provides several research examples for social–personality psychology related to mimicry, prejudice, and emotion.

Terry D. Blumenthal and Joseph C. Franklin, in Chapter 6, discuss the startle eyeblink response, which is a defensive response that occurs in response to sudden and intense external stimulation (e.g., a loud noise).

As Blumenthal and Franklin note, the anatomy and chemistry underlying the startle eyeblink have been well identified in animal research, and as such the measure can be used to index neurological functioning in various areas, including the brainstem, limbic system, and frontostriatal areas. In addition to presenting details on measuring this response, they review the findings of research using this method in social and personality psychology, and consider important issues in experimental design.

In Chapter 7, Wendy Berry Mendes covers the methodologies surrounding measurement of autonomic nervous system (ANS) activity in social and personality psychology. Because ANS responses can indicate changes in emotion, motivation, attention, and preferences, measures of these responses have been widely used in social and personality psychology, as Mendes reviews. In particular, Mendes focuses on electrodermal activity, cardiovascular activity (e.g., heart rate variability, respiration, and cardiac output), and blood pressure responses. She discusses issues related to measuring, scoring, editing, and interpreting these responses. She ends by discussing several important future directions for ANS research, such as research aimed at examining the dynamic nature of ANS changes during ambulatory monitoring of responses during individuals' daily lives.

Jennifer S. Beer begins Chapter 8 with a discussion of how studies of patients can help social and personality psychologists (1) by enabling them to clarify the relation between physical and psychological deficits, and (2) by permitting the manipulation of psychological variables that are otherwise difficult to control in an experimental setting. The chapter then considers the practical concerns of categorization, capability, comorbidity, availability, and control when researchers are designing patient studies. The final section then grounds these principles in the specific examples of designing studies of patients with lesions, patients with psychiatric disorders, or patients with neurological disorders.

In Chapter 9, Eddie Harmon-Jones and Carly K. Peterson provide details regarding electroencephalography (EEG), which is electrical activity generated by the brain and recorded from the scalp. The two most common methods of processing EEG are temporal analyses and frequency analyses. Chapter 10, by Bartholow and Amodio, covers temporal analyses (see below); the chapter by Harmon-Jones and Peterson covers frequency analysis. It involves decomposing the complex EEG signal into its underlying frequencies (cycles per second) and assessing how activity in different frequency bands (e.g., alpha) over different brain regions relate to psychological phenomena. After describing the physiology underlying the EEG, they provide practical details concerning the collection of EEG signals and the preparation of the participant. Then they describe methods of handling artifacts, as well as data-processing issues (e.g., frequency analyses). Finally, they provide some research examples and discuss how EEG compares to other brain imaging methods.

In Chapter 10, Bruce D. Bartholow and David M. Amodio cover ERPs, which are indices of brain activity derived from examining the temporal or time-dependent properties of the EEG. As we have noted earlier, ERPs are especially noteworthy for their ability to measure changes in brain function on the order of milliseconds. The chapter provides lucid discussions of the measurement of ERPs, ways of interpreting ERP data, and examples of using ERPs to address important theoretical questions in social and personality psychology.

Dennis J. L. G. Schutter, in Chapter 11, discusses transcranial magnetic stimulation (TMS)—particularly rTMS, mentioned earlier, which is a relatively new neuroscience methodology that has been used to study social and personality processes. The repetitive, continuous application of magnetic stimulation through the scalp can either decrease or increase neural excitability in the area being stimulated, and thereby permits scientists to understand how temporary impairment or enhancement of a brain region leads to changes in behavior. The chapter discusses the history of this approach; it also provides practical advice about how to conduct a study with rTMS and other variants of TMS, such as which brain regions are well suited to this approach and what kinds of information can be collected. Finally, the chapter illustrates these principles with examples of research that examines social and personality processes.

In Chapter 12, Stephen J. Read and Brian M. Monroe discuss using neural networks to understand social and personality processes. This approach is based on theory about neuroanatomical connectivity and function, but does not require any measurement of neural activity. The authors illustrate how neural network modeling permits social and personality psychologists to build models of the relationships between and among different psychological processes. The chapter provides practical advice about neural modeling, and illustrates these principles with such examples as the virtual personality model and the iterative reprocessing model.

In Chapter 13, Turhan Canli provides practical advice for social and personality psychologists who want to investigate the interrelations among genetic predisposition, brain activation, and psychological variables. The chapter illustrates these benefits in relation to personality characteristics such as neuroticism and genes such as the serotonin transporter gene. Canli also discusses considerations about baseline conditions when emotional processes are being imaged. Finally, the chapter provides for social and personality psychologists advice about how to gain a working understanding of genetics.

Tom Johnstone, M. Justin Kim, and Paul J. Whalen, in Chapter 14, provide background and practical advice for one of the most popular neuroscience methods used by social and personality psychologists: fMRI. This approach allows scientists to identify brain activations in relation to psychological processes. The chapter also illustrates the practical concerns and uses of fMRI with examples of emotional processing.

Acknowledgments

Thanks to David M. Amodio and Ziggy Bialzik for helpful comments on this chapter.

References

Adolphs, R. (Ed.). (2003). Investigating the cognitive neuroscience of social behavior. *Neuropsychologia* [Special issue], *41*(2), 119–126.

Beer, J. S., Mitchell, J. P., & Ochsner, K. N. (2006). Multiple perspectives on the psychological and neural bases of social cognition. *Brain Research* [Special issue], *1079*(1), 1–3.

Cacioppo, J. T., & Visser, P. S. (2003). Political psychology and social neuroscience: Strange bedfellows or comrades in arms? *Political Psychology* [Special issue], *24*(4), 647–656.

Cacioppo, J. T., Visser, P. S., & Pickett, C. L. (Eds.). (2006). *Social neuroscience: People thinking about thinking people.* Cambridge, MA: MIT Press.

Frith, C., & Wolpert, D. (Eds.). (2004). *The neuroscience of social interaction: Decoding, influencing, and imitating the actions of others.* New York: Oxford University Press.

Harmon-Jones, E., & Devine, P. G. (Eds.). (2003). Introduction to the special section on social neuroscience: Promise and caveats. *Journal of Personality and Social Psychology* [Special issue], *85*(4), 589–593.

Harmon-Jones, E., & Winkielman, P. (Eds.). (2007). *Social neuroscience: Integrating biological and psychological explanations of social behavior.* New York: Guilford Press.

Heatherton, T. F. (2004). Introduction to special issue on social cognitive neuroscience. *Journal of Cognitive Neuroscience* [Special issue], *16*, 1681–1682.

Insel, T. R. (2002). Social anxiety: From laboratory studies to clinical practice. *Biological Psychiatry* [Special issue], *51*(1), 1–3.

Lieberman, M. D. (2005). Principles, processes, and puzzles of social cognition: An introduction for the special issue on social cognitive neuroscience. *NeuroImage* [Special issue], *28*(4), 745–756.

2

Collaborations in Social and Personality Neuroscience

Cindy Harmon-Jones
Jennifer S. Beer
Eddie Harmon-Jones

Those with neuroscience skills often find themselves in high demand as collaborators. Psychological scientists without these skills turn to neuroscientists to help them test their ideas. In addition, because neuroscience techniques are multiplying quickly and it is nearly impossible to be skilled in all such techniques, neuroscientists may also form collaborative relationships with other neuroscientists who have different skill sets.

Successful collaborative relationships can greatly increase one's productivity. Collaborating with colleagues who have different backgrounds can bring fresh perspectives and insights to one's work. Collaborating with colleagues who are enthusiastic and energetic can be inspiring and fun. Unfortunately, it is also possible for collaborations to turn out badly, and when this happens the collaborative relationship can become a time and energy drain instead of the productivity boost that it should be. This chapter contains suggestions for fostering healthy collaborations in social–personality neuroscience, preventing unpleasant situations from occurring, and getting derailed collaborations back on track.

Communicating Expectations Clearly from the Start

Collaborations often germinate in a social situation, when scientists are talking about their current projects and sharing ideas, and they get excited about the connections between their individual areas of work. In this initial excitement phase, scientists often jump into collaborations with high hopes and no clearly communicated plans. This is a bit like the infatuation stage of a romantic relationship. It is important to discuss each person's expectations and create a plan early in the process, before the work gets underway, as beginning to collaborate without clearly communicating expectations is likely to lead to disappointment later (this might not be bad romantic relationship advice, either). Even though it may seem "unromantic," putting these plans and mutual expectations in writing is a good idea. Although a collaborative relationship can be friendly and enjoyable, it can also have an impact on each person's career, and thus should be an exchange relationship that is fair to all participants. During this planning phase, it is essential that the participants agree on what each will contribute to the project.

Of all the things that can sour a collaborative relationship, disagreements about authorship are probably the worst and longest-lasting. Even during the planning phase, before the real work gets started, the collaborators should discuss authorship and agree on how authorship will be determined. Authorship is handled somewhat differently across fields, and such differences are important to include in discussions of authorship. For example, a social psychologist may offer to be the last author on a paper going to a neuroscience journal. Although the psychologist may think that he or she is offering to take a position in the author list that indicates a minimal contribution, this position in neuroscience journals is usually reserved for the most senior author, and the work is considered to have taken place in that person's lab. Although the recommendation to plan ahead and reach agreement on authorship (and all other matters) before beginning to work together applies to any collaboration, it is particularly important in neuroscience collaborations, because neuroscience is especially time-consuming, expensive, and effortful.

Non-neuroscientists may have no idea of the time, effort, and expense involved in collecting and processing neuroscience data. Indeed, these factors have several implications for setting up a collaboration. First, when a collaboration is being considered, the first thing a neuroscientist will probably want to know is why studying a particular neurobiological system will reveal anything new about the proposed phenomena. Neuroscientists are not likely to want to invest time and money just "to see" what happens in the brain or with hormones. It is also important to recognize that it is much more difficult to add exploratory conditions to neuroscience experiments without clear and meaningful predictions for those conditions. In addition, some (but not all) neuroscience methodologies are not optimal for studying individual differences, so adding personality questionnaires may not be likely to help ensure that there will be significant results. Therefore, the research plan should be much more straightforward than is often the case in exploratory behavioral research. Furthermore, some neuroscience techniques can be unfamiliar or slightly uncomfortable for human subjects. This may add variance to results, making significant results more difficult to obtain. Thus it is important to demonstrate strong, consistently replicable behavioral results during pilot testing, before attempting to use neuroscience to examine the phenomena further.

Even if non-neuroscientist collaborators do not plan to learn neuroscience techniques, they need to become familiar with the processes. Otherwise, the neuroscientists are likely to feel unappreciated when the non-neuroscientists do not seem to understand how much work has been done to collect and process the data. Neuroscience projects often involve more lab resources than strictly behavioral projects do. For example, a collaborative project is likely to require time on special equipment, and to rely on personnel with technical expertise, special software, and data processing and storage in the neuroscience lab. Furthermore, the non-neuroscientists will be able to give better-informed talks about the project if they have a basic understanding of how the research was conducted.

Developing a Mutually Beneficial Relationship

As the preceding discussion suggests, neuroscience carries a monetary cost that is often greater than the cost of non-neuroscience psychological research. All collaborators on a project need to discuss the cost of the research and to reach agreement on how it will be paid for. When non-neuroscientists collaborate with neuroscientists, money may be what they bring to the relationship. Neuroscientists always need more money to keep their research going; thus a neuroscientist may be willing to collaborate with someone, even if he or she is not particularly interested in that person's research, if that person has grant money to contribute to the project. In neuroscience, each subject often participates in more than one study per experimental session, because preparing to collect and collecting the data are so time-consuming and expensive. A non-neuroscientist who has money to help pay for running the subjects may be able to collect data from the same subjects that the neuroscientist is using for a separate project. Many neuroscience facilities offer time on equipment to faculty members who are new to the technology (i.e., internal "pilot hour" grants). A non-neuroscientist may be able to contribute to the project by applying for this type of support, even if he or she does not have other grant money available.

Another asset that a non-neuroscience collaborator may bring to a project is a special population of subjects. Special populations can make research more clinically relevant and more fundable. Some neuroscientists collect a lot of data, but have trouble getting them written up and submitted; they may benefit by collaborating with someone who is a good, and fast, writer. Other scientists enjoy the technical aspects of neuroscience, but have trouble thinking up new research ideas to test; these scientists could benefit by joining with a creative collaborator who has many interesting ideas. However, neuroscientists who have plenty of research ideas will want to avoid collaborating with people who may treat them merely as technicians, and will expect to be given credit for their creative as well as technical contributions.

A collaboration between faculty members often works best when it is conducted through a graduate student who is interested in both research lines, and who is willing to learn the neuroscience techniques and the relevant literatures. Most faculty members do not have the time or interest to learn new neuroscience techniques, whereas graduate students have more time to devote to learning new techniques and to reading the associated literatures. A neuroscientist who collaborates with both a faculty member and a motivated graduate student can teach the neuroscience techniques to the graduate student, and then the student can take responsibility for carrying out the data collection and processing. This prevents a situation where the neuroscientist is "collaborating," but in fact doing almost all of the work on the project. The payoff for the graduate student is that he or she will become very marketable. Students who develop expertise in neuroscience as well as another aspect of social or personality psychology are attractive hires because of their abilities to integrate different areas in psychological science. For a neuroscientist who is considering a complex, high-commitment collaboration, having a graduate student who is willing and interested can make the project much more attractive.

Just as neuroscientists want to be appreciated by non-neuroscientists for their expertise and creative input, it is important for neuroscientists to respect and appreciate their non-neuroscience collaborators. A neuroscientist should avoid disparaging non-neuroscience methods of conducting research and people who lack technical expertise, particularly in the presence of a non-neuroscientist collaborator (we have seen this happen). This behavior does not foster a positive relationship with the less technically savvy collaborator. If the neuroscientist can find a way to appreciate the collaborator's strengths, the collaborator is more likely to give respect in return. Researchers with different perspectives and different backgrounds should bring more insights to the project, even when they challenge the way their collaborators usually do things. However, this will happen only if those involved are open to those different perspectives.

Evaluating a Potential Collaboration

It can be very flattering to be asked to collaborate, and scientists sometimes agree to work on projects that they are not really interested in, simply because someone asked them to. Sometimes scientists agree to collaborate with a colleague because they believe they can assist with the individual's research and/or they want to help the person to succeed. Helping other people can be rewarding, but sometimes in an unequal exchange relationship, the person who is giving more comes to resent it over time. When one is considering collaborating with someone who is not likely to be able to make an equal contribution, it is important to consider how one will feel months later, after spending money and time on the project, when the collaborator has not been able to contribute much because he or she does not have the resources.

In cases where one is considering a new collaboration, and is unsure about how much the potential collaborator will be able to contribute, it may be a good idea to start *very* small, with a low-stress, low-investment project. Working together on piloting the behavioral portion of the study can be very informative about whether collaborative work is a good idea for the parties involved. It is wise to do careful pilot testing before beginning to collect the neuroscience data, to make sure that the behavioral effects are strong and easily replicable. Behavioral pilot data can be collected and analyzed much faster than neuroscience data can be, and doing so will provide good information about each potential collaborator's commitment to the project, work habits, and idiosyncrasies. The collaborators can find out whether they are compatible without risking the frustration of finding out that they are not compatible while in the midst of a major effort. This also gives a neuroscientist a chance to find out whether the non-neuroscientist collaborator is willing and able to develop the skills necessary to become a more highly contributing partner in the future. If a small initial collaboration goes well, the partnership can move on to something bigger and better.

Another way to find out important information about a potential collaborator before making a commitment to a big project is talking to others who have worked with the person in the past. Since everyone has a different personality and working style, it is important to know one's own needs and priorities in order to consider the questions to ask. Some people like to communicate frequently, while others prefer to work more independently. Some like to finish projects quickly, whereas others are frustrated by collaborators who nag them to work faster. Thus a collaborator who is a great fit for one person may not be right for another. Specific, nonjudgmental questions about the issues that are important to the questioner (e.g., "How quickly did so-and-so respond to your e-mails?") are more likely to yield useful and honest answers than questions that are more vague and subjective (e.g., "How did you like working with so-and-so?").

What If Problems Develop?

Following the suggestions above can get collaborative relationships off to a good start and prevent many problems. But what can be done if things go wrong? If a problem seems to be developing, honest communication may get things back on track. A collaborator may not have had any idea that certain issues were of concern to another collaborator, and may be very willing to make changes. In the midst of a collaboration, resentment sometimes develops because one partner perceives that the other is not doing his or her share of the work. This perception may or may not be accurate, since individuals tend to be highly aware of the work they themselves are doing, but much less aware of the work that others are doing. Sometimes it is unavoidable that one person needs to do the bulk of work on a particular part of the project, and that person only needs acknowledgment and appreciation.

In other cases, a collaborator truly is not moving the project forward. When this happens, it may be necessary to rethink the original plan. The collaborators may need to have a hard conversation about each individual's expectations and about authorship. If one collaborator is no longer willing or able to contribute, the other may need to take over finishing the project. If this can be handled in a cooperative, professional way, the situation has the potential to remain positive. If the individual who is committed to completing the project does not have the skills to do the part of the project that the former collaborator was originally supposed to do, it may be necessary to recruit someone else to do it, and the former collaborator may be able to help with finding that person.

A collaboration that does not go as planned can be a valuable learning experience, helping a scientist to develop more fruitful collaborations in the future. If the suggestion to begin with a commitment to a small project has been followed, then these learning experiences do not have to be terribly costly.

Conclusion

We hope that this chapter will provide useful suggestions for neuroscientists who are considering collaborations with non-neuroscientists, non-neuroscientists who hope to collaborate with neuroscientists, and neuroscientists who choose to collaborate with other neuroscientists who have expertise in a different set of techniques. As neuroscience methods multiply, it has become practically impossible to be an expert in every kind of neuroscience method. Developing expertise in a few areas, along with fostering collaborations with other neuroscientists, can give a neuroscientist access to multiple techniques for answering important questions in psychological science.

3

Assessment of Salivary Hormones

Oliver C. Schultheiss
Steven J. Stanton

A Primer on Concepts and Measurement Issues in Behavioral Endocrinology

"Hormones" are messenger molecules that are released by specialized neurons in the brain and by glands into the bloodstream, and that carry a signal at the speed of blood to other parts of the body. Which specific responses they trigger in target organs depends on the receptors involved and the functions of the organs. For instance, the peptide hormone arginine vasopressin (AVP) regulates water retention in the body when it binds to receptors in the kidneys, but enhances episodic memory when it binds to receptors in the brain (e.g., Beckwith, Petros, Bergloff, & Staebler, 1987). Thus one hormone can drive several different physiological and psychological functions through its effects on several target organs.

Generally, two broad classes of hormonal effects on physiology and behavior are differentiated. "Organizational effects" are lasting influences that hormones exert on the organism, thus changing its shape and functional properties in subtle (and sometimes not so subtle) ways. Organizational hormone effects often occur during development or at times of significant hormonal flux, such as puberty. For instance, the development of the female and male body morphology is largely under hormonal control during fetal development, and deviations from typical-gendered body morphology are frequently the result of deviations in hormone production, conversion, or receptor action. In contrast to organizational effects, "activational effects" are those that hormones exert temporarily, without effecting lasting changes in the organism. For instance, due to peaking estradiol levels around the time of ovulation, women become more sensitive to sexual stimuli, as indicated by an enhanced pupillary response. This effect vanishes again after ovulation, when estradiol levels decrease (Laeng & Falkenberg, 2007). Psychologists interested in the role of hormones in psychological functions and phenomena most frequently study such activational effects of hormones on the brain, although the much more difficult documentation of organizational hormone effects on behavior is also gaining traction (e.g., Baron-Cohen, Lutchmaya, & Knickmeyer, 2006).

The relationship between hormones and behavior is *bidirectional*. Hormones can have a facilitating effect on behavior, such as when high levels of testosterone facilitate learning a behavior that elicits an angry face (Wirth & Schultheiss, 2007), increase cardiac responses to angry faces (van Honk et al., 2001), or increase aggressive responses on a point subtraction game (Pope, Kouri, & Hudson, 2000). Such hormone → behavior effects can be most conclusively demonstrated through experimental manipulation of hormone levels—a method that is covered in detail by van Honk (Chapter 4, this volume). Conversely, the situational outcome of a person's behavior, as well as the stimuli and events impinging on the person, can influence current hormone levels. This is the case when winning or losing a contest raises or lowers testosterone levels in male mammals, including humans (e.g., Gladue, Boechler, & McCaul, 1989; Mazur, 1985; Oyegbile & Marler, 2005); when encounters with an attractive member of the other sex have an impact on an individual's sex hormones (e.g., Graham & Desjardins, 1980; Roney, Lukaszewski, & Simmons, 2007); or when watching romantic movies leads to an increase in viewers' progesterone levels (Schultheiss, Wirth, & Stanton, 2004).

Because hormones have far-reaching and broad effects on physiology and behavior, their release is tightly controlled and monitored, primarily through negative feedback loops. For instance, circulating levels of the steroid hormone cortisol are monitored by the brain. If levels fall below a critical threshold, the hypothalamus releases corticotropin-releasing hormone (CRH), which in turn triggers the release of adrenocorticotropic hormone (ACTH). ACTH travels from the brain to the cortex of the adrenals (small glands that sit on top of the kidneys), where it stimulates the release of cortisol. If rising levels of cortisol exceed a certain threshold, CRH release—and thus the subsequent release of ACTH and cortisol—are curtailed until cortisol levels fall below the critical threshold again, due to metabolic clearance. As a consequence of this negative-feedback-loop mechanism, many hormones are released in repeated bursts occurring every 30–120 min. Notably, hormones can also influence the release of different hormones. The quick (i.e., within minutes) testosterone increase in response to dominance challenges sometimes observed in men and other male primates (Mazur, 1985) is a good example. These rapid changes are the result of the stimulating effects of epinephrine and norepinephrine (NE), which are released within seconds after the onset of a situational challenge, on the testes (which produce testosterone in men). This effect is independent of the hypothalamic–pituitary–gonadal feedback mechanism normally involved in testosterone release (Sapolsky, 1987).

Besides acquiring a basic understanding of endocrine function, two issues are of particular concern to behavioral scientists who want to include endocrine measures in their research. First, current hormone levels are *multiply determined*, and in order to tease out the effects of interest (i.e., relationships between hormones and behavior), it is almost always necessary to control for, or hold constant, other influences on hormone levels. Chief among those influences is the strong circadian variation observed in many endocrine systems. Hormones like testosterone, estradiol, and cortisol start out at high levels in the morning and then decline through the course of the day. The variance generated by this effect can easily drown out whatever between-subjects differences one hopes to observe in an experiment if it is not taken into account—either by recording and adjusting for time of day, or by conducting all testing only at one time of day (e.g., in the afternoon). Effects of experimental factors on hormone levels are more likely to be observed in the afternoon than in the morning, presumably because hormone levels are still too close to their physiological ceiling and too variable earlier in the day (see Dickerson & Kemeny, 2004; Wirth, Welsh, & Schultheiss, 2006). On the other hand, individual differences in peak hormone levels measured in the morning may be a better predictor of behavioral responses to emotional stimuli than hormone measurements later in the day may be (Wirth & Schultheiss, 2007; see also Schultheiss et al., 2005).

Another important chronobiological influence on observed hormone levels is the menstrual cycle. The gonadal steroids estradiol and progesterone vary strongly as a function of cycle phase, and researchers therefore try to control hormone variance due to cycle stage—either by testing only women in a particular stage (e.g., the follicular phase), or by asking female research participants to report the onset date of the last menses and average cycle length, in order to make a rough calculation later of what cycle phase each participant was in during the time of testing.

Besides chronobiological effects on hormone levels, drug status of research participants should also be taken into account (e.g., Daly et al., 2003; Hibel, Granger, Kivlighan, & Blair, 2006; Nadeem, Attenburrow, & Cowen, 2004). Probably the drug most frequently used by female participants is the oral contraception pill, which keeps endogenous gonadal steroid levels low throughout the menstrual cycle. Other, less frequently encountered drugs with profound effects on hormone levels include anabolic steroids, steroid-based anti-inflammatory medications, antidepressants, or drugs influencing the body's fluid levels. Appendix 3.1 is a screening questionnaire we frequently use in behavioral endocrinology studies to control for the most important extraneous influences on hormone levels.

The second issue of concern to a behavioral scientist who wants to use endocrine measures is how easy or difficult it is to assess a particular hormone. This in turn depends primarily on the biochemical properties of the hormone. *Peptide hormones* (i.e., short protein molecules composed of a small number of amino acids), such as insulin, AVP, ACTH, NE, and oxytocin (OXY), are large structures by molecular standards and therefore do not easily pass through cell membranes. As a consequence, they can only be measured in the medium or body compartment into which they have been released or actively transported. For instance, OXY released by the pituitary into the bloodstream can only be assessed in blood, but not in saliva (Horvat-Gordon, Granger, Schwartz, Nelson, & Kivlighan, 2005; but see Carter et al., 2007). Also, OXY concentrations measured in the body may not accurately reflect OXY levels in the brain, because they are released by different hypothalamic sites. Moreover, peptide hormones break down easily, and special precautions are necessary to stabilize their molecular structure after sampling. The other major class of hormones besides the peptides are *steroid hormones*, which are synthesized in the body from cholesterol. In contrast to peptide hormones, steroid hormones are highly stable, and in their free, bioactive form (i.e., not bound to larger proteins) they can pass through cell membranes, leading to roughly similar levels of the free fraction of a hormone across body compartments. This means that, for instance, cortisol levels measured in saliva are similar to (free) cortisol levels measured in blood or cortisol levels in the brain. For this reason, and because saliva sampling is much easier and less stressful for research participants than the collection of blood samples or spinal fluid samples (to get at hormone levels within the central nervous system [CNS]), salivary hormone assessment has become the method of choice among behavioral endocrinologists and psychologists working with human populations (Dabbs, 1992; Hofman, 2001; Kirschbaum & Hellhammer, 1994).

One of the most frequently used methods for the assessment of salivary hormone levels is the radioimmunoassay (RIA). Although RIAs for many hormones can be purchased from commercial vendors, and a researcher therefore does not necessarily have to know how they are manufactured, we think it is useful to know what the term "radioimmunoassay" actually means. An "assay" is a procedure by which the concentration of an analyte (a hormone, in this case) is measured. "Immuno-" signifies that hormonal assays exploit the property of an organism's immune system to produce antibodies (i.e., proteins that adhere in a highly specific manner to alien compounds entering the body) in response to the injection of alien organic matter (antigens); in the case of a hormonal RIA, animals are injected with the human form of a given hormone, and the antibodies produced in response to the injected hormone are harvested from the animal's blood, purified, and used in the RIA to bind to the hormone content added to the assay. "Radio-" signifies that in RIAs, a fixed quantity of hormone molecules with radioactive labels (typically radioiodine [^{125}I]) is added to the assay, and these molecules compete with molecules from samples collected in participants for antibody-binding sites (see Figure 3.1 for a schematic overview of an RIA).

An RIA is therefore a special case of a competitive immunoassay, in which labeled and unlabeled hormones compete for binding sites until they settle into a binding equilibrium that depends only on the concentration of unlabeled hormone in the sample, since the amounts of labeled hormone and antibodies are fixed across the entire assay. Assays have also been developed that use enzymatic labels whose relative presence in a given sample is indicated by degrees of coloration, fluorescence, or luminescence. The chief advantage of such enzymatic immunoassays (EIAs) is that they do not require the use of radioactivity and thus licensing of the assay facility, personnel training, and precise bookkeeping associated with the use of radioactive substances. The drawbacks of EIAs include complex assay protocols and relatively less accuracy and sensitivity than RIAs (see Raff, Homar, & Burns, 2002).

Using Salivary Hormone Assays in Psychological Research: A Guided Tour

In this section, we illustrate the use of a hormonal assay in social neuroscience by describing, from start to finish, the procedures in a study

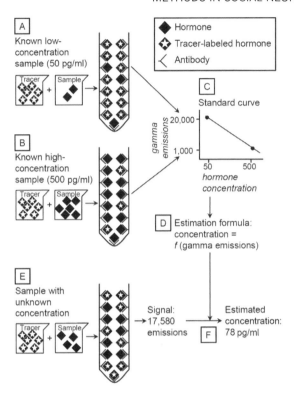

FIGURE 3.1. Schematic overview of a competitive radioimmunoassay (RIA). Each RIA contains, besides the samples whose hormone concentrations need to be determined, standards (or calibrators) with known amounts of hormone concentrations that cover the entire range of the hormone levels expected in the given medium (e.g., saliva) and population studied. In this simplified schematic, a standard with a low concentration (A) and a standard with a high concentration (B) are added to assay tubes containing antibodies that react with the hormone of interest. Radioactive tracer with a fixed concentration of radioisotope-labeled hormone is also added to the assay. Labeled and unlabeled hormones compete for antibody-binding sites until equilibrium is reached. Sample and tracer fluid is then discarded, leaving only antibody-bound hormone, both labeled and unlabeled, in the tube. Tubes are measured in a gamma counter, which provides a high gamma signal for the low-concentration sample (because tracer-labeled hormone is bound to the majority of antibodies) and a low gamma signal for the high-concentration sample (because more unlabeled than tracer-labeled hormone is bound to the antibodies). Interpolation between standards yields a standard curve (C) that allows estimating a given sample's concentration from the number of gamma emissions measured. The relationship between gamma emissions and sample concentration can be calculated and expressed through an estimation formula (D), based on a regression of concentration on gamma signal after appropriate linearization of both variables. This formula can then be applied to samples with unknown concentrations (E; e.g., participants' saliva samples), for which hormone concentrations can be estimated on the basis of the gamma signal (F).

on the joint effects of implicit power motivation and winning or losing a dominance contest on testosterone changes in men (Schultheiss et al, 2005, Study 1). In the course of a 2-hour experiment, three saliva samples were collected before a dominance contest and three after the contest was over. Precontest samples were collected to obtain a baseline at the very start of the session (0 min); after the experimenter had announced that participants would compete against each other on a speed-based task (T2, 52 min); and after participants had imagined the ensuing contest from the winner's perspective through a guided imagery exercise (T3, 64 min, immediately before the contest). Samples at T2 and T3 were taken to examine the effects of verbal instructions versus experiential elaboration of these instructions, respectively (see Schultheiss & Brunstein, 1999; Schultheiss, Campbell, & McClelland, 1999). The T3 sample also served as the baseline covariate closest to the actual contest in later analyses. Postcontest samples were taken immediately after the contest (T4, 78 min) and then, at intervals of 15 min, twice more (T5 and T6) to explore the time course of power motivation × contest outcome effects. Sampling intervals of 15 min and longer were chosen because of the time it takes for steroid hormones to transfer from blood into saliva and be cleared out of it again; the relative sluggishness of the process does not allow for greater temporal resolution (see Riad-Fahmy, Read, Walker, Walker, & Griffiths, 1987). Both pre- and postcontest samples were collected while participants completed other tasks (e.g., mood questionnaires) on a personal computer (PC).

Sample Collection

The goal of the saliva collection phase is to collect high-quality samples (i.e., samples free of contaminants) in a precisely identified sequence and with a sufficient amount of saliva to allow the measurement of all targeted hormones later on. To eliminate contaminants like blood or residues from a meal, we asked participants to refrain from eating and brushing their teeth for at least 1 hour before coming to the lab. After they had arrived, they were asked to rinse their mouths with some water over a sink. During the experimental session, the collection of each sample was coupled to the completion of a noncritical task (e.g., providing mood ratings on the PC). Precise instructions about which tube to use and how much saliva to collect were given by instruction screens on the PC that also featured illustrative pictures (see Figure 3.2). After participants had completed the task, the following instruction was presented on the screen: "Have you filled the tube to the marked line? If not, please continue to collect more saliva before moving on to the next task. If the tube is filled to the line, please put the lid on the tube, place it back on the desk, and spit out the chewing gum. Press a key to move on to the next task." Similar instructions were given for each of the six saliva collections. Of course, these instructions can also be given orally by an experimenter if no computers are used. Whichever method is used, care should be taken that every participant fully understands what he or she is expected to do and that no mistakes creep into the collection of saliva samples (e.g., using the tube for another time point for a given collection time; participants depleting their saliva glands because they continue to chew on a gum instead of taking it out after sample collection). Having participants collect saliva while they are completing a questionnaire or similar task helps keep them occupied during the collection phase, and also reduces the slight embarrassment associated with collecting saliva in front of an experimenter and other participants.

For the collection of saliva, we use skirted 50-ml tubes. The size of the tubes makes it easy for participants to drool directly into a tube; the skirt ensures that the tube can stand on the desk without the use of a holding rack; and the design of the tubes allows us to use them for storage, freezing, and centrifuging. To stimulate saliva flow, we use Trident Original Flavor chewing gum, which has been shown to yield the least bias in steroid levels as compared to unaided saliva flow (Dabbs, 1991; see also Shirtcliff, Granger, Schwartz, & Curran, 2001, for problems

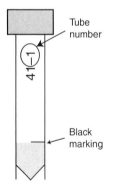

PLEASE LOCATE THE PLASTIC COLLECTION TUBE NUMBERED "1".

While you are working on the first questionnaire, we would like to collect some saliva from you. This will be the first of six saliva samples.

Tube number

To collect saliva, please chew on the **CHEWING GUM** that we put on your desk and spit the saliva that accumulates in your mouth into the PLASTIC COLLECTION **TUBE NUMBERED "1"**.

Please continue to collect saliva in this way until the CLEAR SALIVA FLUID in the tube stands as high as the **BLACK MARKING** on the side of the tube. Then screw the lid back on tightly to prevent any saliva from evaporating or spilling.

Black marking

AFTER YOU HAVE FILLED THE PLASTIC TUBE, PLEASE SPIT OUT THE CHEWING GUM.

If you have questions about this, please ask the experimenter at any time.

* Please press any key *

FIGURE 3.2. Sample computer instruction screen for the collection of saliva in a numbered 50-ml plastic tube.

associated with the use of cotton rolls for saliva collection). Before the start of data collection, all tubes had been properly labeled (using a water-proof permanent marker) with each participant's identification number; an additional number indicating the time point during the experiment at which the sample was taken (e.g., 101-1, 101-2, 101-3, 101-4, 101-5, 101-6); and a line at the 7.5-ml mark to indicate the desired fluid level. In our experience, a sample of this size can be collected quickly and provides enough material for the assessment of up to three different hormones.

After all samples had been collected in a session and participants had left the lab, the experimenter checked whether all tubes were properly sealed and put them into a freezer for storage. A regular chest freezer or upright freezer from a household appliance store is sufficient for this purpose. Frozen samples can last up to a year at −20°C and possibly longer without noticeable changes in the samples' steroid hormone concentration (Dabbs, 1991).

Sample Processing

The goal of the second phase—saliva processing—is to make the saliva samples amenable to precise pipetting in the actual assay. To achieve this goal, all samples are first thawed and frozen three times after all data collection has been completed for the study. This procedure helps to break down the long molecule chains that make saliva sticky and viscous, and to turn it into a more watery (and thus precisely pipettable) fluid. The breakdown of molecular chains can be enhanced by speeding up freezing and thawing through the use of dry ice and a warm water bath; the stronger shearing forces associated with the fast temperature differential induced by the use of these aids facilitates the degradation of the molecule chains. After the third thaw, samples are spun for 10 min at 1000 g in a refrigerated centrifuge to push all coarse content to the bottom of the tube (this process is similar to the separation of serum and plasma in blood samples). After centrifugation, the "supernatant" (i.e., the watery part of the sample that stays on top after centrifugation) of each sample is transferred from the 50-ml tube to an identically labeled, or set of identically labeled, aliquot tube(s) (e.g., 5-ml, 2-ml, or 1.5-ml tubes). Care must be taken to avoid stirring up and transferring the coarse, sticky contents of saliva from the bottom of the tube during transfer. For this reason, we recommend centrifuging and aspirating only small batches of tubes (≤ 12) at a time, because coarse and watery components of saliva tend to mingle again after long waits between centrifugation and sample transfer to aliquots, particularly if samples are not refrigerated during and after centrifugation. After aliquoting, samples can either be assayed right away or refrozen for later assaying.

Sample Assaying

The goal of assaying the samples is to provide a specific, sensitive, accurate, and reliable measurement of their hormone content. Assay quality depends in part on the care taken during the previous steps. For instance, if participants have not been instructed to refrain from eating and brushing their teeth before the experiment, samples may be contaminated with traces of blood from gum lacerations and may therefore yield elevated steroid measurements, thus compromising accuracy (Granger et al., 2007). And if samples have not been processed thoroughly, saliva will be more likely to retain its viscous properties, which makes it difficult to pipette exact amounts of samples into test tubes and compromises measurement reliability.

Assay quality also depends on the properties of the assay itself. A key prerequisite for any assay is that it measures one hormone *specifically* (e.g., testosterone), but not other hormones (e.g., progesterone, estradiol, cortisol; see the first row of Table 3.1). The specificity requirement is sometimes difficult to satisfy, due to the close structural similarities of hormone molecules. An assay that claims to measure testosterone but in fact also responds to other androgens, such as androstenedione, may yield inflated estimates of the actual testosterone content of samples. It is often difficult to evaluate the specificity of a given assay, because running specificity tests in one's own lab requires work, time, and knowledge. But some telltale signs can be used to gauge whether a given assay indeed measures only what it claims to measure. If a sufficient number of subjects have been tested, one can compare the average hormone levels measured to those reported by others who have used high-pressure liquid chromatography (the gold standard in hormone assessment) and other assay methods to measure the same hormone in similar populations in saliva under similar circumstances (e.g., Dabbs et al., 1995). Thus, if one's measured hormone levels are in the same general range as hormone levels reported in the current literature (i.e., within 50–150% of the average levels measured by others), this can serve as an indicator of the assay's specificity. Another indicator is the detection of telltale circadian or group differences, particularly if their magnitude is similar to those observed by others. For instance, on average women typically have one-fourth to one-sixth of the testosterone levels measured in men at the same time of day. It should be a cause for concern if this difference is not observed in one's own samples with a given assay, provided

TABLE 3.1. Overview of the Main Assay Quality Parameters

Assay quality parameter	Definition and estimation
Specificity	Defined as the ability of the assay to maximize measurement of the targeted analyte and minimize measurement of other analytes. Specificity is often established by measuring the degree to which an assay produces measurements different from 0 for nontargeted analytes (e.g., in the case of a cortisol assay, measurements > 0 for progesterone, aldosterone, pregnenolone, and other related steroid hormones). Cross-reactivity with such nontarget analytes is estimated by dividing the measured, apparent concentration of the analyte by the amount added. For example, if 2,000 µg/dL aldosterone is added, and 0.6 µg/dL is measured, (0.6/2000) • 100 = 0.03% cross-reactivity. Measures of specificity are not routinely included in hormone assays, but specificity should at least be carefully examined when a new assay is adopted.
Sensitivity	Defined as the lowest dose of an analyte that can be distinguished from a sample containing no analyte. It is often pragmatically derived by calculating the "lower limit of detection" (LLD), which is defined as signal obtained from a sample with zero analyte (B_0), minus three times the standard deviation of the signal at B_0. Values outside the $B_0 - (3 \times SD)$ range are considered valid nonzero measurements.
Accuracy	Defined as the ability of the assay to measure the true concentrations of the analyte in the samples being tested. Accuracy is measured by including control samples with known amounts of analyte in the assay and then comparing the amount of analyte estimated by the assay (e.g., 95 pg/ml) with the actual amount added (e.g., 100 pg/ml testosterone). The result is expressed as the percentage of the actual amount that is recovered by the assay; for example, accuracy = (95/100) · 100 = 95%. Recovery coefficients between 90% and 110% reflect good accuracy.
Precision	Defined as the closeness of agreement between test results repeatedly and independently obtained under stable conditions. Precision is typically estimated by the "coefficient of variation" (CV), which is calculated as the mean of replicate measurements of a given sample, divided by the standard deviation of the measurements, multiplied by 100. The intra-assay CV is calculated as the average of the CVs of all samples in a given assay or set of assays; the interassay CV is calculated from the between-assay mean and SD of a control sample (e.g., a saliva pool) included in all assays. Intra- and interassays CVs less than 10% are considered good.

that enough subjects from each gender have been tested. Note that these indicators provide at best a rough, indirect test of an assay's ability to measure one specific hormone free of bias from other hormones, and do not constitute positive proof of an assay's specificity. Nonetheless, for a researcher whose interests and expertise lie not in biochemistry but in behavioral endocrinology, close examination of such indicators is imperative if the researcher wants to be able to trust in the validity of his or her hormone data.

Another important determinant of assay quality is the assay's *sensitivity* (see the second row of Table 3.1). Salivary assays for most major steroids are sufficiently sensitive to accurately discriminate even tiny differences—usually in the nanogram (i.e., 1/1,000,000,000 g) or even picogram (i.e., 1/1,000,000,000,000 g) range—in hormone concentrations across the entire range of concentrations usually observed in healthy adult populations. But some hormones and some populations push the limits of what many assays are able to detect and differentiate. For instance, estradiol is a powerful steroid hormone, subserving many different functions in the CNS and peripheral organs. Its enzymatic conversion from hormonal precursors (e.g., testosterone) is therefore tightly constrained, and overall levels in adults are low, with men and women in the follicular phase of the menstrual cycle exhibiting average salivary levels of 1–5 pg/ml. However, most estradiol assays reliably measure only levels of 2 pg/ml and up, and either cannot differentiate levels lower than 2 pg/ml from zero concentrations or yield unreliable or invalid measurements for concentrations below the 2-pg/ml threshold. Likewise, many steroid hormone levels are considerably lower in prepubertal children and in aging or menopausal populations. Assays that are sufficiently sensitive to cover the range of levels typically observed in healthy, fertile, adult populations may therefore not accurately measure the lower levels observed in other populations. Careful consideration of the typical hormone levels reported for such populations in the literature, and the subsequent selection of suitable assays that cover the lower range of hormone levels or the modification of various parameters (e.g., use of a preincubation phase, increase of sample added to assay) of previously used assays, are frequently necessary in such cases.

If an assay is sufficiently specific and sensitive, its *accuracy* over the entire range of measurements needs to be established (see the third row of Table 3.1). This essential validity check can be easily performed by adding control samples with known amounts of an analyte to the assay and monitoring the extent to which the measured concentration matches the expected concentration. Accuracy checks are usually done by including commercially available control samples (e.g., the Lyphochek samples provided by BioRad, Hercules, CA). These frequently contain an array of different hormones and can thus be used for several different hormone assays. However, because they are calibrated to accommodate the hormone levels typically observed in blood, proper dilution is necessary for their use in salivary hormone assays. Accuracy checks should cover the low (25%), medium (50%), and high (75%) range of expected measurements for a given assay type—or, at a minimum, the lower and upper 33% of expected levels. Accuracy checks can and should also be included in batches of samples that are sent out to commercial assay services, and their inclusion should not be indicated to the assay company. They represent the only independent check of an assay's validity that a researcher can perform on the results returned by such companies.

Finally, measurement *reliability* (or *precision*) needs to be established and evaluated (see the fourth row of Table 3.1). This is usually done in two ways. First, all samples are assayed in duplicate, and the degree to which two measurements of the same sample differ, expressed as the "coefficient of variation" (CV), is averaged across all samples and reported as the intra-assay CV. Intra-assay CV is heavily influenced by the consistency of the assayer's pipetting technique; fluctuations in the way samples are pipetted into the assay tubes or plate wells, or improper handling of the pipette itself, increase the intra-assay CV. But other factors also play a role. In our lab, we have found preincubation of salivary testosterone and cortisol RIAs to yield lower CVs, presumably because bonds between salivary hormones and antibodies become more stable during preincubation. We have also observed that CVs for salivary steroid levels drop substantially if the source tube with the aliquoted sample is gently inverted two to three times before the sample is transferred to the assay. This observation suggests that steroid hormones can be unevenly distributed in the fluid column inside a sample tube after prolonged storage, perhaps due to the displacing force of other molecules that differ by size and density.

The intra-assay CV tends to exaggerate lack of reliability at the lower range of the assay, and thus for low-concentration samples, because the same absolute difference (e.g., 14 pg/ml vs. 18 pg/ml) between two duplicate measurements at lower concentrations yields a higher CV than at higher concentrations (e.g., 84 pg/ml vs. 88 pg/ml). It should be noted, too, that rank-order stability of sample concentrations, as estimated by Spearman's correlation coefficient or other measures of between-sample correlation, can be high despite an unsatisfactory intra-assay CV, because the variance between different individuals' hormone levels is frequently substantially higher than the measurement variance within samples (see Stanton & Schultheiss, 2007, for an example).

The second method of establishing measurement reliability is to determine interassay CV. With large batches of samples and many research participants, samples are usually split into several consecutive assays, each with its own set of calibrators for the generation of a standard curve. But if each assay gets its own measurement device (i.e., the calibrators), how can researchers ensure that different consecutive assays yield comparable readings? The solution to this problem is easy: including samples coming from the same source in all assays, and comparing readings for these samples across assays by determining the interassay CV. The sources should be sufficiently large to provide samples for all assays in a given series, and should ideally cover at least two substantially different analyte concentrations. In our own labs, we frequently either pool leftover samples or collect large quantities (> 10 ml) of saliva from lab members, and include these samples in all assays for a given study. To create pools with sufficiently different concentrations, we take known factors that affect hormone concentrations into consideration. For instance, because men and women differ greatly in their testosterone levels, we create separate male and female saliva pools. And to create pools with different cortisol concentrations, we separately pool samples collected early in the morning (when levels are high) and samples collected late at night (when cortisol is close to its circadian low point). When only a small number of samples have been collected that can be accommodated by one single assay for a given hormone, interassay CV cannot be determined. In this case, only the intra-assay CV is reported.

Researchers who would like to employ salivary hormone measures, but do not have the facilities to do the assays themselves, can "outsource" saliva sample analysis to commercial assay labs that specialize in salivary hormone measurement. However, in this case we strongly recommend that researchers not simply trust the claims these labs are making, but actually test their validity before and after sending off the samples. Of course, a thorough understanding of the quality parameters of good endocrine measurement as outlined above and in Table 3.1 is essential for this. One simple way to pick a good assay service is to compare the claims of the assay provider with the published literature. An assay service that uses an assay whose analytical range does not cover the expected hormone concentration range in the tested sample reasonably well (e.g., an estradiol range of 2–40 pg/ml, when average estradiol levels in men and women are typically about 1–4 pg/ml), or that reports excellent recovery coefficients for accuracy checks whose levels are far above the levels typically expected (for the estradiol example, at 10 and 25 pg/ml, which is substantially outside the range of values ordinarily observed in men or normally cycling women), should be viewed with some suspicion. As suggested previously, we also recommend including one's own accuracy checks calibrated for the hormone concentrations expected in the study sample (e.g., cortisol accuracy checks at 1.5 and 3.5 ng/ml, corresponding to low and high salivary levels of this hormone). The investment in a set of commercially available calibrator samples (e.g., the Lyphochek samples mentioned above), a pipette, and a couple of tubes and pipette tips is comparatively minuscule (less than $700) and pays off in the form of an all-important independent verification of the quality of the outsourced assays. Finally, customers of commercial assay services should expect to receive a complete set of data that includes not only the mean hormone level and CV for each sample, but also the values for each individual measurement (for verification of the intra-assay CV); the values for standard pools used across assays (for verification of interassay CVs); and the complete data on the standard curve, including the zero-concentration calibrator, which can be used to verify the service's claims about the sensitivity of the assay. Schultheiss and colleagues (2005) checked assay specificity by comparing salivary testosterone concentrations to levels reported in the literature; determined and reported the "lower limit of detection" (LLD) as a measure of assay sensitivity (1 pg/ml); and also reported interassay CV (6.62%) and intra-assay CV (4.72%). The interassay CV estimate was based on an in-house saliva pool and three Lyphochek control samples, from which assay accuracy was also determined. Accuracy was excellent, with measured levels corresponding closely to expected levels for the low (59 pg/ml: 97%), medium (125 pg/ml: 101%), and high (250 pg/ml: 99%) range of male salivary testosterone levels. The analytical range (i.e., the range from the lowest to the highest nonzero standard) of the assay was 5–400 pg/ml and was sufficient to cover the observed levels of salivary testosterone, which ranged from 7 to 248 pg/ml.

Data Processing

Regardless of whether one uses an RIA or EIA, the actual measurements returned by one's measurement device (be it a gamma counter or a plate reader) are not hormone concentrations but proxy measurements, such as counts per minute in the case of the gamma particles emitted by a decaying isotope. These need to be transformed and interpreted to make sense as hormone concentrations. Of course, many counters and readers come with built-in analysis software that can be programmed to automatically estimate analyte concentrations in samples. In our experience, however, this software is rarely useful for processing data resulting from salivary hormone analysis, because it is usually geared toward the determination of plasma hormone levels. And if it is employed without proper knowledge of the steps involved in assay data processing, and without checking whether all prerequisites are met for the application of the software and the preset parameters, results can be severely biased or simply useless. We therefore advocate using one's preferred statistical software package for the mindful processing of hormone assay data. An excellent, hands-on guide to the steps involved in this process is provided by Nix and Wild (2000); here, we only give a brief overview of the main stepping-stones on the way from the raw measurements to the final concentration estimates.

The first step is usually to put the raw measurements in relation to the known concentrations of the calibrator samples with known concentrations, which constitute the standard curve (see Figure 3.3). This step frequently requires the computational transformation of the calibrator concentrations, the raw measurements, or both to bring calibrator concentrations and measurements into a linear relationship. It also requires the close examination of graphs depicting the relationship between known calibrator concentrations and observed measurements, to control for outliers that might bias the regression equation for the standard curve. In general, a regression of measured signal on calibrator concentrations is expected to exceed 97% of explained variance—a criterion that brings tears to the eyes of many a behavioral scientist, but represents an absolutely reasonable and defensible requirement for the deriva-

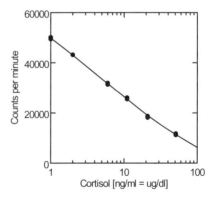

FIGURE 3.3. Standard curve from salivary cortisol assay. Standard concentrations cover the entire range of salivary cortisol levels typically observed in healthy populations (i.e., from 0.05 to 20 ng/ml). The standard with a concentration of 0 ng/ml is not depicted here, but is included in the assay. A distance-weighted least-squares regression line is fitted through the data points. Note that log-transformation of the x axis makes the relationship between hormone concentration (x axis) and gamma emissions (in counts per minute; y axis) approximately linear.

tion of the regression equation that will be used to accurately estimate concentrations in unknown samples. In our experience, including three or more samples for each calibrator concentration greatly facilitates the determination of a robust standard curve, because average concentrations at each level are less likely to be influenced by outliers.

Once a good, linear fit between hormone concentration in the calibrators and measured signal (e.g., counts per minute) has been determined, the relationship between predictor and dependent variable is turned upside down to move from the question "What signal level does a given concentration predict?" to "What concentration can I infer, given a certain signal level?" The flipping of the relationship between predictor and dependent variable entailed in this second step is simplified if the relationship between both variables has been linearized previously, and the regression equation thus becomes symmetrical with regard to the predictor and the criterion. The prediction of calibrator concentrations from the measured signal yields a regression equation that can also be applied to all other, noncalibrator samples—that is, to control samples and samples collected from the research participants.

The application of this formula to the rest of the samples in the assay constitutes the third step. Because the variance around the zero-concentration calibrator and the mean signal levels of control samples can be interpreted in terms of actual analyte concentrations, it is also possible to determine the sensitivity and the accuracy, respectively, of the assay at this point.

In a final step, after data from the calibrators and the control samples have been discarded, the CV of the duplicate measurements for the actual samples collected from research participants is determined, and mean concentration levels for each sample are calculated. These mean estimated concentrations are then used as interval-scale variables in subsequent analyses (regression and correlation analyses, analyses of variance [ANOVAs], analyses of covariance [ANCOVAs], etc.) probing the validity of the research hypothesis.

In the case of the analyses for Study 1 in Schultheiss and colleagues (2005), a repeated-measures ANCOVA design was used. The researchers entered testosterone levels measured immediately before the contest start (T3) as a covariate, postcontest testosterone (T4, T5, T6) as a within-subjects variable, and contest outcome (win vs. lose) and implicit power motivation (z scores) as between-subjects predictors. Schultheiss and colleagues found a power motive × contest outcome × time effect that was consistent with hypotheses: 15 min after the contest (T5) but not earlier (T3) or later (T6), power motivation significantly predicted testosterone increases in winners and decreases in losers (see Figure 3.4).

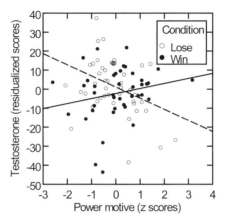

FIGURE 3.4. Effect of dispositional power motivation (*z* scores, *x* axis) and experimentally varied contest outcome (win, lose) on male participants' testosterone levels 15 min after the contest (T5; *y* axis). Postcontest testosterone was residualized for testosterone levels immediately before the contest (T3), which served as baseline. Partial correlations for the effect of power motivation on testosterone changes are .21 for winners and –.38 for losers. From Schultheiss et al. (2005). Copyright 2005 by the American Psychological Association. Reprinted by permission.

Reporting the Results of a Hormone Assay

As the reporting of other findings does, reporting the results of hormone assays involves two steps. First, the method of assessment and its quality should be reported in the "Methods" section. Second, the actual findings are reported in the "Results" section.

Description of the method should include the exact type and make of the assay; a short summary of the sample processing and sample assay protocol, particularly of points where they diverged from routine protocols (e.g., if samples were pretreated in some way or a preincubation period was used); and also the main quality control parameters of the assay—that is, measures of validity (specificity, accuracy, LLD, analytical range) and reliability (intra- and interassay CV). For well-established assay procedures, it is usually sufficient to omit estimates of specificity and accuracy, and to report only analytical range, LLD, and CV. Assay quality parameters provided by the manufacturers of commercially available assays should *not* be reported, as these typically represent best-case scenarios that are included with the assay to promote sales and that may have little to do with the quality of an assay actually conducted in one's own lab.

Reporting of findings should include descriptive data on the hormone levels observed in the sample and their relationship to major influences on endocrine function, such as gender, menstrual cycle stage, use of oral contraceptives, and time of day when samples were collected. In general, the same rules and best practices for analyzing and reporting other kinds of data also apply to hormone measures. Thus hormone data distributions should be examined for skew and, if necessary, transformed to bring them closer to a normal distribution (this is frequently necessary for salivary cortisol data and may be required for other hormones in some cases); if this is done, it should be reported. If outliers are present in the hormone data (e.g., elevated estradiol due to ovulation, high progesterone levels sometimes observed in women in the luteal phase or in the early stages of pregnancy, or extreme levels of cortisol sometimes observed in individuals with undiagnosed endocrine disorders), and they cannot be accommodated through standard data transformations, analyses should be run and reported both with and without the outliers. If the findings hold up to scrutiny either way, nothing is lost by pointing this out; if they emerge only in one or the other case, this needs to be considered in the "Discussion" section and perhaps even before the paper is written.

Advantages and Disadvantages of Salivary Hormone Measures

Toward the end of this chapter's introduction, we have already pointed out that a main advantage of salivary hormone measures is that they are pain-free and thus easy to use in behavioral studies, and that their main disadvantage is the limitation of their use to those hormones that make it into saliva. With regard to the latter issue, it is important to keep in mind that the method should never dictate the research question, and that if it is conceptually reasonable to assess a hormone that is not present in saliva but in other body compartments, a researcher should consider alternative methods. For instance, metabolites of some peptide hormones can be assessed in urine; peptide hormone levels can be varied experimentally through nasal administration of sprays (e.g., Born et al., 2002); and if a hormone of interest can only be assessed in blood, then the researcher could team up with a physician, nurse, or phlebotomist to get the necessary blood samples from participants and take proper care to minimize the effects of venipuncture-induced stress on the measurement of the targeted hormone (e.g., by allowing a sufficient amount of time after venipuncture for the participant to relax and get used to the measurement situation). In this section, we briefly touch on some conceptual advantages and disadvantages of hormone assessment that we think are important for researchers interested in adding endocrine measures to their armamentarium.

A major advantage of salivary hormone measures is that they simultaneously meet personality psychologists' need for rank-order stability and social psychologists' need for measures that are sensitive to the social stimuli impinging on the person. In Study 1 of the data reported by Schultheiss and colleagues (2005), correlations of testosterone concentrations in consecutive saliva samples ranged from .82 to .96, indicating high within-session stability of male testosterone levels. For a testing interval of 48 hours, Sellers, Mehl, and Josephs (2007) recently reported salivary testosterone test–retest correlations of .69 for men and .72 for women. Even for saliva samples taken 2 months apart, Dabbs (1990) reported test–retest correlations between .43 and .59. Comparable findings have been reported for salivary estradiol (Stanton & Schultheiss, 2007) and cortisol (Cieslak, Frost, & Klentrou, 2003). Within-session stability of salivary progesterone levels was high (.80 to .87) in the Schultheiss and colleagues (2004) study, and current investigations in our laboratories suggest that salivary progesterone also shows substantial retest stability over the course of 2 weeks.

Stable differences in salivary hormones in turn are associated with important behavioral differences. Individual differences in salivary testosterone correlate positively with measures of dominant and aggressive behavior (e.g., Dabbs & Hargrove, 1997; Dabbs, Jurkovic, & Frady, 1991; Schaal, Tremblay, Soussigan, & Susman, 1996) and predict attention and learning in response to facial expressions (van Honk et al., 2000; Wirth & Schultheiss, 2007). Likewise, individual differences in salivary cortisol levels are predictive of attentional responding to threat stimuli (van Honk et al., 1998) and can interact with testosterone in shaping behavior (e.g., Dabbs et al., 1991).

In this context, it is remarkable that self-report measures of personality and emotionality notoriously fail to correlate substantially with basal measures of steroid hormones. For instance, salivary and other measures of testosterone have no consistent variance overlap with questionnaire measures of dominance and aggression (Mazur & Booth, 1998). Moreover, a meta-analysis revealed that cortisol, despite its reputation as a "stress hormone," does not correlate with questionnaire measures of negative emotionality (Dickerson & Kemeny, 2004). At the same time, the roles of these hormones in dominance and stress responses are well documented in humans and in a wide variety of nonhuman and even nonmammalian species (see Nelson, 2005), suggesting considerable phylogenetic continuity of the functions these hormones fulfill. Also, the mechanisms through which hormones affect behavior and are affected by situations have been worked out in great detail in many cases (e.g., Albert, Jonik, & Walsh, 1992; Sapolsky, 1987; Schultheiss, 2007a). In contrast, we humans are the only species capable of filling out questionnaires inquiring about our dispositions to dominate, affiliate, experience negative affect, and so on, and the extent to which the beliefs measured through such instruments can be mapped onto the embrained and embodied systems that guide actual dominance behavior, affiliation, stress responses, and so on is often unclear (cf. Gazzaniga, 1985; Kagan, 2002; McClelland, Koestner, & Weinberger, 1989; Schultheiss, 2007b). Therefore, hormonal measures of dominance and other behavioral dispositions have the clear advantage of being more likely to carve nature at its joints than questionnaire measures of the same constructs.

Salivary hormone measures are also sufficiently sensitive to situational stimuli and events to be of use to social psychologists. Examples of the effects of the situation on people's salivary hormone levels include research on the impact of affiliation-arousing movies on progesterone and cortisol (Schultheiss et al., 2004; Wirth & Schultheiss, 2006); competition effects on testosterone (e.g., Gladue et al., 1989; Mazur, Booth, & Dabbs, 1992); and, most thoroughly documented, effects of social-evaluative threat on cortisol changes (Kirschbaum, Pirke, & Hellhammer, 1993; see also the meta-analysis by Dickerson & Kemeny, 2004).

In our view, however, salivary hormone measures are most usefully employed in research that combines dispositional with situational factors, because individuals bring their learning history, genetic makeup, and so forth to a given situation and respond to the situation on the basis of these dispositional factors (cf. also Sapolsky, 1999). Our own worked-out example above has already illustrated the interactive effect of implicit power motivation (disposition) and contest outcome (situation) on testosterone changes. Notably, in this study as in many others, contest outcome per se did not have a main effect on hormonal changes, because the hormonal responses to competitions in individuals who do not seek power are virtually the opposite of the responses in those who do (see also Josephs, Sellers, Newman, & Mehta, 2006; Wirth, Welsh, & Schultheiss, 2006). Work by Josephs and colleagues (2006) illustrates that salivary hormone measures can also be used as predictors, rather than as dependent variables, in person × situation designs. Based on the hypothesis that high levels of salivary testosterone should make people feel comfortable when in a high-power position but uncomfortable in a low-power position, and that low levels of testosterone should be associated with the reverse, Josephs and colleagues showed that low-testosterone participants reported greater emotional arousal and showed worse cognitive functioning in a high-power position, whereas high-power individuals exhibited this pattern in a low-power position. Giving the person × situation design a further twist, Mehta and Josephs (2006) recently demonstrated that men who responded with a salivary testosterone *decrease* to a defeat in a competition were less likely to enter another dominance contest than were men who responded with a testosterone *increase*.

One potential drawback of the use of endocrine measures in social neuroscience is that hormones do not map onto established psychological constructs in a one-to-one fashion, or do so only within certain boundaries. For instance, cortisol increases in response to a public speaking task are readily interpreted as a physiological indicator of stress. But what then about the fact that cortisol also surges after a meal? Or that cortisol reaches its highest peak in the morning, just before people get up? Clearly, cortisol overlaps only partially with the concept of stress, and the energy-regulating functions of cortisol encompass more than just dealing with a stressful situation. As another case in point, high or increasing levels of testosterone are associated with aggression and dominance. But testosterone also regulates libido, energy metabolism, and tissue buildup in the muscles, and many of the central (i.e., brain) effects of testosterone are mediated fully or in part by its powerful metabolite estradiol. Furthermore, the numerous interactions of hormonal systems with each other, as well as with the immune system, brain systems, and peripheral organs, are often complex and intimidating at first glance. The only way to master this complexity and to employ hormone measures successfully in one's research requires a thorough understanding of the endocrine system.

We believe, however, that these apparent disadvantages can be turned into advantages if one is willing (1) to become acquainted with the basic literature on endocrine systems (e.g., Griffin & Ojeda, 2000), their relationships with brain and behavior (e.g., Nelson, 2005), and their assessment (e.g., Gosling, 2000; Riad-Fahmy, Read, Walker, & Griffiths, 1982; Riad-Fahmy et al., 1987); and (2) to be curious about the ramifications of casting one's research hypothesis in endocrinological terms, and to keep an open mind about the findings one obtains from research employing hormonal measures. The apparent disadvantage of complex interactions between hormonal and other systems can quickly turn into an advantage if one realizes that each hormone comes with a rich, multidisciplinary research literature, and that even after relatively coarse perusal this literature can suggest exciting new hypotheses and research directions that would not have been apparent otherwise. For instance, recent research that builds on a knowledge of the organizational effects of testosterone on male facial morphology, and the activational effects of estradiol on female mate choice, demonstrates that women with higher estradiol concentrations exhibit stronger preferences for the faces of men with higher testosterone concentrations—an effect that changes with menstrual cycle stage and thus with circulating estradiol levels (Roney & Simmons, 2008). Because some of the effects of hormones on brain systems mediating specific cognitive functions have been worked out in great detail in animal models, it is no longer far-fetched to postulate and study hormone-mediated effects of stress and social factors on memory and other cognitive processes in humans (e.g., Cahill, 2000; Putman, van Honk, Kessels, Mulder, & Koppeschaar, 2004). And the interface among social psychology, endocrinology, and immunology holds particular promise for a better understanding of how experiential factors affect physical health and illness (e.g., Munck, Guyre, & Holbrook, 1984; Sapolsky, 2004).

In summary, incorporating endocrine measures and concepts in one's research requires work, as all efforts at broadening one's horizon do. But speaking from experience, we believe that it is work well invested, because interfacing psychology with endocrinology makes the study of human behavior more rigorous, intellectually stimulating, and (perhaps most importantly) likely to yield exciting discoveries. And *that* gets our hormones going!

APPENDIX 3.1. PC-Administered Screening Questionnaire Used in Studies with Hormone Assessments

(Time of day is recorded by the PC.)
Please enter your age.
Please enter your gender.
Please enter your weight (in pounds).
Please enter your height.
Have you experienced any gum bleeding over the past day?
Have you experienced any other oral infections and/or oral lacerations over the past day?
How long ago, in hours, has it been since you brushed your teeth?
How many hours ago has it been since you consumed caffeine (coffee, tea, soda, chocolate)?
How many hours ago has it been since you consumed an alcoholic beverage?
Are you currently on any kind of medication? If yes, please provide the name of the prescription.
Do you have a diagnosed endocrine disorder? If yes, please name the disorder.
Do you use any recreational drugs (e.g., marijuana, Ecstasy, speed, cocaine, heroin)?
Do you smoke?
Do you take anabolic steroids?
Are your currently involved in a steady relationship?
Have you had sexual intercourse in the last 24 hours?
Please indicate the hand (left or right) you typically use in activities such as writing, brushing your teeth, holding a glass, etc.

Additional questions for women only:
What was the date on which your last menstrual period started?
What is the average duration of your menstrual cycle (in days)? (By "menstrual cycle," we mean the time from the start of one menstrual period to the start of the next.)
Do you currently take oral contraceptives (i.e., the "pill")?

Acknowledgment

We thank Michelle M. Wirth for her constructive comments and valuable suggestions on an earlier version of this chapter.

References

Recommended introductory readings are marked with an asterisk (*).

Albert, D. J., Jonik, R. H., & Walsh, M. L. (1992). Hormone-dependent aggression in male and female rats: Experiential, hormonal, and neural foundations. *Neuroscience and Biobehavioral Reviews, 16*(2), 177–192.
Baron-Cohen, S., Lutchmaya, S., & Knickmeyer, R. (2006). *Prenatal testosterone in mind: Amniotic fluid studies.* Cambridge, MA: MIT Press.
Beckwith, B. E., Petros, T. V., Bergloff, P. J., & Staebler, R. J. (1987). Vasopressin analogue (DDAVP) facilitates recall of narrative prose. *Behavioral Neuroscience, 101*(3), 429–432.
Born, J., Lange, T., Kern, W., McGregor, G. P., Bickel, U., & Fehm, H. L. (2002). Sniffing neuropeptides: A transnasal approach to the human brain. *Nature Neuroscience, 5*(6), 514–516.
Cahill, L. (2000). Modulation of long-term memory in humans by emotional arousal: Adrenergic activation and the amygdala. In J. P. Aggleton (Ed.), *The amygdala: A functional analysis* (pp. 425–446). New York: Oxford University Press.
Carter, C. S., Pournajafi-Nazarloo, H., Kramer, K. M., Ziegler, T. E., White-Traut, R., Bello, D., et al. (2007). Oxytocin: Behavioral associations and potential as a salivary biomarker. *Annals of the New York Academy of Sciences, 1098,* 312–322.
Cieslak, T. J., Frost, G., & Klentrou, P. (2003). Effects of physical activity, body fat, and salivary cortisol on mucosal immunity in children. *Journal of Applied Physiology, 95*(6), 2315–2320.
Dabbs, J. M. (1990). Salivary testosterone measurements: Reliability across hours, days, and weeks. *Physiology and Behavior, 48,* 83–86.
Dabbs, J. M. (1991). Salivary testosterone measurements: Collecting, storing, and mailing saliva samples. *Physiology and Behavior, 49,* 815–817.(*)
Dabbs, J. M. (1992). Testosterone measurements in social and clinical psychology. *Journal of Social and Clinical Psychology, 11,* 302–321.(*)
Dabbs, J. M., Jr., Campbell, B. C., Gladue, B. A., Midgley, A. R., Navarro, M.

A., Read, G. F., et al. (1995). Reliability of salivary testosterone measurements: A multicenter evaluation. *Clinical Chemistry, 41*(11), 1581–1584.

Dabbs, J. M., & Hargrove, M. F. (1997). Age, testosterone, and behavior among female prison inmates. *Psychosomatic Medicine, 59*, 477–480.

Dabbs, J. M., Jurkovic, G. J., & Frady, R. L. (1991). Salivary testosterone and cortisol among late adolescent male offenders. *Journal of Abnormal Child Psychology, 19*, 469–478.

Daly, R. C., Su, T. P., Schmidt, P. J., Pagliaro, M., Pickar, D., & Rubinow, D. R. (2003). Neuroendocrine and behavioral effects of high-dose anabolic steroid administration in male normal volunteers. *Psychoneuroendocrinology, 28*(3), 317–331.

Dickerson, S. S., & Kemeny, M. E. (2004). Acute stressors and cortisol responses: A theoretical integration and synthesis of laboratory research. *Psychological Bulletin, 130*(3), 355–391.

Gazzaniga, M. S. (1985). *The social brain: Discovering the networks of the mind.* New York: Basic Books.

Gladue, B. A., Boechler, M., & McCaul, K. D. (1989). Hormonal response to competition in human males. *Aggressive Behavior, 15*, 409–422.

Gosling, J. P. (Ed.). (2000). *Immunoassays: A practical approach.* Oxford, UK: Oxford University Press.(*)

Graham, J. M., & Desjardins, C. (1980). Classical conditioning: Induction of luteinizing hormone and testosterone secretion in anticipation of sexual activity. *Science, 210*, 1039–1041.

Granger, D. A., Cicchetti, D., Rogosch, F. A., Hibel, L. C., Teisl, M., & Flores, E. (2007). Blood contamination in children's saliva: Prevalence, stability, and impact on the measurement of salivary cortisol, testosterone, and dehydroepiandrosterone. *Psychoneuroendocrinology, 32*(6), 724–733.

Griffin, J. E., & Ojeda, S. R. (Eds.). (2000). *Textbook of endocrine physiology* (4th ed.). Oxford, UK: Oxford University Press.(*)

Hibel, L. C., Granger, D. A., Kivlighan, K. T., & Blair, C. (2006). Individual differences in salivary cortisol: Associations with common over-the-counter and prescription medication status in infants and their mothers. *Hormones and Behavior, 50*(2), 293–300.

Hofman, L. F. (2001). Human saliva as a diagnostic specimen. *Journal of Nutrition, 131*(5), 1621S–1625S.

Horvat-Gordon, M., Granger, D. A., Schwartz, E. B., Nelson, V. J., & Kivlighan, K. T. (2005). Oxytocin is not a valid biomarker when measured in saliva by immunoassay. *Physiology and Behavior, 84*(3), 445–448.

Josephs, R. A., Sellers, J. G., Newman, M. L., & Mehta, P. H. (2006). The mismatch effect: When testosterone and status are at odds. *Journal of Personality and Social Psychology, 90*(6), 999–1013.

Kagan, J. (2002). *Surprise, uncertainty, and mental structures.* Cambridge, MA: Harvard University Press.

Kirschbaum, C., & Hellhammer, D. H. (1994). Salivary cortisol in psychoneuroendocrine research: Recent developments and applications. *Psychoneuroendocrinology, 19*(4), 313–333.(*)

Kirschbaum, C., Pirke, K. M., & Hellhammer, D. H. (1993). The "Trier Social

Stress Test": A tool for investigating psychobiological stress responses in a laboratory setting. *Neuropsychobiology, 28*(1–2), 76–81.

Laeng, B., & Falkenberg, L. (2007). Women's pupillary responses to sexually significant others during the hormonal cycle. *Hormones and Behavior, 52*(4), 520–530.

Mazur, A. (1985). A biosocial model of status in face-to-face primate groups. *Social Forces, 64*, 377–402.

Mazur, A., & Booth, A. (1998). Testosterone and dominance in men. *Behavioral and Brain Sciences, 21*, 353–397.

Mazur, A., Booth, A., & Dabbs, J. M. (1992). Testosterone and chess competition. *Social Psychology Quarterly, 55*, 70–77.

McClelland, D. C., Koestner, R., & Weinberger, J. (1989). How do self-attributed and implicit motives differ? *Psychological Review, 96*, 690–702.

Mehta, P. H., & Josephs, R. A. (2006). Testosterone change after losing predicts the decision to compete again. *Hormones and Behavior, 50*(5), 684–692.

Munck, A., Guyre, P. M., & Holbrook, N. J. (1984). Physiological functions of glucocorticoids in stress and their relation to pharmacological actions. *Endocrine Reviews, 5*, 25–44.

Nadeem, H. S., Attenburrow, M. J., & Cowen, P. J. (2004). Comparison of the effects of citalopram and escitalopram on 5-HT-mediated neuroendocrine responses. *Neuropsychopharmacology, 29*(9), 1699–1703.

Nelson, R. J. (2005). *An introduction to behavioral endocrinology* (3rd ed.). Sunderland, MA: Sinauer Associates.(*)

Nix, B., & Wild, D. (2000). Data processing. In J. P. Gosling (Ed.), *Immunoassays: A practical approach* (pp. 239–261). Oxford, UK: Oxford University Press.

Oyegbile, T. O., & Marler, C. A. (2005). Winning fights elevates testosterone levels in California mice and enhances future ability to win fights. *Hormones and Behavior, 48*(3), 259–267.

Pope, H. G., Jr., Kouri, E. M., & Hudson, J. I. (2000). Effects of supraphysiologic doses of testosterone on mood and aggression in normal men: A randomized controlled trial. *Archives of General Psychiatry, 57*(2), 133–140 (discussion, 155–156).

Putman, P., van Honk, J., Kessels, R. P., Mulder, M., & Koppeschaar, H. P. (2004). Salivary cortisol and short- and long-term memory for emotional faces in healthy young women. *Psychoneuroendocrinology, 29*(7), 953–960.

Raff, H., Homar, P. J., & Burns, E. A. (2002). Comparison of two methods for measuring salivary cortisol. *Clinical Chemistry, 48*(1), 207–208.

Riad-Fahmy, D., Read, G. F., Walker, R. F., & Griffiths, K. (1982). Steroids in saliva for assessing endocrine function. *Endocrine Reviews, 3*(4), 367–395.(*)

Riad-Fahmy, D., Read, G. F., Walker, R. F., Walker, S. M., & Griffiths, K. (1987). Determination of ovarian steroid hormone levels in saliva: An overview. *Journal of Reproductive Medicine, 32*(4), 254–272.(*)

Roney, J. R., Lukaszewski, A. W., & Simmons, Z. L. (2007). Rapid endocrine responses of young men to social interactions with young women. *Hormones and Behavior, 52*(3), 326–333.

Roney, J. R., & Simmons, Z. L. (2008). Women's estradiol predicts preference for facial cues of men's testosterone. *Hormones and Behavior, 53*(1), 14–19.

Sapolsky, R. M. (1987). Stress, social status, and reproductive physiology in free-living baboons. In D. Crews (Ed.), *Psychobiology and reproductive behavior: An evolutionary perspective* (pp. 291–322). Englewood Cliffs, NJ: Prentice-Hall.

Sapolsky, R. M. (1999). Hormonal correlates of personality and social contexts: From nonhuman to human primates. In C. Panter-Brick & C. Worthman (Eds.), *Hormones, health, and behaviour: A socio-ecological and lifespan perspective* (pp. 18–46). Cambridge, UK: Cambridge University Press.

Sapolsky, R. M. (2004). *Why zebras don't get ulcers* (3rd ed.). New York: Holt.

Schaal, B., Tremblay, R. E., Soussigan, R., & Susman, E. J. (1996). Male testosterone linked to high social dominance but low physical aggression in early adolescence. *Journal of the American Academy of Child and Adolescent Psychiatry, 34,* 1322–1330.

Schultheiss, O. C. (2007a). A biobehavioral model of implicit power motivation arousal, reward and frustration. In E. Harmon-Jones & P. Winkielman (Eds.), *Social neuroscience: Integrating biological and psychological explanations of social behavior* (pp. 176–196). New York: Guilford Press.

Schultheiss, O. C. (2007b). A memory-systems approach to the classification of personality tests: Comment on Meyer and Kurtz (2006). *Journal of Personality Assessment, 89*(2), 197–201.

Schultheiss, O. C., & Brunstein, J. C. (1999). Goal imagery: Bridging the gap between implicit motives and explicit goals. *Journal of Personality, 67,* 1–38.

Schultheiss, O. C., Campbell, K. L., & McClelland, D. C. (1999). Implicit power motivation moderates men's testosterone responses to imagined and real dominance success. *Hormones and Behavior, 36*(3), 234–241.

Schultheiss, O. C., Wirth, M. M., & Stanton, S. J. (2004). Effects of affiliation and power motivation arousal on salivary progesterone and testosterone. *Hormones and Behavior, 46*(5), 592–599.

Schultheiss, O. C., Wirth, M. M., Torges, C. M., Pang, J. S., Villacorta, M. A., & Welsh, K. M. (2005). Effects of implicit power motivation on men's and women's implicit learning and testosterone changes after social victory or defeat. *Journal of Personality and Social Psychology, 88*(1), 174–188.

Sellers, J. G., Mehl, M. R., & Josephs, R. A. (2007). Hormones and personality: Testosterone as a marker of individual differences. *Journal of Research in Personality, 41,* 126–138.

Shirtcliff, E. A., Granger, D. A., Schwartz, E., & Curran, M. J. (2001). Use of salivary biomarkers in biobehavioral research: Cotton-based sample collection methods can interfere with salivary immunoassay results. *Psychoneuroendocrinology, 26*(2), 165–173.

Stanton, S. J., & Schultheiss, O. C. (2007). Basal and dynamic relationships between implicit power motivation and estradiol in women. *Hormones and Behavior, 52*(5), 571–580.

van Honk, J., Tuiten, A., Hermans, E., Putman, P., Koppeschaar, H., Thijssen, J., et al. (2001). A single administration of testosterone induces cardiac accelerative responses to angry faces in healthy young women. *Behavioral Neuroscience, 115*(1), 238–242.

van Honk, J., Tuiten, A., van den Hout, M., Koppeschaar, H., Thijssen, J., de Haan, E., et al. (1998). Baseline salivary cortisol levels and preconscious selective attention for threat: A pilot study. *Psychoneuroendocrinology, 23*(7), 741–747.

van Honk, J., Tuiten, A., van den Hout, M., Koppeschaar, H., Thijssen, J., de Haan, E., et al. (2000). Conscious and preconscious selective attention to social threat: Different neuroendocrine response patterns. *Psychoneuroendocrinology, 25*(6), 577–591.

Wirth, M. M., & Schultheiss, O. C. (2006). Effects of affiliation arousal (hope of closeness) and affiliation stress (fear of rejection) on progesterone and cortisol. *Hormones and Behavior, 50*, 786–795.

Wirth, M. M., & Schultheiss, O. C. (2007). Basal testosterone moderates responses to anger faces in humans. *Physiology and Behavior, 90*(2–3), 496–505.

Wirth, M. M., Welsh, K. M., & Schultheiss, O. C. (2006). Salivary cortisol changes in humans after winning or losing a dominance contest depend on implicit power motivation. *Hormones and Behavior, 49*(3), 346–352.

4

Neuroendocrine Manipulation of the Sexually Dimorphic Human Social Brain

Jack van Honk

The Sexually Dimorphic Social Brain

Social cognition involves highly adaptive abilities, such as the interpretation of social stimuli, social communication, cooperation, empathizing, and mentalizing. Humans excel in all of these, and may stand alone in some of them; indeed, their evolutionary success is suggested to be based on their unrivaled social-cognitive aptitude (Kringelbach & Rolls, 2003). Social-cognitive neuroscience investigates the psychobiology of human social cognition, but research targeting the human social brain is in its early years, and the evident sex and individual differences in social cognition—with their critically implicated neuroendocrine regulatory mechanisms—have received little attention as yet. Nonetheless, both correlational research and causal hormone manipulation in human subjects indicate that the sexually dimorphic neuroendocrine system importantly establishes the individual variation in social cognition (Kosfeld, Heinrichs, Zak, Fischbacher, & Fehr, 2004; Schultheiss, Wirth, & Stanton, 2004; van Honk et al., 1999, 2004), and is responsible for enhanced empathic, mind-reading, and emotion recognition abilities in females (Domes, Heinrichs, Michel, Berger, & Herpertz, 2007; Hampson, van Anders, & Mullin, 2006; Hermans, Putman, & van Honk, 2006b; van Honk & Schutter, 2007a).

In sum, sex differences in emotion and social cognition have received attention in social psychology, but much less in social-cognitive neuroscience; this lack of attention may be problematic, especially in light of the recently observed critical anomaly of the famous "social brain hypothesis" from behavioral biology (Dunbar, 1998). This hypothesis simply holds that increases in social group size underlie increases in the size of the primate neocortex. However, it may apply to females exclusively, since the male primate neocortex may even shrink somewhat when the social group size increases (Lindenfors, 2005). Moreover, in addition to brain measures, recent behavioral data also indicate that male and female social brains differ considerably: Female sociality stems from prosocial motivations, whereas male sociality is often instrumentally driven (van Vugt, De Cremer, & Janssen, 2007). Finally, females tend to outperform males in various aspects of social cognition: the interpretation of social stimuli (e.g., Hampson et al., 2006; Montagne, Kessels, Frigerio, de Haan, & Perrett, 2005), empathizing, and mentalizing (e.g., Voracek & Dressler, 2006). In short, if human evolutionary success is truly based on unrivaled social-cognitive aptitude, the male contribution to this success may be relatively small.

To return to instrumental sociality, it indicates that the male sex hormone testosterone may well be an important endocrine factor in sex differences in the social brain and social cognition. Testosterone levels in blood plasma are 10–15 times higher in males, and, importantly, this hormone does not promote affiliation or sociality that is not repaid with sex, dominance, power, or material gain. Rather, the male sex hormone promotes a superficial form of sociality that mirrors the superficial charm of psychopathic personalities (van Honk & Schutter, 2007a). However, these neural and neuroendocrine mechanisms have been relatively ignored to date in human social-cognitive neuroscience. The hypothalamus, for instance, is a critical structure in the primate social brain (Emery & Amaral, 2000), but it plays only a marginal role in theories of the human social brain and social cognition.

The Neuroendocrine Social Brain

Among the key structures of the human social brain are the anterior cingulate and orbitofrontal cortices (Amodio & Frith, 2007), the superior temporal and fusiform gyrus (Corden, Critchley, Skuse, & Dolan,

2006), the parietal–premotor mirror neuron circuits (Keysers & Gaz-zola, 2006), and the amygdala (Adolphs, 2003). Animal researchers, as noted above, pay much more attention than human researchers do to the hypothalamus; in human social neuroscience, the amygdala often stands in the spotlight (Adolphs et al., 2005) and is even seen as the social-emotional center of the brain (Anderson, 2007). Other researchers in human social-cognitive neuroscience focus their attention on the medial prefrontal cortex or the mirror neuron systems (Amodio & Frith, 2007; Keysers & Gazzola, 2006). However, according to a few theorists (e.g., deCantazaro, 1999), the hypothalamus is the most important structure in motivation and emotion—central in the development of the social brain and in the execution of all aspects of sociality. Ignoring the hypo-thalamus is incongruent with its role as a major interface of the neural and endocrine systems. The hypothalamus belongs to the core limbic cir-cuitry and is located close to the amygdala, which lies in the medial tem-poral lobe of the brain. Hypothalamus dysfunction has a much greater impact on social and emotional behavior than amygdala dysfunction or dysfunction of any other structure of the social brain. Patients with selec-tive bilateral amygdala damage as a result of Urbach–Wiethe disease, for instance, often lead normal social and sexual lives (work, marriage, children), and their general intelligence does not differ from that of con-trols (Siebert, Markowitsch, & Bartel, 2003). Bilateral hypothalamus lesions, on the other hand, lead to deficiencies in testosterone, oxytocin, vasopressin, and cortisol, and thus to major sexual, social, and physical problems, without extensive medical care (i.e., chronic supplementation of the relevant hormones to normal levels). The hypothalamus is the true heart of the social brain (deCantanzaro, 1999).

Nonetheless, the amygdala is definitely a critical structure in social motivation and emotion, because of its unique properties that give social meaning to our environments (Adolphs, 2003). However, the type of social meaning the amygdala endows our world with depends critically on circulating levels of steroid and peptide hormones in the social brain, and thus on the hypothalamus (Huber, Veinante, & Stoop, 2005; Kirsch et al., 2005; van Honk & Schutter, 2007b). The notion that the amygdala is critical for human social cognition is largely based on research involv-ing the processing of emotional facial expressions (e.g., Adolphs et al., 2005; Calder & Nummenmaa, 2007), and emotional responses to and social-cognitive interpretations of facial expressions are highly sensitive to hormonal alterations (Domes, Heinrichs, Gläscher, et al., 2007; van Honk et al., 2001; van Honk, Peper, & Schutter, 2005). Facial expres-sions have pivotal signaling properties that can modify and control the behavior of individuals and social groups. Most critical for survival are the facial expressions of fear and anger, which arguably evolved as social signals capable of changing the onlooker's behavioral strategies quickly and directly. Angry and fearful facial expressions can induce nonconscious preparation for aggressive approach or fearful withdrawal when these signals travel the colliculopulvinar pathway to the amygdala (e.g., Morris, Öhman, & Dolan, 1999; Whalen et al., 1998), but conscious processing may be required for the involvement of emotion-inhibiting cortical control mechanisms that add behavioral flexibility (Reiman, 1997). Nonconsciously processed fearful and angry faces may be more "unconfounded" in activating the brain's primordial defense systems, including the amygdala, hypothalamus, and midbrain, when signaling danger (fear faces) versus aggression (anger faces) (van Honk et al., 2001; Whalen et al., 1998). Facial fear, however, not only acts as a silent danger signal; it can also evoke empathy in bystanders or potential aggressors, thereby eliciting social support and inhibiting violence (Blair, 2003, 2004). In support of this notion, prosocial abilities are accompanied by excellent facial fear recognition, whereas antisocial individuals are obviously impaired in recognizing fearful faces (Marsh & Blair, 2008; Marsh, Kozak, & Ambady, 2007). In all these processes and functions of facial threat, many social brain structures are implicated, but the amygdala is thought to play a crucial role (Amaral, 2003; Blair, 2003; Hermans, Ramsey, & van Honk, 2008; Morris et al., 1999).

This research on facial expressions and the amygdala has importantly defined the theoretical and methodological course in social and affective neuroscience, but it does not incorporate critical issues surrounding amygdala-centered neuroendocrine regulation, including sex-hormone-regulated sexually dimorphic social cognition (Hamann, 2004). Although the knowledge that the amygdala gives social meaning to our world (Adolphs, 2003) is an enormous step forward in social-cognitive neuroscience, we now need to get deeper into this remarkable function of the amygdala. Recent data suggest that the social meaning the amygdala gives to our world is importantly decided by neuroendocrine regulation (Hermans et al., 2008; Huber et al., 2005). Moreover, neuroendocrine factors not only influence our interpretation of the social world; they are also the engineers of the sexually dimorphic social brain from before birth until death.

Sex Steroids and Social Peptides

From the prenatal period onward, the female and male estrogens and androgens, most potently estradiol and testosterone, are busy building, breaking down, and rebuilding the sexually dimorphic social brain

(Schulkin, 2003). The brain's sexually dimorphic plasticity depends vitally on estradiol and testosterone, which regulate neurogenesis, neuronal migration, neurotransmitter plasticity, axonal guidance, synaptogenesis, and cell death (Carter, 2007; Hulshof Pol et al. 2006; Simerly, 2002). Moreover, sex differences in the brain and in social behavior importantly arise from diverging estradiol and testosterone levels during sensitive developmental periods, and can even be sex-reversed by acutely or chronically bringing the levels of circulating sex steroids to those of the other sex (Hermans, Putnam, & van Honk, 2006b; Hulshof Pol et al., 2006; van Honk & Schutter, 2007a). The acute effects of sex hormones on brain function may occur via an enormous number of possible pathways, but the up-regulating action of testosterone and estradiol in vasopressin and oxytocin synthesis is unmistakably critical in their effects on social cognition (Carter, 2007). Note that the social peptides oxytocin and vasopressin are completely dependent on the sex hormones for their actions and synthesis. However, fundamental research using testosterone and estradiol administration to examine social cognition in healthy humans is very limited. Moreover, past research often employed self-reports of mood, which showed little or no effect; this has led to mistaken assumptions about testosterone's relation to aggression, such as that it is meager or nonexistent in humans. In fact, relations between hormones and human behaviors are much more intricate and implicit, and have properties that often cannot be assessed by self-report.

The role of vasopressin and oxytocin in social-cognitive and emotional behaviors has been systematically studied in rats (De Wied, 1984) and voles (Insel & Young, 2000), but the role of these social peptides in human social and emotional behavior was less well understood until recently. However, methodological insights and innovations have recently made it easier to scrutinize the role of vasopressin and oxytocin in human social behaviors. It has been established not only that individual differences in peptide secretion in response to environmental change can reliably be assessed by taking urinary measures (Fries, Ziegler, Kurian, Jacoris, & Pollak, 2005), but that the effects of the peptides on social-emotional processes can be investigated reliably by exploiting the transnasal pathway to the brain for oxytocin and vasopressin (Born et al., 2002). Only a few (though very interesting) studies on the effects of vasopressin and oxytocin on human social cognition have been reported so far, and only one explicitly addresses sex differences. In what follows, I describe a range of recent experiments that have used diverse research strategies and methodologies for investigating the acute effects of the sex steroids estradiol and testosterone, and the social peptides oxytocin and vasopressin, on social cognition in healthy humans.

Estradiol: The Mysterious Female Sex Steroid

The logical hormonal candidates for human neuroscientific research into the acute effects of sex steroids on social cognition are the highly potent male and female sex hormones testosterone and estradiol. Many studies have used estradiol in clinical settings, but it is striking that there has been so very little research on the acute effects of estradiol on social-emotional processing in healthy females or males. I could only find two studies of direct relevance in the literature; one used a single dose of intranasal estradiol and the other a single dose of transdermal estradiol, both in healthy though postmenopausal women (Kaya, Cevrioglu, Onrat, Fenkci, & Yilmazer, 2003; Schleifer, Justice, & de Wit, 2002). Kaya and colleagues (2003) worked from the idea that acute estrogen administration has beneficial effects on autonomic tone in rodents, meaning that it shifts the balance from strained sympathetic to more relaxed parasympathetic function. In a double-blind study, the authors investigated the acute effects of intranasal estradiol administration on autonomic control of heart rate. Nineteen postmenopausal women with normal hormone profiles were tested in a crossover randomized design after intake of 300 µg nasal 17β-estradiol (i.e., the pure form of estradiol) and placebo at least 5 days apart. Compared to placebo, estradiol resulted in a reduced low-frequency-to-high-frequency ratio in the cardiac spectrum 45 min after administration, which points to the expected shift from strained sympathetic to relaxed parasympathetic function. Interestingly, this finding also fits neuroendocrine regulatory mechanisms of social cognition, wherein estradiol promotes oxytocin expression (Schulkin, 2007), and the up-regulating effects of oxytocin on the parasympathetic nervous system are well documented (e.g., Porges, 2003, 2007).

Schleifer and colleagues (2002) based their hypothesis on the observation that chronic treatment with estrogen has been found to produce mood improvement in postmenopausal women. The study was designed to find potential positive mood effects of single dose of transdermal estradiol in healthy postmenopausal women. Twelve women participated in a five-session, within-subjects, double-blind study, in which they received placebo, transdermal estradiol (0.2, 0.4, or 0.8 mg), or D-amphetamine (15 mg, oral) in a randomized order. Amphetamine was included as a positive control. Expected dose-dependent increases in plasma estradiol levels were found, and D-amphetamine produced some stimulant-like effects in these postmenopausal women, but estradiol did not produce any effects on mood. However, the design of the study seems somewhat unusual; in particular, I do not understand what the D-amphetamine condition controlled for, or what it added to the study. Moreover, the use of five sessions with three doses of estradiol, one of D-amphetamine, and one of a placebo put the study statistically at risk, especially since only weak measures such as self-reports of mood were employed. As the later descriptions of oxytocin and testosterone studies make clear, single doses of hormones often change social-affective processes on all levels of behavior, but there are rarely effects on self-report. It is not unlikely that the positive mood effects in clinical estradiol treatment studies are mediated in large part by more chronic increases in oxytocin synthesis, which may reduce anxiety and anger (Schulkin, 2007) but single doses of intranasal oxytocin seem to have no effect on mood (Domes, Heinrichs, Gläscher, et al., 2007; Kosfeld et al., 2004).

In summary, the causal effects of estradiol on social-emotional behavior in healthy populations have received very little attention. There have been many clinical studies, but these tell us little, because they involved malfunctioning social brains and mostly work exclusively with questionnaires or interviews. A few months of steroid hormone treatment in patients will absolutely change the structure and function of their defective brains, and these changes may or may not have clinical relevance, but it will be hard (i.e., time-consuming and expensive) to find fundamentally scientific and interesting data in the course of treatment. Fundamental acute estradiol administration studies in healthy individuals can teach us much more about individual and sex differences in effective social cognition. For instance, estradiol administered to males might induce an acute shift along the continuum of individual differences from male-type instrumental social behavior to female-type affiliative social behavior, which would be completely opposite to the effects of testosterone seen in females (Hermans et al., 2008; van Honk & Schutter, 2007a).

There are many possibilities for administering estradiol, but my method of choice would be to use the pure form, 17ß-estradiol, because all extra substances often have unwanted side effects; such substances can perhaps also be put into the placebo, but may still confound the study. A caveat is that the dosage and time course of estradiol effects on social cognition in males and females need to be established. The Kaya and colleagues (2003) study shows that this steroid hormone works quite fast when administered in females, at least. However, the study of estradiol in males seems of higher relevance for insights into the hormone's effects on affiliative versus instrumental sociality, because healthy females are relatively loaded with estradiol. With respect to the absence of mood effects shown in the Schleifer and colleagues (2002) study, this absence may even be critical, as it precludes criticism in terms of secondary mood-generated effects on social cognition. Note that none of the studies reported below using testosterone and oxytocin found any changes in mood, but there were constant and consistent changes in social-cognitive function. This substantiates my earlier suggestion concerning the applicability of self-reports of mood in hormone behavior research. For research using self-reports, perhaps even the best thing is to find nothing, given the possible explanations in terms of secondary mood-generated effects on social cognition if effects on mood are found.

Testosterone: The Notorious Male Sex Steroid

Testosterone is our most famous and notorious hormone; it has been studied in both animals and humans, and has been used and abused abundantly. There are many methods of administering testosterone (pills, transdermal patches, injections, etc.). However, there is, to my knowledge, only one sublingual administration method. This was developed in our laboratory by Adriaan Tuiten (Tuiten et al., 2000), and it has repeatedly been applied in fundamental settings and shown reliable effects in social-cognitive and affective neuroscience. The success of this method may at least partly be due to pioneering research that established the time course of changes in blood levels of testosterone and physiological responsiveness in healthy young women after a single sublingual administration of 0.5 mg testosterone in a liquid form (Tuiten et al., 2000). In that research, a 10-fold increase in total testosterone was observed (in each individual) 15 min after intake, and testosterone levels returned to baseline within 90 min. These findings indicated that during a 60-min period, the testosterone levels of these women, normally accounting for the biggest hormonal difference between the sexes, approximated male testosterone levels. Crucially, however, the behavioral effect of the drug peaked 2.5 hours after testosterone levels in the blood had returned to baseline: Testosterone significantly elevated vaginal pulse amplitude beginning about 4 hours after administration of the drug (Tuiten et al., 2000). The reliability and generalizability of the 4-hour time course has been successfully established in a dozen studies addressing both cognitive and social-emotional behaviors (e.g., Hermans, Putman, Baas, Koppeschaar, & van Honk, 2006; Hermans et al., 2006a, 2006b; Schutter & van Honk, 2004; van Honk et al., 2001, 2005).

The sublingual administration technique seems an appealing method for fundamental applications in social and affective neuroscience, because it may give critical insights into the role of testosterone in individual differences in social cognition by temporarily inducing an acute sex reversal in the blood levels of testosterone. Of course, this cannot be translated into genuine acute sex reversal of testosterone's brain function level; however, given the effects found in a number of studies addressing cognitive and affective factors, it may come close (e.g., Aleman, Bronk, Kessels, Koppeschaar, & van Honk, 2004; Postma, Meyer, Tuiten, van Honk, & Koppeschaar, 2000; van Honk et al., 2005; van Honk & Schutter, 2007a).

The method uses pure testosterone, in solutions that consist of 0.5 mg testosterone, 5 mg hydroxypropyl-beta-cyclodextrin (the carrier), 5 mg ethanol, and 0.5 ml water. Placebo solutions are similar except for the absence of testosterone. This protocol has been successfully applied in many studies (e.g., Aleman et al., 2004; Hermans, Putman, Baas, et al., 2006; Hermans, Ramsay, & van Honk, 2008; Postma et al., 2000; Schutter, Leitner, Kenemans, & van Honk, 2006; Schutter & van Honk, 2004; Tuiten et al., 2000; van Honk et al., 2001, 2004; van Honk & Schutter, 2007a). Below I discuss a selection of these studies, concentrating on angry facial expressions, in which testosterone administration brings about a revealing dissociation in implicit and explicit processing of social threat.

To begin with, using correlational methods, our group demonstrated that individuals with high levels of testosterone selectively attended to angry facial expressions in an emotional Stroop task (van Honk et al., 1999). This effect was recently replicated by Wirth and Schultheiss (2007), who observed it, more fascinatingly, under masked exposure conditions. As an explanation of the effect, we argued that the angry facial expression evolved in primates to function as a threat signal in dominance encounters (Öhman, 1986), with vigilant responses in terms of an enduring threatening angry gaze signaling dominance, and avoidant responses in terms of eye or gaze aversion signaling submission and preventing aggression (Mazur & Booth, 1998). Depending on the social relation between sender and receiver, angry faces can therefore be responded to with either avoidant, fearful submission or vigilant, aggressive dominance (van Honk & Schutter, 2007b). Furthermore, high levels of testosterone are known to be associated with an aggressive, dominating personality style, and this can be observed as a vigilant attentional response to the angry face in the emotional Stroop task. Thus vigilant responses to angry faces vary positively with testosterone levels (van Honk et al., 1999; Wirth & Schultheiss, 2007). However, since these early findings were correlational in nature, no firm conclusions could be drawn.

To seek more definite evidence, we administered exogenous testosterone and used a physiological measure, the cardiac defense response—an acceleration of heart rate within 5 seconds after stimulus presentation, which signals flight–fight preparation (Öhman, 1986). A double-blind, placebo-controlled design was used to examine whether testosterone would induce cardiac acceleration in response to angry faces. Healthy young women passively viewed neutral, happy, or angry faces. It was hypothesized that testosterone would induce cardiac acceleration in responses to angry faces exclusively. As can be seen in Figure 4.1, testosterone induced a significant increase in only the angry-face condition.

These causal psychophysiological findings strongly support the correlational evidence described above (van Honk et al., 1999; Wirth & Schultheiss, 2007), but there are of course no direct clues as to how, or by what neural mechanisms, testosterone may influence this social-emotional cardiac response to angry faces. It is known that this steroid hormone acts on motivation and emotion by binding to specific steroid-responsive networks in the limbic system (Wood, 1996). A key element in these networks is the amygdala, and, critically, the central nucleus of the amygdala and the hypothalamus innervate brainstem centers that control heart rate. In addition, evidence from neuroimaging studies

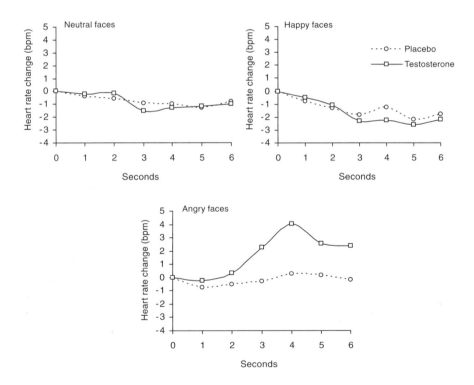

FIGURE 4.1. Mean heart rate changes in beats per minute (bpm) from baseline (1 second before the stimulus) during the 6 poststimulus seconds for neutral, happy, and angry faces.

suggests a critical role of the amygdala in autonomic responsiveness to angry faces (Morris et al., 1999).

One might therefore expect amygdala, hypothalamus, and brainstem involvement in the enhanced cardiac responses to angry faces after testosterone administration. To gather insights in the matter, we recently redesigned the experiment for a neuroimaging application in which the amygdala, hypothalamus, and brainstem were among the regions of interest. However, initially in a design without testosterone, 12 female participants (ages 18–28) underwent functional magnetic resonance imaging (fMRI) while passively viewing angry and happy facial expressions (Hermans et al., 2008). Next, these same participants were retested in a second and a third session, using the literal placebo-controlled sublingual administration of 0.5 mg testosterone from the study above. The findings of the first session demonstrated activation to angry facial expressions (using happy faces as contrast) in the amygdala, hypothalamus, and brainstem, but also in the orbitofrontal cortex (Brodmann's area 47)—a region importantly implicated in the control of human social aggression (Blair, 2004).

Data from the analyses of the second and third sessions (the placebo-controlled testosterone part of the study) revealed enhanced activation of and connectivity among the amygdala, hypothalamus, and brainstem in response to anger faces after testosterone administration. Note that this amygdala–hypothalamus–brainstem circuit is well known in rodent research as being critical for the expression of social aggression. There was, however, also a slight acute effect of testosterone on orbitofrontal reactivity in response to angry faces in the Hermans and colleagues (2008) study. This might reflect increased effort for inhibitory control, given strong subcortical activations. In sum, the Hermans and colleagues data are in tune with other findings on testosterone and responsivity to angry facial expressions (e.g., van Honk et al., 1999, 2001; Wirth & Shultheiss, 2007), and they concur with animal research by demonstrating that testosterone increases activity and connectivity in subcortical neural circuits of social aggression in response to angry facial expressions.

There is also evidence that socially aggressive patients have difficulties in the conscious recognition of angry facial expressions (Best, Williams, & Coccaro, 2002; Blair, 2003). This seems somewhat counterintuitive, because the relationship between testosterone and social aggression is rather convincing (e.g., Dabbs & Hargrove, 1997; Dabbs & Morris, 1990), and the hormone undeniably increases social-emotional responsivity to angry facial expressions (van Honk et al., 1999, 2001; Wirth & Schultheiss, 2007). Note, however, that the conscious recognition of anger acts at explicit, higher levels of processing, whereas the data on testosterone and emotional responses to angry facial expressions indicate that these responses involve implicit processing levels (see Toates, 2006). It has been argued that impairments in the recognition of facial anger may provide insights into the mechanisms underlying the resistance of socially aggressive subjects to social correction. That is, at higher levels of processing, the facial signal of anger serves sociality through its socially corrective properties (Blair, 2003).

Nonetheless, testosterone is clearly capable of increasing implicit social-emotional responses to the angry face, but might the hormone also be able to impair the conscious recognition of facial anger? In a within-subjects design, we administered testosterone (0.5 mg) or placebo to 16 female volunteers ages 19–26 years (van Honk & Schutter, 2007a). Afterward, an emotion recognition task using morphed displays was administered to index the effects of testosterone on subjects' sensitivity to facial expressions indicating threat (fear, anger, and disgust) and nonthreat (happiness, sadness, and surprise). This emotion recognition task measures "sensitivity" as the percentage of intensity at which a subject is able to correctly identify an emotional facial expression. Gradually morphing expressions instead of static ones used for ecological validity, since expressions in everyday life are also dynamic. The sensitivity point is defined as the morphing percentage at which an emotion is consistently correctly recognized (Montagne et al., 2005). Results showed that testosterone induced a significant reduction in the conscious recognition of facial threat (see Figure 4.2). Separate analyses for the three categories of threat faces indicated that this effect was reliable for angry facial expressions exclusively.

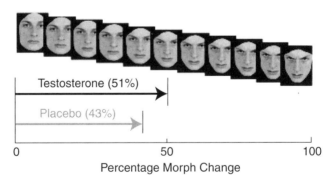

FIGURE 4.2. Example of the morphing of facial expressions from neutrality to full-blown anger. The difference between the amount of morphing needed for the emotion to be recognized in the placebo and testosterone conditions indicates the percentage of recognition sensitivity lost after administration of testosterone. From Hermans, Ramsay, and van Honk (2008). Copyright 2008 by Elsevier. Reprinted by permission.

In summary, testosterone augments physiological and cognitive–affective responses to angry facial expressions (van Honk et al., 1999, 2001), and it increases activity in the brain structures critically involved in the impulsive aggressive response: the amygdala, the hypothalamus, and the brainstem (Hermans et al., 2008). On the other hand, the hormone impairs the conscious recognition of anger.

How can these seemingly divergent findings be explained in terms of the brain mechanisms involved? Importantly, steroid hormones have properties that enable them to influence social brain processing locally (i.e., by inducing peptide synthesis), but in particular they alter brain communication. Critically, cross-frequency analyses that provide indices for cortical–subcortical communication in the human electroencephalogram (Schutter, Kenemans, & van Honk, 2006) have revealed that testosterone decreases information transfer among subcortical and cortical regions (Schutter & van Honk, 2004). Cortical–subcortical communication is not only of vital importance for top-down cognitive control over social-aggressive tendencies (Kringelbach & Rolls, 2003; Reiman, 1997; van Honk et al., 2005); it also mediates bottom-up transmission of information conveying angry threat value, which is speedily spotted by the amygdala (Morris et al., 1999), to the orbitofrontal cortex, where higher-level modulation of emotion occurs (Reiman, 1997; van Honk et al., 2005). Thus a feasible neurobiological mechanism for the observed testosterone-induced reductions in the conscious recognition of angry facial expressions is the testosterone-induced reduction in cortical–subcortical communication (Schutter & van Honk, 2004), which blocks information transfer between the amygdala and orbitofrontal cortex. Subcortical activation in aggression circuits, in combination with the reduced cortical–subcortical communication, introduces a neurobiologically realistic two-layered mechanism by which testosterone would incline an individual toward a socially aggressive outburst.

In conclusion, testosterone has great potential for research in social neuroscience—not only because the hormone may explain much of the variance in sex differences in social cognition, but also because testosterone specifically sets the balance between social and asocial forms of cognition through its actions on the peptides of love and war, oxytocin and vasopressin (see Debiec, 2005). Note again that in none of the reported testosterone studies were effects on mood found; as noted earlier, this is critical, because it precludes top-down cognitive explanations in terms of secondary mood-generated changes or response biases. For further research on acute effects of testosterone, social neuroscience research investigating social cooperation, fairness, and morality is of interest.

Vasopressin: The Peptide of War

Neurohormones or peptides such as oxytocin and vasopressin differ from the gonadal steroid hormones estradiol and testosterone in numerous ways, but the most important of these with respect to social behavior is that the peptides are the so-called "goal setters" of the social brain, whereas the steroid hormones are "play makers" that set the pace of communication (Schulkin, 2003). Oxytocin and vasopressin receptors perform their social-emotional actions on highly localized places in the limbic system (e.g., on the amygdala, hypothalamus, and brainstem), but depend on the steroid hormones for synthesis and thus for action. Reflecting the male and female properties of all chemicals involved, testosterone is critical for vasopressin synthesis, while estradiol is important for oxytocin synthesis (Carter, 2007).

It is furthermore of methodological importance that steroid hormones easily pass the blood–brain barrier, but that for the social peptides this is much more problematic. Also, social peptides circulating in peripheral blood have an enormous range of side effects that we are not looking for in social neuroscience studies. Changing the blood levels of these peptide hormones to induce alterations in social cognition by way of injection or sublingual administration is therefore not preferable. Intranasal peptide administration, however, seems to work quite well. This method may not be completely novel, but a groundbreaking methodological paper published in *Nature Neuroscience* demonstrated that a range of neuropeptides (including melanocortin, vasopressin, and insulin) when administered intranasally achieve access to the brain's cerebrospinal fluid within 30 min, without affecting peptide blood levels (Born et al., 2002). It thus seems that intranasal administration of peptides gives access to the social brain and that side effects are precluded. These findings opened up opportunities not only for fundamental causally controlled research on the effects on social peptides on emotion and social cognition in normal populations, but also for possible clinical applications. Especially with respect to oxytocin, this research is on the rise. Research on the acute effects of intranasal vasopressin on human social-emotional behavior is much more limited, at least in nonclinical populations. This is probably due to the fact that this social peptide is less well known than oxytocin and may also be more unpredictable in terms of sex and environmental differences, as the research described below reveals.

Two studies of interest using acute intranasal vasopressin have been reported in the literature by Thompson and colleagues (Thompson, George, Walton, Orr, & Benson, 2006; Thompson, Gupta, Miller,

Mills, & Orr, 2004). These two studies may have some common characteristics, but the 2006 study is unique because it explicitly addressed sex differences in the effects of vasopressin on social-emotional behavior in humans. Thompson and coworkers demonstrated that intranasal vasopressin differentially influences certain forms of social communication in males and females, and discussed a possible mechanism for this sexually dimorphic effect of vasopressin on social cognition. The earlier study (Thompson et al., 2004) showed that electromyographic (EMG) responses of the corrugator supercilii to neutral faces were increased in men by intranasal vasopressin administration—a finding interpreted as preparation for aggressive defense (but see Hermans et al., 2006b). The second study was extended to women, because sexual dimorphisms of vasopressin function have been established throughout species. To address this fundamental question, Thompson and colleagues (2006), investigated whether social responses are influenced by intranasal vasopressin in a sexually dimorphic manner.

In a double-blind, placebo-controlled design, subjects received a 1-ml solution containing 20 units of arginine vasopressin (AVP; American Reagent Laboratories, Shirley, NY), which counts up to 50 µg, by means of self-administered intranasal sprays over a 2-min period in the presence of the experimenter. The placebo, which was applied in the same manner, was a sterile saline (see Born et al., 2002). Facial EMG was measured in response to pictures of facial expressions of emotion (see Thompson et al., 2006, for details). Subjects also rated the approachability/friendliness of the facial expressions and filled out an anxiety questionnaire. It was hypothesized that vasopressin would influence EMG responses to the facial expressions, but especially in males, because the peptide of defense is most strongly associated with the regulation of male-type social communication (Carter, 2007). Results showed that vasopressin influenced the facial EMG to facial expressions differentially in males and females, as well as ratings of the approachability of these faces (see Figure 4.3). Vasopressin increased corrugator supercilii (brow) activity to neutral faces in males. This was explained as an agonistic reflex, and it specifically decreased the friendliness/approachability ratings of pictures of other unfamiliar men displaying happy, affiliative expressions. It seems that in males, as argued by Thompson and colleagues (2006), vasopressin promotes agonistic responses in male-to-male encounters. On the other hand, females showed affiliative responses toward the emotional faces of same-sex models in response to vasopressin. In females, vasopressin inhibited corrugator responses to angry and happy faces, and stimulated zygomaticus (cheek) responses that have been associated with smiling. Moreover, the pictures were rated as more friendly and approachable.

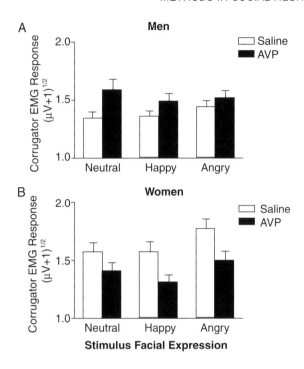

FIGURE 4.3. Changes in corrugator activity in response to facial expressions after vasopressin and placebo. Vasopressin increased responses to neutral faces in men, but it decreased activity to happy and angry faces in women ($p < .05$). From Thompson, George, Walton, Orr, and Benson (2006). Copyright 2006 by the National Academy of Sciences, U.S.A. Reprinted by permission.

Finally, contrary to many of the data reported earlier, the self-reported mood scales used in the Thompson and colleagues (2006) study showed that vasopressin increased anxiety in both sexes. Especially given the sexually dimorphic effects of vasopressin on social behavior, increased anxiety in both sexes seems counterintuitive at first sight. However, the authors have elegantly fitted this result within Taylor's evolutionary framework, wherein anxiety or stress prompts defense states or "fight-or-flight" behaviors in males, and social affiliation or the "tend-and-befriend" response in females (Taylor et al., 2000). Thompson and colleagues have suggested that vasopressin induces aggression proneness in males in same-sex encounters, and peacemaking in females in such encounters.

The sexually dimorphic effects of vasopressin on human social cognition found by Thompson and colleagues (2006) are in agreement with findings from animal research, and although there may be some uncertainties in the data and the interpretations, this research is truly groundbreaking.

Studying the effects of vasopressin on human social cognition seems to introduce complexities similar to those that have been shown in animal research. Vasopressin administration can teach us much about the evolution and neurobiology of individual and sex differences in social cognition. However, as noted earlier, oxytocin is currently the most popular hormone in social neuroscience.

Oxytocin: The Peptide of Love

The remarkable selective social-behavioral properties of oxytocin with respect to human sociality became public after the famous study of Kosfeld and colleagues (2005) was published in *Nature*. These authors demonstrated that intranasal administration of oxytocin increased trusting behavior in an economic game among male human subjects. This is a landmark result, as it represents the first causal evidence that a controlled hormone manipulation can increase prosocial behavior in humans.

In the Kosfeld and colleagues (2005) experiment, male participants received internasally either 24 IU oxytocin (Syntocinon-Spray, Novartis; three puffs of 4 IU per nostril) or placebo 50 min before the start of the experiment in a randomly assigned double-blind fashion. The placebo contained all ingredients of the drug except for the neuropeptide itself. Participants then played a prisoner's dilemma variant called the "trust game." In the trust game, each player receives an amount of money and must decide whether to invest any of that money with another, unknown player. When a player does invest in the other player, the amount of money is tripled, but it's up to the other player to share the money or not. In short, trust is needed for investment. In their double-blind study design, Kosfeld and coworkers simply compared the trusting behavior of subjects who received intranasal oxytocin with that of subjects receiving placebo. It was hypothesized that investors in the oxytocin group would transfer more money than investors in the placebo group would. As expected, oxytocin increased subjects' trusting behavior significantly. The average transfer was 17% higher in the oxytocin group, and nearly half of the subjects in this group showed maximum trust, whereas in the placebo group maximum trust was observed in only 21% of the subjects.

Importantly, to exclude the alternative explanation that the oxytocin group transferred more because oxytocin had made these subjects less risk-averse, a second experiment was performed wherein an investment game was played without the element of trust, to see whether risk-taking behavior was influenced by oxytocin. No evidence that oxytocin influenced risk taking was found, indicating that oxytocin specifically influences trust in social interactions. Notably, these findings not only concur with results from animal research in terms of relations among oxytocin, affiliation, and bonding, but point to a critical role for oxytocin in the psychobiology of human prosocial communication.

In another recent oxytocin administration study, fMRI was employed to investigate a possible role of oxytocin in neural responses to facial threat (Kirsch et al., 2005). Rodent research has established that oxytocin reduces fearfulness, and in particular the findings of Huber and colleagues (2005) in rodents have indicated that the neuropeptide may establish such effects by way of amygdala-centered limbic pathways. Kirsch and coworkers used fMRI to investigate the effects on amygdala activation to angry and fearful faces in right-handed healthy males after intranasal administration of oxytocin or placebo in a double-blind, counterbalanced, within-subjects design. Thirty minutes before the start of the fMRI sessions, subjects intranasally self-administered five puffs of oxytocin (27 IU total) or placebo (only the carrier substance) under the supervision of the experimenter. In line with the evidence of Huber and colleagues in rodents, the data showed that oxytocin not only reduced activation of the amygdala, but, more importantly, reduced amygdala–brainstem functional connectivity. These findings are quite opposite to the data from the Hermans and colleagues (2008) study, wherein enhanced amygdala and brainstem activity in response to angry faces was found after testosterone administration. In conclusion, the data of Kirsch and colleagues (2005) and Hermans and colleagues fit a framework in which sexually dimorphic neuroendocrine pathways lead toward prosocial and asocial behavior.

More evidence comes from oxytocin and testosterone studies on mind reading (Domes, Heinrichs, Michel, et al., 2007). Domes and colleagues (2007) found that oxytocin increased the ability to read the mind of social others in Baron-Cohen's "Reading the Mind in the Eyes" task (Baron-Cohen, Wheelwright, Hill, Raste, & Plumb, 2001). In an unpublished study by van Honk and colleagues, testosterone administration had exactly the opposite effect: This hormone impaired mind reading in the Baron-Cohen task. Taken together, these results suggest that in certain conditions or social environments, testosterone and oxytocin may well operate antagonistically. In sum, not only does testosterone facilitate the effects of vasopressin through the up-regulation of this peptide's synthesis, but it seems from behavioral data that the steroid may have additional properties for the inhibition of sociality through inducing reductions in oxytocin synthesis.

A Neuroendocrine Framework for Social Cognition

Animal research has established that the social-emotional functions of the social peptides vasopressin and oxytocin, and the sex steroids estradiol and testosterone, depend on a multiplicity of variables. However, within a neuroendocrine framework for social cognition (see Figure 4.4), the male-type vasopressin peptide seems to have augmenting properties on the inherently antagonistic motives of aggression and fear, whereas the female-type oxytocin peptide down-regulates both fear and aggression and enhances prosocial functions. Sex and social-environmental differences must be considered within this framework, as must the structural similarity of vasopressin and oxytocin, which gives the peptides the opportunity to influence each other's actions. The sex hormones play a defining role in the synthesis of these social peptides, with the female sex hormone estradiol sustaining oxytocin synthesis, and the male sex hormone testosterone sustaining vasopressin synthesis.

Many crucial findings and theoretical considerations from human social-cognitive neuroscience are in tune with neurobiological research on animals' social-emotional behavior. Importantly, testosterone induces limbic–midbrain predominance in social brain processing, whereas estradiol seems to foster frontal social brain power. Depending on conditions, testosterone increases activity in limbic brain regions especially and seems to inhibit neurotransmitter function in the medial prefrontal cortex, whereas estradiol contrariwise increases neurotransmitter function (Handa, Hejna, & Lorens, 1997). At the amygdala, the male and female sex steroids regulate the genetic expression of the male- and female-type

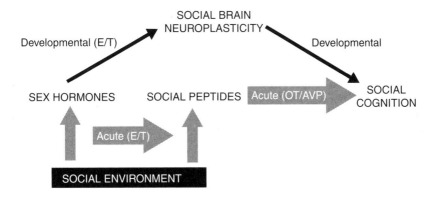

FIGURE 4.4. A neuroendocrine framework for sexually dimorphic social cognition. E, estradiol; T, testosterone; AVP, arginine vasopressin; OT, oxytocin.

social peptides vasopressin and oxytocin, respectively, which may well be a key mechanism underlying sexually dimorphic social cognition (Carter, 2007; Curley & Keverne, 2005; Schulkin, 2003). Importantly, testosterone increases the genetic expression of vasopressin, the peptide of defense (Debiec, 2005; Schulkin, 2003), while estradiol increases the genetic expression of oxytocin, the peptide of affiliation (Carter, 2007). In unsafe conditions, vasopressin prepares an individual for flight or fight by increasing activity and connectivity in the brain defense circuits (which include the amygdala, hypothalamus, and brainstem) and by breaking down cortical–subcortical communication (Huber et al., 2005; Porges, 2003). Oxytocin works in the opposite manner: It seeks to protect, reduce stress, increase social communication, and heighten trust (Kosfeld et al., 2005). Oxytocin promotes cortical control by inactivating the social limbic structures (amygdala, hypothalamus) and increasing communication between the limbic system and neocortical social brain regions (Domes, Heinrichs, Gläscher, et al., 2007), while decreasing limbic–midbrain communication (Domes, Heinrichs, Michel, et al., 2007; Huber et al., 2005; Kirsch et al., 2005; Porges, 2007). In sum, the sex steroids estradiol and testosterone are not only the engineers of the social brain from early development onward, but they also regulate synthesis of the social peptides oxytocin and vasopressin, thereby critically defining sexually dimorphic social-cognitive aptitude in humans.

Interestingly, the neuroendocrine regulation of social cognition indicates that the sex differences in sociality are of ancient origin. Data from neuroendocrine paleontology point to a very early date for the preadaptations that may underlie them. Many hundred million years ago, a gene duplication of a primordial peptide gave rise to two peptide lineages. First, the vasotocin–isotocin complex evolved in bony fish, followed millions of years later by the mammalian peptides vasopressin and oxytocin (Insel & Young, 2000). These social peptides also regulate many peripheral bodily processes, but the differences and deviations in functionality of the peptides on the level of the brain account defensibly for many important sex differences in social cognition (Carter, 2007; Taylor et al., 2000). In conclusion, neuroendocrine administration studies hold great promise in human social-cognitive neuroscience, because they can provide the causal data that are necessary to set theoretical boundaries in this promising scientific discipline. This is especially important because causal comparative data cannot easily be drawn from animal research, since human and animal social cognition are not always comparable. Particularly critical insights into individual and sex differences in social cognition may be gathered by research lines that combine estradiol and testosterone or vasopressin and oxytocin in combinations of behavioral and neuroimaging studies.

References

Adolphs, R. (2003). Cognitive neuroscience of human social behaviour. *Nature Reviews Neuroscience, 4*, 165–178.

Adolphs, R., Gosselin, F., Buchanan, T. W., Tranel, D., Schyns, P., & Damasio, A. R. (2005). A mechanism for fear recognition after amygdala damage. *Nature, 433*, 68–72.

Aleman, A., Bronk, E., Kessels, R. P. C., Koppeschaar, H. P., & van Honk, J. (2004). A single administration of testosterone improves visuospatial ability in young healthy women. *Psychoneuroendocrinology, 29*, 612–617.

Amaral, D. G. (2003). The amygdala, social behavior, and danger detection. *Annals of the New York Academy of Sciences, 1000*, 337–347.

Amodio, D. M., & Frith, C. D. (2007). Meeting of minds: The medial frontal cortex and social cognition. *Nature Reviews Neuroscience, 7*, 268–277.

Anderson, A. K. (2007). Feeling emotional: The amygdala links emotional perception and experience. *Social, Cognitive, and Affective Neuroscience, 2*, 71–72.

Baron-Cohen, S., Wheelwright, S., Hill, J., Raste, Y., & Plumb, I. (2001). The "Reading the Mind in the Eyes" Test, Revised Version: A study with normal adults, and adults with Asperger syndrome or high-functioning autism. *Journal of Child Psychology and Psychiatry, 42*(2), 241–251.

Best, M., Williams, J. M., & Coccaro, E. F. (2002). Evidence for a dysfunctional prefrontal circuit in patients with an impulsive aggressive disorder. *Proceedings of the National Academy of Sciences USA, 99*, 8448–8453.

Blair, R. J. (2003). Facial expressions, their communicatory functions and neuro-cognitive substrates. *Philosophical Transactions of the Royal Society of London, Series B, 358*, 561–572.

Blair, R. J. (2004). The roles of orbital frontal cortex in the modulation of antisocial behavior. *Brain and Cognition, 55*, 198–208.

Born, J., Lange, T., Kern, W., McGregor, W. P. Bickel, U., & Fehm, H. L. (2002). Sniffing neuropeptides: A transnasal approach to the human brain. *Nature Neuroscience, 5*, 514–516.

Calder, A. J., & Nummenmaa, L. (2007). Face cells: Separate processing of expression and gaze in the amygdala. *Current Biology, 17*, 371–372.

Carter, C. S. (2007). Sex differences in oxytocin and vasopressin: Implications for autism spectrum disorders? *Behavioural Brain Research, 176*(1), 170–186.

Corden, B., Critchley, H. D., Skuse, D., & Dolan, R. J. (2006). Fear recognition ability predicts differences in social cognitive and neural functioning in men. *Journal of Cognitive Neuroscience, 18*, 889–897.

Curley, P. J., & Keverne, E. B. (2005). Genes, brains and mammalian bonds. *Trends in Ecology and Evolution, 10*, 561–567.

Dabbs, J. M., & Hargrove, M. F. (1997). Age, testosterone, and behavior among female prison inmates. *Psychosomatic Medicine, 59*, 477–480.

Dabbs, J. M., & Morris, R. (1990). Testosterone, social class, and antisocial behavior in a sample of 4,462 men. *Psychological Science, 1*, 209–211.

Debiec, J. (2005). Peptides of love and fear: Vasopressin and oxytocin modulate the integration of information in the amygdala. *Bioessays, 27,* 869–873.

deCantanzaro, D. A. (1999). *Motivation and emotion.* Upper Saddle River, NJ: Prentice Hall.

De Wied, D. (1984). Central target for the behavioral effects of vasopression peptide. *Nature, 308,* 276–278.

Domes, G., Heinrichs, M., Gläscher, J., Büchel, C., Braus, D. F., & Herpertz, S. C. (2007). Oxytocin attenuates amygdala responses to emotional faces regardless of valence. *Biological Psychiatry, 62*(10), 1187–1190.

Domes, G., Heinrichs, M., Michel, A., Berger, C., & Herpertz, S. C. (2007). Oxytocin improves "mind-reading" in humans. *Biological Psychiatry, 61*(6), 731–733.

Dunbar, R. I. M. (1998). The social brain hypothesis. *Evolutionary Anthropology, 183,* 178–190.

Emery, N. I., & Amaral, D. G. (2000). The role of the amygdala in social cognition. In R. D. Lane & L. Nadel (Eds.), *Cognitive neuroscience of emotion*(pp. 156–191). New York: Oxford University Press.

Fries, A. B., Ziegler, T. E., Kurian, J. R., Jacoris, S., & Pollak, S. D. (2005). Early experience in humans is associated with changes in neuropeptides critical for regulating social behavior. *Proceedings of the National Academy of Sciences USA, 102,* 17237–17240.

Hamann, S. (2004). Sex differences in the responses of the human amygdala. *The Neuroscientist, 11,* 288–293.

Hampson, E., van Anders, S. M., & Mullin, L. I. (2006). A female advantage in the recognition of emotional facial expressions: Test of an evolutionary hypothesis. *Evolution and Human Behavior, 27,* 401–416.

Handa, R. J., Hejna, G. M., & Lorens, S. A. (1997). Androgen inhibits neurotransmitter turnover in the medial prefrontal cortex of the rat following exposure to a novel environment. *Brain Research, 751,* 131–138.

Hermans, E. J., Putman, P., Baas, J. M., Koppeschaar, H. P., & van Honk, J. (2006). A single administration of testosterone reduces fear-potentiated startle in humans. *Biological Psychiatry, 59,* 872–874.

Hermans, E. J., Putman, P., & van Honk, J. (2006a). Testosterone acutely reduces the fear potentiated startle. *Biological Psychiatry, 59,* 872–874.

Hermans, E. J., Putman, P., & van Honk, J. (2006b). Testosterone reduces empathic mimicking in healthy young women. *Psychoneuroendocrinology, 31,* 859–866.

Hermans, E. J., Ramsey, N. F., & van Honk, J. (2008). Exogenous testosterone enhances responsiveness to social threat in the neural circuitry of social aggression in humans. *Biological Psychiatry, 63*(3), 263–270.

Huber, D. R., Veinante, P., & Stoop, R. (2005). Vasopressin and oxytocin excite distinct neuronal populations in the central amygdala. *Science, 308,* 245–248.

Hulshoff Pol, H. E., Cohen-Kettenis, P. T., Van Haren, N. E. M., Peper, J. S., Brans, R. G. H., Cahn, W. E., et al. (2006). Changing your sex changes your brain: Influences of testosterone and estrogen on adult human brain structure. *European Journal of Endocrinology, 155,* 107–114.

Insel, T. R., & Young, L. J. (2000). Neuropeptides and the evolution of social behavior. *Current Opinion in Neurobiology, 10,* 784–789.

Kaya, D., Cevrioglu, S., Onrat, E., Fenkci, I. V., & Yilmazer, M. (2003). Estradiol acutely reduces sympathovagal balance to the heart in postmenopausal women. *Journal of Obstetrics and Gynaecology Research, 29,* 406–411.

Keysers, C., & Gazzola, V. (2006). Towards a unifying neural theory of social cognition. *Progress in Brain Research, 156,* 379–401.

Kirsch, P., Esslinger, C., Chen, Q., Mier, D., Lis, S., Siddhanti, S., et al. (2005). Oxytocin modulates neural circuitry of social cognition and fear in humans. *Journal of Neuroscience, 25,* 11489–11493.

Kosfeld, M., Heinrichs, M., Zak, P. J., Fischbacher, U., & Fehr, E. (2005). Oxytocin increases trust in humans. *Nature, 435,* 673–676.

Kringelbach, M. L., & Rolls, E. T. (2003). Neural correlates of rapid reversal learning in a simple model of human social interaction. *NeuroImage, 20,* 1371–1383.

Lindenfors, P. (2005). Neocortex evolution in primates: The social brain is for females. *Biology Letters, 1,* 401–410.

Marsh, A. A., & Blair, R. J. (2008). Deficits in facial affect recognition among antisocial populations: A meta-analysis. *Neuroscience and Biobehavioral Reviews, 32*(3), 454–465.

Marsh, A. A., Kozak, M. N., & Ambady, N. (2007). Accurate recognition of facial fear expressions predicts prosocial behavior. *Emotion, 7,* 239–251.

Mazur, A., & Booth, A. (1998). Testosterone and dominance in men. *Behavioral Brain Sciences, 21,* 353–397.

Montagne, B., Kessels, R., Frigerio, E., de Haan, E., & Perrett, D. (2005). Sex differences in the perception of affective facial expressions: Do men really lack emotional sensitivity? *Cognitive Processing, 6*(2), 136–141.

Montagne, B., van Honk, J., Kessels, R. P., Frigerio, E., Burt, M., Perrett, D. I., et al. (2005). Reduced efficiency in recognising fear in subjects scoring high on psychopathic personality characteristics. *Personality and Individual Differences, 6,* 136–141.

Morris, J. S., Öhman, A., & Dolan, R. J. (1999). A subcortical pathway to the right amygdala mediating "unseen" fear. *Proceedings of the National Academy of Sciences USA, 96,* 1680–1684.

Öhman, A. (1986). Face the beast and fear the face: Animal and social fears as prototypes for evolutionary analyses of emotion. *Psychophysiology, 23,* 123–145.

Öhman, A. (1997). A fast blink of the eye: Evolutionary preparedness for pre-attentive processing of threat. In P. J. Lang, R. F. Simons, & M. T. Balaban (Eds.), *Attention and orienting: Sensory and motivational processing* (pp. 165–184). Mahwah, NJ: Erlbaum.

Porges, S. W. (2003). The polyvagal theory: Phylogenetic contributions to social behavior. *Physiology and Behavior, 79,* 503–513.

Porges, S. W. (2007). The polyvagal perspective. *Biological Psychology, 74,* 116–143.

Postma, A., Meyer, G., Tuiten, A., van Honk, J., & Koppeschaar, H. F. (2000). Effects of testosterone administration on selective aspects of object location memory in healthy young women. *Psychoneuroendocrinology, 25,* 563–575.

Reiman, E. M. (1997). The application of positron emission tomography to the study of normal and pathologic emotions. *Journal of Clinical Psychiatry, 58,* 4–12.

Schleifer, L. A., Justice, A. J. H., & de Wit, H. (2002). Lack of effects of acute estradiol on mood in postmenopausal women. *Pharmacology, Biochemistry and Behavior, 71,* 71–77.

Schulkin, J. (2003). *Rethinking homeostasis.* Cambridge, MA: MIT Press.

Schulkin, J. (2007). Autism and the amygdala: An endocrine hypothesis. *Brain and Cognition, 65,* 87–99.

Schultheiss, O. C., Wirth, M. M., & Stanton, S. J. (2004). Effects of affiliation and power motivation arousal on salivary progesterone and testosterone. *Hormones and Behavior, 46,* 592–599.

Schutter, D. J. L. G., Kenemans, J. L., & van Honk, J. (2006). Electrophysiological correlates of cortico–subcortical interaction: A cross-frequency spectral EEG analysis. *Clinical Neurophysiology, 17,* 381–387.

Schutter, D. J. L. G., & van Honk, J. (2004). Decoupling of midfrontal delta–beta oscillations after testosterone administration. *International Journal of Psychophysiology, 53,* 71–73.

Siebert, M., Markowitsch, H. J., & Bartel, P. (2003). Amygdala, affect and cognition: Evidence from 10 patients with Urbach–Wiethe disease. *Brain, 126,* 2627–2637.

Simerly, R. B. (2002). Wired for reproduction: Organization and development of sexually dimorphic circuits in the mammalian forebrain. *Annual Review of Neuroscience, 25,* 507–536.

Taylor, S. E., Klein, L. C., Lewis, B. P., Gruenewald, T. L., Gurung, R. A., & Updegraff, J. A. (2000). Biobehavioral responses to stress in females: Tend-and-befriend, not fight-or-flight. *Psychological Review, 107,* 411–429.

Thompson, R., George, K., Walton, J. C., Orr, S. P., & Benson, P. (2006). Sex-specific influences of vasopressin on human social communication. *Proceedings of the National Academy of Sciences USA, 103,* 7889–7894.

Thompson, R., Gupta, S., Miller, K., Mills, S., & Orr, S. (2004). The effects of vasopressin on human facial responses related to social communication. *Psychoneuroendocrinology, 29,* 35–48.

Toates, F. (2006). A model of the hierarchy of behaviour, cognition, and consciousness. *Consciousness and Cognition, 15,* 75–118.

Tuiten, A., van Honk, J., Koppeschaar, H., Bernaards, C., Thijssen, J., & Verbaten, R. (2000). Time course effects of testosterone on sexual arousal in women. *Archives of General Psychiatry, 57,* 149–153.

van Honk, J., Peper, J. S., & Schutter, D. J. L. G. (2005). Testosterone reduces unconscious fear but not consciously experiences anxiety. *Biological Psychiatry, 58,* 218–225.

van Honk, J., & Schutter, D. J. L. G. (2007a). Testosterone reduces conscious detection of signals serving social correction: Implications for antisocial behavior. *Psychological Science, 18,* 663–667.

van Honk, J., & Schutter, D. J. L. G. (2007b). Vigilant and avoidant responses to angry facial expressions: Dominance and submission motives. In E. Harmon-Jones & P. Winkielman (Eds.), *Social neuroscience* (pp. 197–223). New York: Guilford Press.

van Honk, J., Schutter, D. J. L. G., Hermans, E. J., Putman, P., Tuiten, A., & Koppeschaar, H. P. F. (2004). Testosterone shifts the balance between sensitivity for punishment and reward in healthy young women. *Psychoneuroendocrinology, 29*, 937–943.

van Honk, J., Tuiten, A., Hermans, E., Putman, P., Koppeschaar, H. F., & Verbaten, R. (2001). A single administration of testosterone induces cardiac accelerative responses to angry faces in healthy young women. *Behavioral Neuroscience, 115*, 238–242.

van Honk, J., Tuiten, A., Verbaten, R., Van den Hout, M., Koppeschaar, H., Thijssen, J., et al. (1999). Correlations among salivary testosterone, mood, and selective attention to threat in humans. *Hormones and Behavior, 36*, 17–24.

van Vugt, M., De Cremer, D., & Janssen, D. P. (2007). Gender differences in cooperation and competition: The male-warrior hypothesis. *Psychological Science, 18*, 19–23.

Voracek, M., & Dressler, S. G. (2006). Lack of correlation between digit ratio (2D:4D) and Baron-Cohen's "Reading the Mind in the Eyes" test, empathy, systemising, and Autism-Spectrum Quotients in a general population sample. *Personality and Individual Differences, 41*, 1481–1491.

Whalen, P. J., Rauch, S. L., Etcoff, N. L., McInerney, S. C., Lee, M. B., & Jenike, M. A. (1998). Masked presentations of emotional facial expressions modulate amygdala activity without explicit knowledge. *Journal of Neuroscience, 18*, 411–418.

Wirth, M. M., & Schultheiss, O. C. (2007). Basal testosterone moderates responses to anger faces in humans. *Physiology and Behavior, 28*, 496–505.

Wood, R. I. (1996). Functions of the steroid responsive network in control of the hamster's sexual behavior. *Trends in Endocrinology and Metabolism, 7*, 338–344.

5

Facial EMG

Ursula Hess

Electromyography (EMG) is a measure of the electric activity (action potentials) generated during muscle contraction. This measure is directly related to the force produced by muscles (Lawrence & DeLuca, 1983). Facial EMG is the measurement of the activity of facial muscles.

In what follows, I first briefly describe the EMG signal, the factors that influence measurement, and the procedures used for recording. I then discuss data treatment as it is typically carried out in psychology. Both of these sections are designed as general overviews; for additional details, see Tassinary and Cacioppo (2000); for many more details, the reader is referred to Loeb and Gans (1986). Finally, I present some examples of the use of EMG in psychology. In this context, I also discuss the advantages and disadvantages of EMG as a measure of facial activity compared to other methods.

What Does Facial EMG Measure?

Striated muscles consist of groups of bundles of individual muscle fibers. These are packed with myofibrils, with interdigitated sets of the proteins actin and myosin (see Figure 5.1). The release of calcium allows small extensions from the myosin protein (the "cross-bridges") to pull the actin over the myosin, which results in muscle contraction. The muscle fibers are activated in groups called "motor units." Each motor unit is inner-

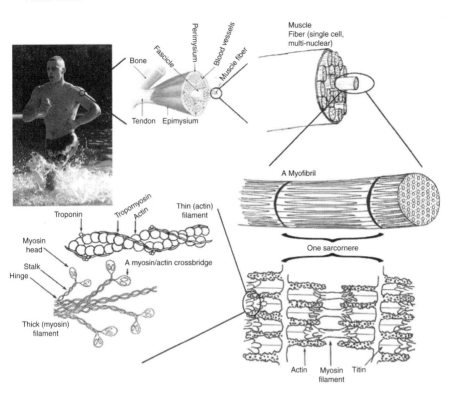

FIGURE 5.1. Top-down view of skeletal muscle. From Wikipedia (2008).

vated by a single motor axon; hence when a motor neuron is activated, all of the muscle fibers in that motor unit are enervated. EMG records the changes in electrical potential that result from the conduction of action potentials along the muscle fibers, or rather the motor units, during muscle contraction (motor unit action potentials, or MUAPs).

An EMG signal recorded by electrodes attached to the skin overlying a muscle consists of the electrical activity from numerous individual motor units within the detection region and therefore represents the sum of numerous MUAPs, where some are canceled out and others are intensified, as the different motor units are not aligned. The frequency of the EMG ranges from a few hertz to about 500 Hz and across a wide span of amplitudes. These characteristics of the EMG overlap with the characteristics of other electrical signals generated by the body (e.g., the electrocardiogram and electroencephalogram), as well as with ambient signals such as the 50- to 60-Hz electrical noise emitted by alternating current (AC)–powered equipment.

Recording the Signal

Electrodes

EMG can be recorded via a number of means. In medical settings, needle electrodes placed directly into the muscle are often used. In psychological research, surface electrodes are preferred. Several different types of surface electrodes exist, with different advantages and disadvantages (Loeb & Gans, 1986). For the recording of facial EMG in psychological experiments, bipolar Ag/AgCl surface electrodes are most commonly used. Bipolar surface electrodes measure the voltage difference between two closely spaced locations, using two contact surfaces. A differential amplifier takes the difference in electrical potential between the two signals and amplifies it. This difference signal is referred to a third signal obtained from a monopolar reference electrode or ground, which is located at an electrically neutral place (for facial EMG, usually the middle of the forehead, but earlobes are also an option). Referring the signal from the two measurement electrodes to the reference electrode allows the rejection of extraneous electrical signals mentioned above, as these signals, but not the potential difference from the muscle of interest, are picked up by the reference electrode as well. The differential amplifier then rejects signals that are common with respect to the reference electrode, such that only the difference in potential between the bipolar electrodes is retained. As in all psychophysiological applications, only one reference should be used.

The amplitude of the recorded signal depends on the muscle fiber diameter, on the distance between the fiber and the detection site, and on electrode properties. In principle, a larger surface area allows better measurement, as impedance is lower; however, two considerations demand that electrode size be kept small when facial EMG is measured. First, the larger the surface, the more likely is it that activity from other muscles is recorded as well ("cross-talk"); second, larger electrodes may impede the movement of the face. For facial EMG, 4-mm-diameter minielectrodes are a good choice.

Electrode Placements and Skin Preparation

For best results, the two electrodes should be placed near the middle of the muscle, on a line parallel to the muscle fiber (Loeb & Gans, 1986). The head and face have over 30 bilaterally symmetrical muscle pairs (Gray, 1918/2000). Figure 5.2 highlights the muscles commonly assessed in psychological research. One challenge is to place an electrode so as to have a good measure of the muscles' activity in combination with

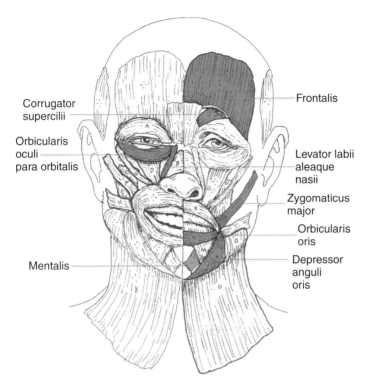

FIGURE 5.2. The muscles commonly assessed in psychophysiological research. From Kapit and Elson (2001). Copyright 2001 by Benjamin Cummings. Adapted by permission.

as little cross-talk as possible from other muscles. The Society for Psychophysiological Research guidelines for human EMG research (Fridlund & Cacioppo, 1986) suggest the placements shown in Figure 5.3 (the placement for levator labii aleaque nasii has been added; also, the placement for orbicularis oculi is slightly modified to reduce eyeblink artifact). The guidelines also provide a detailed description of how to locate these placements on the skin. However, there are individual variations in muscle trajectories and even in the presence of certain muscles. Gray (1918/2000) notes, for example, that zygomaticus major is sometimes absent or can be fused with zygomaticus minor.

Two additional EMG placements are of interest when EMG is used to assess startle modification (see below). Eyeblink startle modification can be assessed via EMG of the orbicularis oculi. The placement for

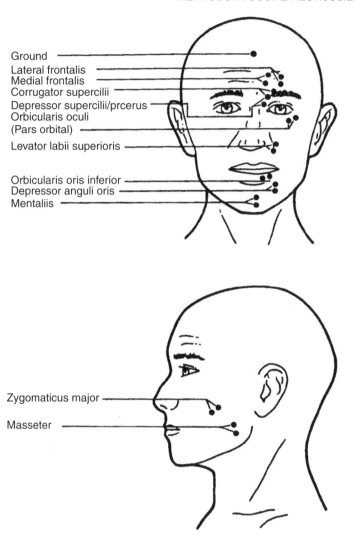

Ground
Lateral frontalis
Medial frontalis
Corrugator supercilii
Depressor supercilii/prcerus
Orbicularis oculi
(Pars orbital)
Levator labii superioris

Orbicularis oris inferior
Depressor anguli oris
Mentaliis

Zygomaticus major
Masseter

FIGURE 5.3. Suggested electrode placements for surface EMG recording. Top: Front view. Bottom: Side view. From Fridlund and Cacioppo (1986). Copyright 1986 by the Society for Psychophysiological Research. Adapted by permission.

orbicularis oculi shown in Figure 5.3 refers to orbicularis oculi pars lateralis. For the assessment of eyeblinks, the electrodes are placed more medially. More recently, interest in the use of the postauricular reflex (PAR) has developed (e.g., Benning, Patrick, & Lang, 2004; Hess, Sabourin, & Kleck, 2007). For PAR measurement, electrodes are placed near the tendon of insertion of the postauricular muscle behind the ear (see Figure 5.4). The auricularis posterior (which draws the ear backward) is a vestigial muscle in humans and has been found to be absent in 5% of cadavers examined (Guerra et al., 2004). Even when it is present, not all participants show measurable muscle activity in response to a sound.

Usually electrodes are attached to the skin with double-sided adhesive tape. The cups of the electrodes are filled with a conductive medium (paste or gel). This medium allows contact of the electrode surface with the skin, which is not disrupted by movement. The medium also penetrates the skin to some degree and increases its conductive properties. It is quite important (despite the increased amplification abilities of modern equipment) to clean the skin carefully, to remove oils and dead skin cells; both reduce the conductivity of the skin. A paste containing pumice or pumice/alcohol pads can be used for this purpose. As the skin below the eye and behind the ear is very sensitive, it is important to take extra care in abrading the skin. Also, alcohol can irritate the eye and hence should be applied carefully for orbicularis oculi skin preparation.

The guidelines (Fridlund & Cacioppo, 1986) suggest that impedances should be between 5 and 10 kΩ. With modern amplifiers, higher impedances can be tolerated; however, one should note that the overall impedance of the electrode–cable–amplifier circuit determines its sensitivity to stray capacitive coupling of extraneous noise sources—

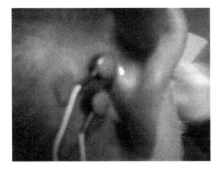

FIGURE 5.4. Electrode placement for the postauricular reflex (PAR).

that is, how much extraneous noise will be captured by the electrode (see Loeb & Gans, 1986, Ch. 20). Hence impedances should probably not exceed 30 kΩ. For some specific applications (e.g., recording of the PAR; see below), lower impedances should be aimed for, as this muscle is extremely weak and the electrical signal is correspondingly small.

An additional practical consideration with regard to skin preparation is that the adhesive on the electrode collars does not stick well on oily skin, and there is a risk that electrodes detach during the experiment. It is important to note that some people are allergic to this adhesive. As this is the same adhesive used for Band-Aids, screening for allergies to Band-Aids is one way to limit such adverse reactions. Also, some individuals show adverse skin reactions to alcohol. In some rare cases, the use of alcohol swipes may trigger panic reactions from people who have had traumatic medical experiences; hence one should also ask people about possible reactions to alcohol.

Sources of Ambient Noise

As mentioned above, the logic of a differential amplifier is to consider the difference between the two bipolar electrodes as the EMG signal and common signal as noise. However, stray signals can affect the two bipolar electrodes differentially and hence will not be rejected as common noise, but rather interpreted as signal. The problem is that this noise— once the signal is filtered, rectified, and integrated—tends to masquerade as signal. Noise is therefore best recognized from the raw EMG signal. Possible sources of noise are power supplies, neon lights, heaters, nearby AC lines, and even local radio stations. Although not all noise is immediately visible, unphysiologically fast components and slow undulations are usually noise.

The best approach is to make sure to minimize noise as much as possible by identifying and removing sources of noise. Some noise is generated by the building (e.g., cables in the walls, elevators). If a Faraday cage is not an option—and often it is not—one should check the available laboratory space with an oscilloscope. It is often the case that some rooms are much noisier than others, depending on the location of the noise sources (e.g., elevators) and the cabling in the building.

The content of the laboratory should also be inspected for sources of noise. For example, electrical leads other than electrode cables should be well shielded. Neon lights emit more noise than simple light bulbs. Transformers (e.g., halogen lamps!) are usually very noisy and should not be placed in the vicinity of the participant. Fortunately, flat-screen monitors pose considerably fewer problems than cathode ray tube monitors do.

Some Methodological Considerations

Baselines

There are different strategies to obtain baselines for EMG recordings. In principle, the true baseline for EMG activity is zero, such that what constitutes the baseline would be the noise level of the recording system. However, a number of factors—such as tonic muscle activity throughout the experiment—may raise this baseline. A commonly used approach to obtain a baseline measure consists of including a preexperiment resting period during which baseline EMG is recorded. This procedure has, however, the requirement that the participant is actually resting. In reality, participants are often somewhat stressed when first entering a psychophysiology laboratory. The unfamiliarity of both the procedure and the environment leads to increased alertness; over time, this effect wears off. But if the resting baseline is taken before this is the case, the experimenter may end up with baseline levels that are higher than trial levels obtained late in the experiment. Alternatively, if the resting period lasts too long, a participant may show relaxation levels that are considerably lower than during normal alertness, thereby inflating differences between trial and baseline. In any case, it is advisable to allow participants to become familiar with their environment, and to create an atmosphere in the laboratory that is conducive to reducing anxiety. Much can be achieved with comfortable chairs, non-clinical-looking furniture, and pleasantly colored walls.

McHugo and Lanzetta (1983) advocate a closed-loop baseline procedure, in which baselines are taken prior to each trial. As Tassinary and Cacioppo (2000) point out, this procedure can have the disadvantage that the regular taking of baselines may shape the participants' reactions in undesirable ways. However, it is often possible to take baselines during the natural course of the experiment—for example, during interstimulus intervals while a participant looks at a blank screen. In another example, Blairy, Herrera, and Hess (1999) recorded facial EMG in response to emotional facial expressions and used the recording during a preceding presentation of the neutral face as baseline, in order to control for all expressive aspects except those directly linked to the emotional stimulus. This procedure does not so much assess a true baseline for muscle activity as it does a reference situation in which emotional stimulation is absent. In short, the choice of baseline depends on the specifics of the experimental procedure. However, it is important to carefully consider the implications of this choice for the validity and generalizability of the experiment.

Communication

Participants should be free to discontinue their participation at any time. However, participants in experiments using psychophysiological measures, including EMG, are attached to equipment via the captors that are used for recording. This may lead participants to the impression that their freedom is curtailed. It is therefore important to assure that participants can communicate freely with the experimenter—for example, via an intercom. It is also advisable to observe each participant during the experiments, as some individuals may experience malaise during the experiment but hesitate to contact the experimenter.

Artifact Removal

Gross motor movements, as well as participants' touching the electrodes, can lead to artifact in EMG recording. Gross motor movements such as sneezing are usually readily discernible as large signals across all channels. But some movements, especially the touching of electrodes, can masquerade as signal. A video record allows the researcher to detect these and to reject the relevant part of the signal. In any case, the record should be screened for unphysiological signal components. Depending on the length of the record versus the length of the artifact, either the record can be rejected entirely, or the artifact can be selectively removed.

Analyzing EMG Data

To some degree, the choice of data analysis strategy is limited by the sampling procedure used. However, modern equipment easily samples at 1000 Hz and higher, making it possible for the researcher to collect raw EMG data and to treat the data offline. Offline treatment of data sampled at lower rates may be problematic, as the frequency range of the EMG data is up to 500 Hz. However, according to Van Boxtel, Boelhouwer, and Bos (1996, cited in Berg & Balaban, 1999), the energy above 250 Hz is negligible. The Nyquist–Shannon sampling theorem states that a continuous-time baseband signal can be reconstructed from its samples if the signal is band-limited and the sampling frequency is greater than twice the signal bandwidth. Hence in order to sample a 500-Hz signal adequately, at least a sampling rate higher than 1000 Hz is needed. Given the frequency range of the EMG signal, a 30- to 500-Hz bandpass filter allows a researcher to remove extraneous signals with frequencies that are unlikely to represent true EMG signal.

The raw EMG signal is a pseudorandom signal around an electrical zero point. As averaging such a signal yields a mean of 0, the signal has to be first rectified before it can be further quantified (see Figure 5.5). The most common method of quantifying the EMG response is to use the mean across a time window of either the unsmoothed or smoothed rectified EMG. Sometimes the root mean square of samples across the relevant time window is employed for this. The mean amplitude of the integrated EMG covaries linearly with muscle contraction, as long as the contraction is not close to the muscle's limit and the muscle does not become fatigued (Goldstein, 1972; Lippold, 1967).

Yet mean amplitude is not the only means of quantifying the EMG signal. Although uncommon in psychophysiological applications, analyses of the frequency domain based on fast Fourier transforms are used in other fields such as kinanthropology, as a down-shifting in frequency is a good indicator of muscle fatigue (e.g., Murata, Uetake, Matsumoto, & Takasawa, 2003).

Cacioppo, Marshall-Goodell, and Dorfman (1983) have proposed a topographical analysis of the EMG signal. This approach represents the temporal information contained in the EMG signal, which is lost when mean EMG amplitudes are analyzed. For example, both theoretical distributions in Figure 5.6a have the same mean amplitude, but they differ in the timing of the onset. Also, both theoretical distributions in Figure 5.6b have the same variance, but one is more variable than the other. The time domain mean and variance, respectively, capture these differ-

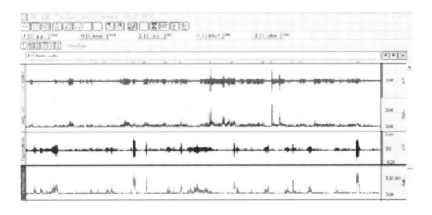

FIGURE 5.5. Raw and rectified/integrated EMG signals.

(a)

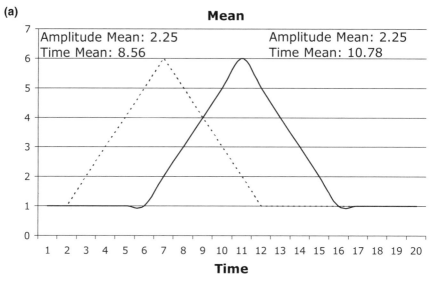

(b)

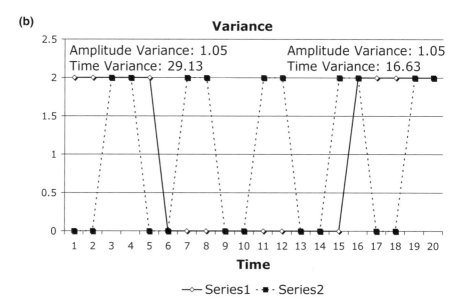

FIGURE 5.6. Theoretical distributions demonstrating the difference between time and amplitude mean (a) and variance (b).

ences. In an early study, Hess, Kappas, McHugo, Kleck, and Lanzetta (1989) demonstrated the usefulness of combining amplitude and temporal information to distinguish between posed and spontaneous smiles.

In another example, Lanctôt and Hess (2007) analyzed EMG onsets with an algorithm for pause detection developed by W. Hess (1973). For this, a frequency analysis was conducted to distinguish noise from signal. Noise was defined as small-amplitude values that occurred frequently. Then signal threshold was defined as values larger than noise values. The EMG onset then corresponded to the point in time where the signal exceeded the threshold.

Mean EMG amplitudes are not distributed normally. Thus, unless the N is relatively large, the data will have to be transformed for use with parametric statistics. Bush, Hess, and Wolford (1993) conducted a Monte Carlo study comparing a range of frequently used transformations in a simple pre–post repeated-measures design. They concluded that the z statistic yielded overall the best result. However, nonlinear data transformations have been known to create surprising effects when real data are used. Hence, Fridlund and Cacioppo (1986) note that such transformations should be applied with caution and well justified. It is also recommended to consider both transformed and nontransformed data, and to inspect the data for inversions in ordering caused by the transformation.

When EMG is used to assess startle modification, the peak magnitude of the EMG is the measure of interest (see Blumenthal & Franklin, Chapter 6, this volume). As the signal recorded from the PAR is very weak, it can be useful to use the aggregate waveform across trials for the baseline-to-peak measures (Hackley, Woldorff, & Hillyard, 1987; Sollers & Hackley, 1997).

Some Research Examples

EMG and Alternatives for the Assessment of Facial Expression

One common use of facial EMG is the study of emotional reactions as signaled by facial expressions. In general, there are three methods to assess facial expressions: observer ratings, the systematic coding of facial expressions, and facial EMG.

Observer ratings have the advantage of not requiring either specialized equipment or highly trained observers. However, it is generally recognized that raters can "vary dramatically in their reliability" (Rosenthal, 2005, p. 199). Hence a considerable number of observers may often be needed, especially as observers fatigue rapidly and can only rate a small set of expressions before desisting.

Cohn and Ekman (2005) list 14 systems for measuring facial action, starting with that of Landis (1924). Of these, the Facial Action Coding System (FACS; Ekman & Friesen, 1978) is the most commonly used technique for the systematic coding of expressions. FACS allows the reliable description (Sayette, Cohn, Wertz, Perrott, & Parrott, 2001) of almost any conceivable facial movement based on appearance changes (action units, or AUs). Most AUs describe the action of a single muscle (such as AU12, the lip corner puller, which describes the action of the zygomaticus major), but FACS also includes such actions as sticking the tongue out. Since FACS is based on the observation of visible appearance changes, it requires overt expressions to be present. This is why it is less useful in situations where only very subtle facial activity can be expected, such as research on facial mimicry. The use of FACS requires the face to be filmed with good resolution and at least a three-quarters profile. FACS is not easy to use and requires trained coders. It takes about 100 hours to learn, and coders are certified by passing a test. FACS is also not very fast to use; a general estimate is about 1 hour of coding for 1 min of facial behavior. There have been advances in the automatic coding of certain AUs (for a review, see Tian, Kanade, & Cohn, 2003), but so far no system can automatically code the full set. The main advantage of FACS is that it offers a comprehensive description of all appearance changes. By contrast, when EMG is used, only a small number of muscles can be assessed at a time (see below).

Facial EMG has been used for the assessment of affective state based on facial expressions in a large number of contexts. Starting with a paper by Cacioppo, Petty, Losch, and Kim (1986), who asserted that "facial EMG activity differentiated both valence and intensity of the affective reaction,"[1] facial EMG has become an accepted index of affective reactions to a variety of visual (e.g., Davis, Rahman, Smith, & Burns, 1995; Larsen, Norris, & Cacioppo, 2003), auditory (e.g., Dimberg, 1990), gustatory (e.g., Hu et al., 1999), and olfactory (e.g., Jäncke & Kaufmann, 1994) emotional stimuli; emotional faces (e.g., Dimberg, 1982; Dimberg & Öhman, 1996); human (e.g., Hess, 2007) or virtual (e.g., Mojzisch et al., 2006) interaction partners; nicotine (e.g., Robinson, Cinciripini, Carter, Lam, & Wetter, 2007) and other drugs (e.g., Newton, Khalsa-Denison, & Gawin, 1997); as well as an index of attitudes toward others (e.g., Brown, Bradley, & Lang, 2006; Dambrun, Desprès, & Guimond,

---

[1]However, a number of studies (e.g., Fridlund, Schwartz, & Fowler, 1984; McHugo, Lanzetta, Sullivan, Masters, & Englis, 1985) had used this index prior to Cacioppo and colleagues (1986).

2003; Vanman, Saltz, Nathan, & Warren, 2004) and oneself (e.g., Buck, Hillman, Evans, & Janelle, 2004); in children as well as in adults (e.g., Armstrong, Hutchinson, Laing, & Jinks, 2007); and has been used with subliminal as well as supraliminal stimuli (e.g., Arndt, Allen, & Greenberg, 2001).

For certain questions, facial EMG measures of affect have been found to be more reliable and revealing than self-report measures, making this method specifically attractive (e.g., Hazlett & Hazlett, 1999; Vanman, Paul, Ito, & Miller, 1997; see also below). In addition, facial EMG has been used to assess attention (e.g., Cohen, Davidson, Senulis, & Saron, 1992) and fatigue (e.g., Veldhuizen, Gaillard, & de Vries, 2003).

As regards the use of facial EMG to assess specific emotions rather than simply positive–negative affect, a number of efforts have been made to describe distinct facial expressions of certain emotions (e.g., Vrana, 1993; Wolf, Mass, et al., 2005) and pain (Crombez, Baeyens, & Eelen, 1997; Wolf, Raedler, et al., 2005). The problem with using facial EMG to identify specific emotional expressions is twofold. First, it cannot be systematically demonstrated that individuals show clear, well-defined, specific facial expressions when experiencing specific emotions (see, e.g., Parkinson, 2005). Rather, as Motley and Camden (1988) have noted, spontaneous facial expressions tend to be weak, partial, and (to some degree) idiosyncratic. Hence, whether facial EMG or FACS is used for the assessment of emotion expressions, the main problem rests in specifying which specific pattern is considered indicative of a specific emotion. Second, the researcher who uses facial EMG is limited by the fact that no more than four or five pairs of electrodes can be affixed to the face before the measure becomes obtrusive and hence likely to inhibit facial action. To this, one needs to add that the same muscle may subserve several expressions. Thus, corrugator supercilii activity is found as a component of both angry and sad faces (Hess & Blairy, 2001), as well as a sign of attention and goal obstruction (Lanctôt & Hess, 2007; Pope & Smith, 1994). In addition, cross-talk between muscles can muddle patterns. For example, the masseter, a muscle that is often engaged in anger (clenching of the teeth) is one of the strongest muscles in the body and can in fact carry a person's full body weight. In contrast, the zygomaticus major muscle is a relatively weak muscle that pulls the corners of the lips up in a smile. As seen in Figure 5.3, the electrode placements for these two muscles are close to each other. Hence it is possible that absolute higher values of *zygomaticus major* activity are observed during anger than during happiness, not because the participants smile when angry, but rather because of cross-talk from the masseter. This problem can be addressed by measuring the activity of both muscles and controlling for presence of masseter activity when analyzing zygomaticus major activity. Overall, the usefulness of facial EMG for the assessment of specific emotional expressions depends on how much the experimental situation can be constrained to limit the range of possible expressions and hence the likelihood of misidentification.

A specific advantage of facial EMG compared to other procedures is its high spatial resolution (Tassinary & Cacioppo, 1992). Facial EMG can be used to assess facial reactions too subtle to be seen reliably with the naked eye. This is why facial EMG is particularly useful in research assessing subtle reactions. One example of such research is the study of facial mimicry.

Facial Mimicry

Dimberg and colleagues have conducted extensive research on people's tendency to imitate the emotional facial expressions they observe (e.g., Dimberg, 1982, 1988; Dimberg & Öhman, 1996). This tendency is fast and usually automatic (e.g., Dimberg, Thunberg, & Grunedal, 2002). However, whereas the phenomenon as such is well established, its function remains unclear. Proponents of simulationist accounts of face-based emotion recognition (Gallese & Goldman, 1998; Goldman & Sripada, 2005) have suggested that mimicry aids emotion recognition, but Blairy and colleagues (Blairy et al., 1999; Hess & Blairy, 2001) did not find any direct link between mimicry as measured via EMG and emotion recognition. The Hess and Blairy (2001) study is a good example of how EMG is used in facial mimicry research.

Hess and Blairy (2001) showed participants videos with dynamic emotional expressions of anger, sadness, disgust and happiness. Facial EMG was assessed at the corrugator supercilii, orbicularis oculi, and levator labii aleaque nasii sites. In addition, an unobtrusive measure of emotional contagion was taken after one of the emotion expressions of each type, and decoding accuracy was assessed. Participants showed the expected pattern of increased orbicularis oculi activity in combination with decreased corrugator supercilii activation for happiness, and the reverse pattern for sadness and anger. Importantly, they did not show the same pattern when viewing disgust images, which suggests that the increased corrugator supercilii and decreased orbicularis oculi activation shown when participants were viewing sadness and anger did not simply signify negative affect. Furthermore, evidence for emotional contagion of happiness and sadness was found, as participants reported higher levels of feeling sad when watching sad expressions and higher levels of feeling cheerful when watching happy expressions. However, mediational analyses could not confirm any relation between mimicry and emotional contagion, or between mimicry and emotion recognition.

Prejudice

Vanman and colleagues (2004) employed facial EMG as a measure of prejudice. Specifically, they measured EMG at the zygomaticus major (smile) and corrugator supercilii (frown) sites to assess positive and negative affective reactions of white university students to pictures of black and white individuals. In a separate task on a different day, the same university students were asked to choose the best of three applicants (two were white and one was black) for a prestigious teaching fellowship. Individuals who showed less zygomaticus major activity when looking at photos of black individuals were found to be more likely to show a bias against selecting a black applicant. Interestingly, the Implicit Association Test (IAT) (Greenwald, McGhee, & Schwartz, 1998)—an implicit measure of racial bias—did not predict selection bias. Furthermore, motivation to control prejudice influenced the IAT but not the EMG measure, suggesting that facial EMG can be used as an implicit measure of prejudice related to discrimination.

Startle

Another popular use of facial EMG is for the assessment of the potentiation of eyeblinks in reaction to a startling sound (see Blumenthal & Franklin, Chapter 6, this volume). Ample research has demonstrated that the startle eyeblink reflex to a sudden acoustic probe is modulated by the individual's emotional state (e.g., Lang, 1995; Lang, Bradley, & Cuthbert, 1990; Vrana, Spence, & Lang, 1988). According to Lang (1995; Lang et al., 1990), when an individual is exposed to an unpleasant stimulus, the relevant subcortical aversive system circuitry is activated; this leads to the augmentation of defensive reflexes, such as the eyeblink reflex. As appetitive and aversive/defensive states are opponent states, the opposite effect can be observed when the individual is exposed to pleasant stimuli.

More recently, Benning and colleagues (2004) obtained a pattern opposite to that for the eyeblink reflex for the PAR—the reflexive contraction of the postauricular muscle, which serves to pull the ear back and up (Berzin & Fortinguerra, 1993). The PAR can be observed in response to nonstartling sounds as well. This reflexive reaction to a sound is augmented when individuals are exposed to pleasant stimuli and is reduced when they are exposed to unpleasant stimuli.

Using both reflexes as indices of approach and withdrawal tendencies, respectively, Hess, Sabourin, and Kleck (2007) explored people's reaction to male and female anger and happiness expressions. Specifically, we tested a prediction based on the functional equivalence hypothesis (Hess, Adams, & Kleck, 2007), which postulates that facial expressive behavior and morphological cues to dominance and affiliation are similar in their effects on emotional attributions. The cues linked to perceived dominance (e.g., square jaw, heavy eyebrows, high forehead) are more typical for men, and men are generally perceived as more dominant than are women. In contrast, baby-facedness, a facial aspect more closely linked to perceived affiliation, is more common in women. This leads to the hypothesis that anger in men should be seen as more threatening, due to the double association of dominance with anger and male features. Likewise, because of the double association with happiness and female features, smiling women should be perceived as more appetitive. Hess, Sabourin, and Kleck assessed both eyeblink startle and the PAR while participants were viewing happy and angry expressions shown by men and women. The PAR was potentiated during happy expressions and inhibited during anger expressions; however, as predicted, this pattern was more clearly found for female expressers. Also as predicted, eyeblink startle was potentiated during viewing of angry faces and inhibited during happy faces only for expressions shown by men.

Summary

Facial EMG provides many advantages for the measurement of facial behavior. In particular, the high temporal and spatial resolution of facial EMG allows the measurement of fleeting and subtle movements, which may easily escape the naked eye. However, the use of facial EMG demands that the researcher can specify in advance which of a few muscles will be of interest in a given context. For certain applications, such as the use of EMG to assess startle potentiation, this requirement does not pose a problem. However, when facial EMG is used to assess emotional expressions, the potential for misidentification is higher. This said, for many applications facial EMG is certainly the measure of choice. Studies like those by Vanman and colleagues (2004) point to its use as an implicit measure that is not easily influenced by voluntary action—not because participants can not produce expressions voluntarily, but simply because they are not aware of the expressions they show.

In addition, facial EMG has unprobed potential. Most studies that have used facial EMG have quantified the signal by using mean amplitude over a certain time period. Yet such additional measures as the parameters of the temporal domain suggested by Cacioppo and colleagues (1983) have not yet been well explored with regard to their potential for the measurement of facial behavior. However, recent research has shown that the temporal dynamics of facial expressions contain valuable information (see, e.g., Yoshikawa & Sato, 2006), and hence it may be time to exploit the temporal information provided by facial EMG.

References

Armstrong, J. E., Hutchinson, I., Laing, D. G., & Jinks, A. L. (2007). Facial electromyography: Responses of children to odor and taste stimuli. *Chemical Senses, 32*, 611–621.

Arndt, J., Allen, J. J. B., & Greenberg, J. (2001). Traces of terror: Subliminal death primes and facial electromyographic indices of affect. *Motivation and Emotion, 25*, 253–277.

Benning, S. D., Patrick, C. J., & Lang, A. R. (2004). Emotional modulation of the post-auricular reflex. *Psychophysiology, 41*, 426–432.

Berg, W. K., & Balaban, M. T. (1999). Startle elicitation: Stimulus parameters, recording techniques, and quantification. In M. E. Dawson, A. M. Shell, & A. H. Böhmelt (Eds.), *Startle modification: Implications for neuroscience, cognitive science, and clinical science* (pp. 21–50). Cambridge, UK: Cambridge University Press.

Berzin, F., & Fortinguerra, C. R. (1993). EMG study of the anterior, superior, and posterior auricular muscles in man. *Anatomischer Anzeiger, 175*, 195–197.

Blairy, S., Herrera, P., & Hess, U. (1999). Mimicry and the judgment of emotional facial expressions. *Journal of Nonverbal Behavior, 23*, 5–41.

Brown, L. M., Bradley, M. M., & Lang, P. J. (2006). Affective reactions to pictures of ingroup and outgroup members. *Biological Psychology, 71*, 303–311.

Buck, S. M., Hillman, C. H., Evans, E. M., & Janelle, C. M. (2004). Emotional responses to pictures of oneself in healthy college age females. *Motivation and Emotion, 28*, 279–295.

Bush, L. K., Hess, U., & Wolford, G. (1993). Transformations for within-subject designs: A Monte Carlo investigation. *Psychological Bulletin, 113*, 566–579.

Cacioppo, J. T., Marshall-Goodell, B., & Dorfman, D. D. (1983). Skeletal muscular patterning: Topographical analysis of the integrated electromyogram. *Psychophysiology, 20*, 269–283.

Cacioppo, J. T., Petty, R. E., Losch, M. E., & Kim, H. S. (1986). Electromyographic activity over facial muscle regions can discriminate the valence and intensity of affective reactions. *Journal of Personality and Social Psychology, 50*(2), 260–268.

Cohen, B. H., Davidson, R. J., Senulis, J. A., & Saron, C. D. (1992). Muscle tension patterns during auditory attention. *Biological Psychology, 33*, 133–156.

Cohn, J. F., & Ekman, P. (2005). Measuring facial action. In J. A. Harrigan, R. Rosenthal, & K. R. Scherer (Eds.), *The new handbook of methods in nonverbal behavior research* (pp. 9–64). Oxford, UK: Oxford University Press.

Crombez, G., Baeyens, F., & Eelen, P. (1997). Changes in facial EMG activity related to painful heat stimuli on the hand. *Journal of Psychophysiology, 11*, 256–262.

Dambrun, M., Després, G., & Guimond, S. (2003). On the multifaceted nature of prejudice: Psychophysiology responses to ingroup and outgroup ethnic stimuli. *Current Research in Social Psychology, 8*, 200–204.

Davis, W. J., Rahman, M. A., Smith, L. J., & Burns, A. (1995). Properties of human affect induced by static color slides (IAPS): Dimensional, categorical and electromyographic analysis. *Biological Psychology, 41*, 229–253.

Dimberg, U. (1982). Facial reactions to facial expressions. *Psychophysiology, 19*(6), 643–647.

Dimberg, U. (1988). Facial expressions and emotional reactions: A psychobiological analysis of human social behavior. In H. L. Wagner (Ed.), *Social psychophysiology and emotion: Theory and clinical applications* (pp. 131–150). Chichester, UK: Wiley.

Dimberg, U. (1990). Perceived unpleasantness and facial reactions to auditory stimuli. *Scandinavian Journal of Psychology, 31*, 70–75.

Dimberg, U., & Öhman, A. (1996). Behold the wrath: Psychophysiological responses to facial stimuli. *Motivation and Emotion, 20*(2), 149–182.

Dimberg, U., Thunberg, M., & Grunedal, S. (2002). Facial reactions to emotional stimuli: Automatically controlled emotional responses. *Cognition and Emotion, 16*, 449–472.

Ekman, P., & Friesen, W. V. (1978). *The Facial Action Coding System: A technique for the measurement of facial movement.* Palo Alto, CA: Consulting Psychologists Press.

Fridlund, A. J., & Cacioppo, J. T. (1986). Guidelines for human electromyographic research. *Psychophysiology, 23*, 567–589.

Fridlund, A. J., Schwartz, G. E., & Fowler, S. C. (1984). Pattern recognition of self-reported emotional state from multiple-site facial EMG activity during affective imagery. *Psychophysiology, 21*, 622–637.

Gallese, V., & Goldman, A. (1998). Mirror neurons and the simulation theory of mind-reading. *Trends in Cognitive Sciences, 2*, 493–501.

Goldman, A. I., & Sripada, C. S. (2005). Simulationist models of face-based emotion recognition. *Cognition, 94*, 193–213.

Goldstein, B. (1972). Electromyography: A measure of skeletal muscle response. In N. S. Greenfield & R. A. Sternbach (Eds.), *Handbook of psychophysiology* (pp. 329–366). New York: Holt, Rinehart & Winston.

Gray, H. (2000). *Anatomy of the human body.* Retrieved from *www.bartleby.com/107/* (Original work published 1918)

Greenwald, A. G., McGhee, D. E., & Schwartz, J. L. K. (1998). Measuring individual differences in implicit cognition: The Implicit Association Test. *Journal of Personality and Social Psychology, 74*, 1464–1480.

Guerra, A. B., Metzinger, S. E., Metzinger, R. C., Xie, C., Xie, Y., Rigby, P. L., et al. (2004). Variability of the postauricular muscle complex: Analysis of 40 hemicadaver dissections. *Archives of Facial Plastic Surgery, 6,* 342–347.

Hackley, S. A., Woldorff, M., & Hillyard, S. A. (1987). Combined use of microreflexes and event-related brain potentials as measures of auditory selective attention. *Psychophysiology, 24,* 632–647.

Hazlett, R. L., & Hazlett, S. Y. (1999). Emotional response to television commercials: Facial EMG vs. self-report. *Journal of Advertising Research, 39,* 7–23.

Hess, U. (2007, May 31–June 1). *Smiling in dyadic interactions: The influence of status and gender.* Paper presented at the NCCR Workshop "Power, Gender, and Emotion," University of Neuchâtel, Neuchâtel, Switzerland.

Hess, U., Adams, R. B., Jr., & Kleck, R. E. (2007). When two do the same it might not mean the same: The perception of emotional expressions shown by men and women. In U. Hess & P. Philippot (Eds.), *Group dynamics and emotional expression* (pp. 33–52). New York: Cambridge University Press.

Hess, U., & Blairy, S. (2001). Facial mimicry and emotional contagion to dynamic emotional facial expressions and their influence on decoding accuracy. *International Journal of Psychophysiology, 40,* 129–141.

Hess, U., Kappas, A., McHugo, G. J., Kleck, R. E., & Lanzetta, J. T. (1989). An analysis of the encoding and decoding of spontaneous and posed smiles: The use of facial electromyography. *Journal of Nonverbal Behavior, 13*(2), 121–137.

Hess, U., Sabourin, G., & Kleck, R. E. (2007). Postauricular and eye-blink startle responses to facial expressions. *Psychophysiology, 44,* 431–435.

Hess, W. (1973). Digitale Segmentation von Signalen im Zeitbereich [Digital segmentation of signals in time interval]. In M. Beckmann, G. Goos, & H. P. Kunzi (Eds.), *Lecture notes in economic and mathematical systems* (pp. 161–171). Berlin: Springer.

Hu, S., Player, K. A., Mcchesney, K. A., Dalistan, M. D., Tyner, C. A., & Scozzafava, J. E. (1999). Facial EMG as an indicator of palatability in humans. *Physiology and Behavior, 68,* 31–35.

Jäncke, L., & Kaufmann, N. (1994). Facial EMG responses to odors in solitude and with an audience. *Chemical Senses, 19,* 99–111.

Kapit, W., & Elson, L. M. (2001). *The anatomy coloring book* (3rd ed.). San Francisco: Benjamin Cummings.

Lanctôt, N., & Hess, U. (2007). The timing of appraisals. *Emotion, 7,* 207–212.

Landis, C. (1924). Studies in emotional reactions: II. General behavior and facial expression. *Journal of Comparative Psychology, 4,* 447–509.

Lang, P. J. (1995). The emotion probe: Studies of motivation and attention. *American Psychologist, 50,* 372–385.

Lang, P. J., Bradley, M. M., & Cuthbert, B. N. (1990). Emotion, attention, and the startle reflex. *Psychological Review, 97,* 377–395.

Larsen, J. T., Norris, C. J., & Cacioppo, J. T. (2003). Effects of positive and negative affect on electromyographic activity over zygomaticus major and corrugator supercilii. *Psychophysiology, 40,* 776–785.

Lawrence, J. H., & DeLuca, C. J. (1983). Myoelectric signal versus force relationship in different human muscles. *Journal of Applied Physiology, 54,* 1653–1659.

Lippold, O. C. J. (1967). Electromyography. In P. H. Venables & I. Martin (Eds.), *A manual of psychophysiological methods* (pp. 245–297). Amsterdam: North-Holland.

Loeb, G. E., & Gans, C. (1986). *Electromyography for experimentalists.* Chicago: University of Chicago Press.

McHugo, G. J., & Lanzetta, J. T. (1983). Methodological decisions on social psychophysiology. In J. T. Cacioppo & R. E. Petty (Eds.), *Social psychology: A sourcebook* (pp. 630–665). New York: Guilford Press.

McHugo, G. J., Lanzetta, J. T., Sullivan, D. G., Masters, R. D., & Englis, B. G. (1985). Emotional reactions to a political leader's expressive displays. *Journal of Personality and Social Psychology, 49,* 1513–1529.

Mojzisch, A., Schilbach, L., Helmert, J. R., Pannasch, S., Velichkovsky, B. M., & Vogeley, K. (2006). The effects of self-involvement on attention, arousal, and facial expression during social interaction with virtual others: A psychophysiological study. *Social Neuroscience, 1,* 184–195.

Motley, M. T., & Camden, C. T. (1988). Facial expression of emotion: A comparison of posed expressions versus spontaneous expressions in an interpersonal communications setting. *Western Journal of Speech Communication, 52,* 1–22.

Murata, A., Uetake, A., Matsumoto, S., & Takasawa, Y. (2003). Evaluation of shoulder muscular fatigue induced during VDT tasks. *International Journal of Human Computer Interaction, 15,* 407–417.

Newton, T. F., Khalsa-Denison, M. E., & Gawin, F. H. (1997). The face of craving?: Facial muscle EMG and reported craving in abstinent and nonabstinent cocaine users. *Psychiatry Research, 73,* 115–118.

Parkinson, B. (2005). Do facial movements express emotions or communicate motives? *Personality and Social Psychology Review, 9,* 278–311.

Pope, L. K., & Smith, C. A. (1994). On the distinct meanings of smiles and frowns. *Cognition and Emotion, 8,* 65–72.

Robinson, J. D., Cinciripini, P. M., Carter, B. L., Lam, C. Y., & Wetter, D. W. (2007). Facial EMG as an index of affective response to nicotine. *Experimental and Clinical Psychopharmacology, 15,* 390–399.

Rosenthal, R. (2005). Conducting judgment studies: Some methodological issues. In J. A. Harrigan, R. Rosenthal, & K. R. Scherer (Eds.), *The new handbook of methods in nonverbal behavior research* (pp. 199–234). Oxford, UK: Oxford University Press.

Sayette, M. A., Cohn, J. F., Wertz, J. M., Perrott, M. A., & Parrott, D. J. (2001). A psychometric evaluation of the Facial Action Coding System for assessing spontaneous expression. *Journal of Nonverbal Behavior, 25,* 167–185.

Sollers, J. J., III, & Hackley, S. A. (1997). Effects of foreperiod duration on reflexive and voluntary responses to intense noise bursts. *Psychophysiology, 34,* 518–526.

Tassinary, L. G., & Cacioppo, J. T. (1992). Unobservable facial actions and emotion. *Psychological Science, 3*, 28–33.

Tassinary, L. G., & Cacioppo, J. T. (2000). The skeletomotor system: Surface electromyography. In J. T. Cacioppo, L. G. Tassinary, & G. G. Berntson (Eds.), *Handbook of psychophysiology* (2nd ed., pp. 163–199). Cambridge, UK: Cambridge University Press.

Tian, Y., Kanade, T., & Cohn, J. F. (2003). Facial expression analysis. In S. Z. Li & A. K. Jain (Eds.), *Handbook of face recognition* (pp. 247–276). New York: Springer.

Vanman, E. J., Paul, B. Y., Ito, T. A., & Miller, N. (1997). The modern face of prejudice and structural features that moderate the effect of cooperation on affect. *Journal of Personality and Social Psychology, 73*, 941–959.

Vanman, E. J., Saltz, J. L., Nathan, L. R., & Warren, J. A. (2004). Racial discrimination by low-prejudiced whites facial movements as implicit measures of attitudes related to behavior. *Psychological Science, 15*, 711–714.

Veldhuizen, I. J. T., Gaillard, A. W. K., & de Vries, J. (2003). The influence of mental fatigue on facial EMG activity during a simulated workday. *Biological Psychology, 63*, 59–78.

Vrana, S. R. (1993). The psychophysiology of disgust: Differentiating negative emotional contexts with facial EMG. *Psychophysiology, 30*, 279–286.

Vrana, S. R., Spence, E. L., & Lang, P. J. (1988). The startle probe response: A new measure of emotion? *Journal of Abnormal Psychology, 97*, 487–491.

Wikipedia. (2008). Muscle contractions. Retrieved from *en.wikipedia.org/wiki/Muscle_contractions*

Wolf, K., Mass, R., Ingenbleek, T., Kiefer, F., Naber, D., & Wiedemann, K. (2005). The facial pattern of disgust, appetence, excited joy and relaxed joy: An improved facial EMG study. *Scandinavian Journal of Psychology, 46*, 403–409.

Wolf, K., Raedler, T., Henke, K., Kiefer, F., Mass, R., Quante, M., et al. (2005). The face of pain: A pilot study to validate the measurement of facial pain expression with an improved electromyogram method. *Pain Research and Management, 10*, 15–19.

Yoshikawa, S., & Sato, W. (2006). Enhanced perceptual, emotional, and motor processing in response to dynamic facial expressions of emotion. *Japanese Psychological Research, 48*, 213–222.

6

The Startle Eyeblink Response

Terry D. Blumenthal
Joseph C. Franklin

The purpose of this chapter is to describe the various methodological issues that researchers should consider when using the startle response as a way to investigate personality and social psychology. Although this chapter is not a review of variations in startle as a function of personality and social psychological factors, it does provide a summary and assessment of the methods used in these areas. Understanding these methods not only will be useful when investigators are deciding how to utilize startle as a measure, but also will be vital to interpreting the findings in this area. Even though the purpose of this chapter is not to persuade readers to add startle to their own research programs, it is our hope that the methods and ideas reviewed here will facilitate the effective application of startle to the study of problems and processes that have not traditionally been examined with startle. Readers may wish to use startle in their own research for any of several reasons: (1) Startle is sensitive to many things and can therefore be used as a measure of those things; (2) the anatomy and chemistry underlying startle have been largely identified, due to the fact that this response is available across many animal species—a fact that supports both translational research and a more complete understanding of the mechanisms underlying those things that startle measures; and (3) startle is relatively easy to measure, and the data are relatively easy to reduce into an understandable form.

With that said, we remind our readers that the intention of this chapter is to make their use of startle more informed and dynamic.

What Is Startle, and Why Use It?

Defensive Activation

Startle is considered to be a defensive response, with skeletal muscle activity serving to protect the back of the neck, facial muscle activity serving to protect the eyes, and increased sympathetic nervous system activity serving to ready the organism for further action (Yeomans, Li, Scott, & Frankland, 2002). The startle response generally functions either to protect the organism from bodily harm or to propel the organism from a situation in which such harm may occur. This defensive startle response may be viewed as an index of the organism's ability to respond to danger, and can be expected to increase in situations in which danger (either real or perceived) is more likely. This makes startle a useful measure of relatively automatic reactivity to such situations, with this reactivity expected to vary as social and personality characteristics differ.

With variations in methodology, the startle response can be utilized to index a variety of neurocognitive processes, including arousal, emotion, attention, and information processing. Likewise, depending on the specific methods used, the startle response can also be employed to index neurological functioning in various areas, including the brainstem, limbic system, and frontostriatal areas. It should be noted that the specificity and reliability of the startle response as a measure of these processes and functions is strongly tied to the type and quality of the methods utilized.

Advantages and Disadvantages of Startle

Ironically, the primary disadvantage of startle as a measure is also its primary advantage: the fact that it is so sensitive to so many things. This sensitivity allows us to use startle in a wide variety of experimental situations to investigate an equally wide variety of research questions. However, this sensitivity also requires us to control extraneous factors that could add error or confusion to our results. In order to reliably and validly measure specific factors of interest, we must be mindful of our specific methods and their ability to control or eliminate as many of these extraneous factors as possible. Alternatively, these extraneous factors may actually be used in the design of new experiments, becoming independent or classification variables. The error in one study may be the effect in another.

Relative to many other neurobiological measures, startle has a short and precise onset latency. The eyeblink component of the startle response has a latency of approximately 50 msec, which means that the blink has already occurred by the time a person is consciously aware that a stimulus has been presented. Consequently, a researcher can be confident that the blink is a response to the eliciting stimulus (although spontaneous eyeblinks fall inside the scoring window for reflex blinks on 1–3% of trials). This allows the researcher to monitor the participant and withhold the startle stimulus until the participant is sitting still, for example. This also allows the blink to be elicited at a specific time, such as following a change in the social environment, or 0.5 sec after some other stimulus has been presented.

Startle also has the advantage of being available across the lifespan, in that it can be measured in the same manner in infants, adolescents, younger adults, and older adults. This allows one to look at developmental progressions of the factor of interest with a measurement methodology (eyeblink electromyography [EMG]) that is consistent across ages. For example, with the paradigm involving prepulse inhibition of startle, it may be possible to evaluate the developmental course of frontostriatal functioning in introverted versus extraverted personalities, or to examine the impact of social stressors on this developmental course. A related advantage is the fact that startle can be elicited from participants when they are either awake or asleep, making it a useful measure in neonatal research (Blumenthal, Avendano, & Berg, 1987).

Just as startle is available across the lifespan, it is also measurable across much of the phylogenetic spectrum, allowing for the application of startle in the investigation of animal models of human conditions and processes. Analogous responses, and in some cases the same responses, can be used to investigate the mechanisms underlying factors across species. The startle response and its underlying neuroanatomy are relatively simple (Davis, 2006); however, the fact that the startle pathway receives input from, and projects to, a number of other locations in the central nervous system makes this response useful in evaluating activity in a variety of other systems. For example, startle can be used to measure activation of the amygdala, the frontal cortex, various sensory systems, the tegmentum, and many other locations (Swerdlow, Geyer, & Braff, 2001). This allows us to use startle to quantify emotion, arousal, attention, perceptual sensitivity, and many other factors, including personality and social psychological factors.

Like many other psychophysiological measures, startle is more automatic than self-report measures; consequently, it has the advantage of being able to provide information that is less likely to be tainted by response bias. For example, the magnitude of the startle response is larger when state anxiety is greater (Grillon, 2002), and this may be true even if the participant from whom startle is being measured is not aware of that increased anxiety (Grillon & Davis, 1997). The point here is that startle may be more sensitive than some self-report measures are to variations that are below the level of awareness. In this way, startle may be a useful way to access variables related to personality and social functioning that may be unavailable to or obscured by other methods.

Measuring the Startle Response

Overview

Startle can be affected by three categories of factors: (1) situational factors external to the participant, such as stimulus parameters or contextual cues; (2) characteristics of the participant, such as clinical diagnosis, the presence of drugs, conditioning history, or social and personality traits; and (3) information-processing methods by which the participant takes in and integrates information from the environment, such as attention, emotion, and arousal. A great deal of overlap and interaction occurs among these three categories, and, accordingly, to the extent that certain variables are controlled or manipulated, researchers may examine these factors as either independent or interactive factors. For instance, emotional modulation of startle may vary as a function of personality characteristics (Patrick, Bradley, & Lang, 1993); these personality characteristics may interact with environmental stimuli (Grillon & Baas, 2003); and stimulus parameters may interact with all of these (Britt & Blumenthal, 1992). These relationships can also depend on how the situation is perceived (Flaten & Blumenthal, 1999; Haerich, 1994). Although it may seem as if this intertwining of factors would make any research outcome uninterpretable, the fact that startle is sensitive to all of these factors means that we can use startle to tease apart these interrelated issues. However, this requires experimentally stabilizing as many factors as possible, in order to allow variations in startle reactivity to reflect variations in the single factor of interest. Startle is not unique in this respect; isolating the variable of interest is necessary in any research design whenever the dependent variable can be affected by more than one factor. Such methodological control increases the extent to which results can be compared across studies, following the minimization of confounds. Whereas more methodological rigor may limit the degree to which results can be generalized to other situations, this rigor is necessary for internal validity. This issue is somewhat more important in startle research than in some other paradigms, due to the exquisite sensitivity of startle to a variety of influences (Blumenthal et al., 2005). Accordingly, for the sake of interpretability of results, it is essential that methodological decisions be scrupulously reported.

Specific Methodology

Basic Methods

The startle response in humans consists of several components, including skeletal muscle activity, facial muscle activity, changes in heart rate and skin conductance, and cortical evoked potentials (Berg & Balaban, 1999). In humans, the eyeblink component of the startle response is the component most often recorded because it is easy to measure, exceedingly sensitive to a wide variety of parameters, and the earliest and most habituation-resistant component of the startle response. Correspondingly, measuring eyeblinks allows startle to be reliably measured, even after over 100 trials (Blumenthal et al., 2005). The startle eyeblink reflex is quantified by recordings of the electrical activity (EMG) of the facial muscle that closes the eyelid, the orbicularis oculi (Blumenthal et al., 2005). This muscle activity, recorded from electrodes taped to the surface of the skin (see Figure 6.1), provides a measure of the output of the facial motor nucleus in the brainstem, allowing for a relatively noninvasive measure of central nervous system activity. The facial motor nucleus is activated by the startle center—the nucleus reticularis pontis caudalis, located in the pons (Lee, Lopez, Meloni, & Davis, 1996). This startle center receives input from many structures, and projects to a variety of response-activating locations. The facts that the startle response is similar across species, and that these anatomical pathways are similar across species, mean that we can use the startle response in translational research to identify the physiological mechanisms underlying those factors resulting in differences in startle reactivity. For example, a great

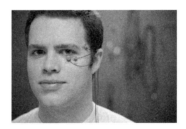

FIGURE 6.1. Placement of EMG recording electrodes. Photo by Ken Bennett.

deal has been learned about the physiology of anxiety in humans by studying fear-potentiated startle in rats (Davis, 2006).

One important consideration in evaluating startle eyeblink responses is the fact that there is a wide range of baseline startle reactivity across participants (Blumenthal, Elden, & Flaten, 2004). It is not unusual for the most reactive participant in a study to have average baseline startle responses 50 times larger than those of the least reactive individual. This means that comparing startle reactivity across individuals without compensating for these variations in baseline startle magnitudes may be misleading. Fortunately, there are several ways to deal with this problem (see Blumenthal et al., 2004). For example, a researcher may convert startle magnitudes to standard scores, either within an individual or across individuals within a group. Of course, this should not be done across groups if a group effect is the actual research question under study. Alternatively, a few preliminary trials may be presented in order to determine the baseline reactivity of each participant, with subsequent reactivity in the various experimental conditions then being a ratio of that initial baseline reactivity. If premanipulation baseline trials are used, the researcher must consider the fact that startle normally habituates, so one of the experimental conditions should involve an absence of the factor under study. For example, if the experiment calls for comparing two levels of a variable within participants, the study would have four blocks of trials: a first block of startle-alone trials, followed by three test trial blocks (one with each level of the variable in question, and one block with just startle stimuli again). If the order in which conditions are presented is counterbalanced, then the block of startle-alone trials can be used to index the extent of habituation, and this can then be used to more accurately evaluate the impact of the actual experimental variables.

Methodological considerations for determining the way in which eyeblink EMG is used to quantify the startle response are explained in detail by Blumenthal and colleagues (2005). Briefly, two recording electrodes are attached to the face below the eye, with a ground electrode placed elsewhere (often on the temple or the forehead), and the EMG activity of the orbicularis oculi muscle is recorded for a specified period of time following the presentation of an eliciting stimulus. That EMG activity is then processed in specific ways (see Blumenthal et al., 2005) to extract such response parameters as magnitude, amplitude, onset latency, and probability. These can then be analyzed across the factors of experimental interest (e.g., stimulus intensity, personality classification, experimental condition). Hess (Chapter 5, this volume) also discusses EMG signal processing.

Importance of Experimental Control

A researcher must also be careful to control as many parameters of the testing situation as possible, because startle is so exquisitely sensitive to so many things. For example, an increase in startle may occur because of attention being directed toward the modality in which the startle stimulus is presented (Neumann, Lipp, & McHugh, 2004), because of an increase in general arousal (Dillon & LaBar, 2005), or because of an increase in negative affect (Vrana, Spence, & Lang, 1988). If the parameter under investigation is emotional modulation of startle, then failing to control for attention and arousal may yield misleading results. In fact, in emotional-modulation-of-startle studies, pleasant and unpleasant slides both result in an increase in arousal, although they have opposite effects on startle reactivity if the inherent arousal level of the slide is sufficiently high (Cuthbert, Bradley, & Lang, 1996). For example, startle sessions are often boring for the participant, so variations in arousal can be minimized by keeping the session as short as possible, by asking the participant to sit still, and by avoiding such instructions as "Relax" or "Don't blink." Attentional variability can be minimized by removing interesting and potentially distracting objects from the testing space, although attentional wandering is impossible to eliminate completely. The point is that variations in startle may be due to a number of variables, with attention, arousal, and affect interacting with each other. Furthermore, these interactions may vary as a function of stimulus intensity, baseline arousal, personality, clinical characteristics, or a host of other factors. This means that methodology in a startle study must be very finely tuned and strictly controlled.

Using the Startle Response in Social and Personality Research

Overview

The startle response can be a useful measure in social and personality research. The fact that startle is affected by a variety of factors means that startle can be used to measure those factors. Startle provides a measure that is different from, but often correlated with, information provided from self-report questionnaires. Startle is a defensive response, and it has been effectively applied to the study of issues related to defensive motivation, such as fear and negative valence (Bradley, Codispoti, & Lang, 2006; Davis, 2006). However, startle is also an interruptive response, allowing for its application in research dealing with information processing, attention, and inhibitory processes (Braff, Geyer, & Swerdlow, 2001; Dawson, Schell, & Böhmelt, 1999; Graham, 1992). In the realm of personality research, startle has been employed to study many issues, including traits of extraversion and neuroticism (Eysenck & Eysenck, 1985), harm avoidance (Cloninger, 1988), sensation seeking (Zuckerman, 1994), anxiety (Spielberger, Gorsuch, Lushene, Vagg, & Jacobs, 1983), and a variety of subclinical personality traits (Grillon & Baas, 2003). In the realm of social psychological research, startle has been used to study social phobia/social anxiety disorder (Larsen, Norton, Walker, & Stein, 2002; Marcin & Nemeroff, 2003), rejection sensitivity (Downey, Mougious, Ayduk, London, & Shoda, 2004), antisocial behaviors (Benning, Patrick, & Iacono, 2005), racial bias (Amodio, Harmon-Jones, & Devine, 2003), and anti-gay bias (Mahaffey, Bryan, & Hutchison, 2005). In addition, prepulse inhibition of the startle response has been used to investigate the effects of social isolation (Weiss & Feldon, 2001) and maternal care (Zhang, Chretien, Meaney, & Gratton, 2005) in rats, and social perception in humans with schizophrenia (Wynn, Sergi, Dawson, Schell, & Green, 2005). Similar methodology is used across many studies; we describe examples that are meant to be representative, but not comprehensive, of the work in this area.

Startle Reactivity

In studies using startle as a measure, we can look at the processing of the startle stimulus itself to see how this processing differs for different stimulus parameters, or between people with different characteristics. This constitutes a measurement of "startle reactivity," which is the measurement of the magnitude, amplitude, probability, and/or onset latency of the startle response. We can then compare measures of startle reactivity across stimulus parameters, participant groups, and so forth. One way in which startle has been used in the area of personality research involves simply measuring startle reactivity in people who score either high or low on certain personality questionnaires. For example, startle has been used to test Eysenck's hypothesis of differential excitability of the central nervous system in extraversion, by presenting startle stimuli to participants identified as introverts or extraverts. Blumenthal (2001) showed that startle responses were larger in introverts than in extraverts, and that direction of attention resulted in differential effects on startle as a function of extraversion (see Figure 6.2). As another example, patients with high levels of anxiety (Grillon, Ameli, Foot, & Davis, 1993) and with social phobia and panic disorder (Larsen et al., 2002) tend to have larger startle responses than nonanxious control participants do. This design involves simply comparing startle reactivity across groups, or across levels of a personality construct.

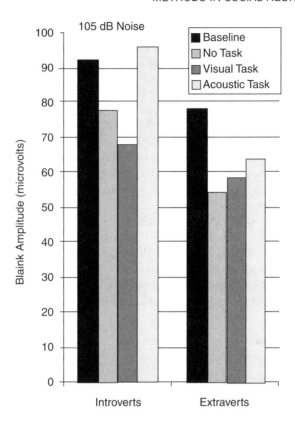

FIGURE 6.2. Difference in acoustic startle reactivity in introverts and extraverts as a function of attention directed to acoustic or visual tasks. From Blumenthal (2001). Copyright 2001 by the International Society for the Study of Individual Differences. Reprinted by permission.

A further step might involve quantifying the extent to which startle reactivity habituates across a session, by comparing startle reactivity on early and late trials. This can allow for the assessment of the degree to which habituation rate varies as a function of personality construct (LaRowe, Patrick, Curtin, & Kline, 2006). One caveat specifically related to the use of startle to investigate anxiety is the finding that potentiated startle is often not seen in patients with anxiety during baseline recordings; it is only seen when they are under a specific threat or contextual stress (Grillon & Morgan, 1999; Grillon, Morgan, Davis, & Southwick, 1998). This is an example of a personality construct interacting with the stimulus environment.

All of these cases involve measuring reactivity to the startle stimulus itself. However, we can complicate such a design by measuring startle in participants at different levels of a personality construct while presenting different intensities of startle stimuli, for example (Britt & Blumenthal, 1991, 1993). Alternatively, we can modify the pharmacological environment by administering caffeine or amphetamines to participants in one test session, but not in another (Flaten & Blumenthal, 1999; Hutchison, Wood, & Swift, 1999), or we can test clinical patients while they are or are not medicated (Duncan et al., 2006; Hamm, Weike, & Schupp, 2001). In all of these cases, differential reactivity to the startle stimulus can tell us something about the levels of the independent or classification variables of interest.

Fear-Potentiated Startle

If startle is elicited in the presence of a stimulus that has previously been repeatedly paired with an aversive unconditional stimulus, the startle response tends to be larger than if elicited in the presence of a neutral stimulus—a phenomenon referred to as "fear-potentiated startle" (Brown, Kalish, & Farber, 1951). In the original report of this effect, a light was repeatedly paired with a foot shock in rats, and when startle was subsequently elicited in the presence of that light, the response was larger in rats that had received the conditioning than in those that had not. This fear potentiation is an example of classical conditioning, with a previously neutral stimulus gaining conditional power based on its pairing with an unconditional aversive stimulus. The anatomical pathways underlying this effect have been identified (see Davis, 2006, for a review); as mentioned earlier, they involve a projection from the central nucleus of the amygdala to the brainstem startle center, the nucleus reticularis pontis caudalis. Using a conditioning procedure in humans very similar to that used in rats, Grillon and Davis (1997) showed that the eyeblink startle response could also be potentiated by stimuli that had been paired with shock. In fact, Grillon, Ameli, Woods, Merikangas, and Davis (1991) showed that presenting shock was not necessary, the threat of shock was sufficient to induce fear-potentiated startle. Importantly, to the extent that an experimenter's interaction with participants signifies a social situation, measuring startle reactivity as a function of social phobia (Larsen et al., 2002) may represent fear-potentiated startle. Similarly, researchers have experimentally induced fear of negative evaluation by having participants engage in an actual (Panayiotou & Vrana, 1998) or virtual (Cornwell, Johnson, Berardi, & Grillon, 2006) public speech task. Likewise, the emotion/valence studies described below may also partially represent fear-potentiated startle.

Startle can also be potentiated by corticotropin-releasing hormone (CRH), and this effect seems to be due to CRH reception in the bed nucleus of the stria terminalis (BNST), an area that is closely related to the amygdala (Alheid, deOlmos, & Beltramino, 1995). This led Walker and Davis (1997) to conduct experiments that resulted in their proposal of an animal model of anxiety that they referred to as "light-enhanced startle," caused by exposing rats to bright light for 20 min. Davis and colleagues (see Davis, 2006) showed that fear-potentiated startle depends on the amygdala, whereas anxiety-related startle depends on the BNST. Fear-potentiated startle appears to be faster and more stimulus-specific, whereas anxiety-enhanced startle develops more slowly, but remains in effect for a much longer time. The involvement of CRH in the enhancement of startle occurs outside the hypothalamic–pituitary–adrenocortical axis (Walker & Davis, 1997), and may be an indicator of the degree to which stress contributes to anxiety—an effect that can be measured with the startle response (Grillon & Baas, 2003). In fact, startle is enhanced by the conditional stimulus in fear conditioning (an example of cue conditioning), but also by the environment in which the conditioning took place (an example of context conditioning). This means that researchers may use startle as an indicator of the effectiveness of desensitization or extinction therapy, simply by measuring startle before and after such therapy in the presence of trigger (conditional) stimuli (de Jong et al., 1996; Vrana, Constantine, & Westman, 1992). This makes the measurement of the startle response a useful index of anxiety in patients dealing with various anxiety disorders, such as generalized anxiety disorder and posttraumatic stress disorder (Grillon & Baas, 2003). Startle is also a useful measure of state anxiety in nonpatients, in whom anxiety levels can be manipulated in the experimental setting (Britt & Blumenthal, 1993). The sensitivity of startle to variations in state anxiety means that researchers who are not specifically studying anxiety must be very careful to minimize anxiety-provoking stimuli in their testing environments.

The Emotion Probe: The Valence Match–Mismatch Hypothesis

The startle stimulus can be used to probe or evaluate ongoing processing, such as in the study of emotion, or to investigate the impact of social interaction on information processing. Here the startle probe is being used to evaluate the processing of information or situations that we researchers present to the participants. That is, we are not testing the stable characteristics of the participants, nor are we testing the various levels of an independent variable that we administer to modulate those characteristics. Instead, we are evaluating one process (e.g., defensive motivation) by eliciting an automatic response that is sensitive to that process. Many studies in this area use the valence-matching method described by Vrana and colleagues (1988). This involves presenting startle stimuli while participants view slides that have been rated affectively positive, neutral, or negative. Startle is expected to be larger in the presence of negative slides than in the presence of positive slides. Some studies in this area compare startle reactivity during negative and positive slide conditions, while others compare startle reactivity during negative and neutral slide conditions, and also reactivity during positive and neutral slide conditions (see Lang, 1995, for more information about this procedure). Increased startle during negative slides can be thought of as a reaction to threat, similar to fear-potentiated startle (described above), and it involves the activation of aversive or avoidance motivation. Startle is a defensive response and can be used to index the activity of protective or avoidance motivation as follows: If a participant is experiencing a negatively valenced situation (which should be accompanied by an evaluation of unpleasantness) and a startle stimulus is presented, the ensuing startle response can be expected to be larger than the startle response elicited during a positively valenced, or pleasant, situation. When defensive motivation is increased by the unpleasant slide, the subsequent presentation of a startle stimulus will further increase activity in defensive responses, such as startle (Lang, Bradley, & Cuthbert, 1997). This affective modulation of startle has been used to investigate many personality constructs, including extraversion, harm avoidance, sensation seeking, and a host of others (Corr et al., 1995; Corr, Tynan, & Kumari, 2002). Similarly, this paradigm has also been employed to investigate such socially relevant constructs as rejection sensitivity (Downey et al., 2004), racial bias (Amodio et al., 2003), anti-gay bias (Mahaffey et al., 2005), and anti-social personality disorder (Benning et al., 2005).

In a study investigating the emotional modulation of startle, the interval between picture onset and startle stimulus presentation is an important consideration. The slide must be on for at least 500 msec before the startle stimulus is presented, in order to see differential startle reactivity as a function of slide content (Bradley et al., 2006). At shorter stimulus onset asynchrony, no valence effect is seen. Another important consideration is the degree to which the slides are rated as arousing. Studying the impact of a slide's valence on startle requires a slide with a relatively high level of rated arousal (Cuthbert et al., 1996). If slides are not rated as sufficiently arousing, startle will not vary as a function of the valence rating of the slides. This is a very important consideration, because the failure to find a valence effect may be due to some property of the participants or stimuli under study, but such a failure may also be due to insufficiently arousing slides. Many researchers in this area use a standardized set of slides (Lang, Bradley, & Cuthbert, 2005) with arousal and valence ratings that have been empirically established.

Prepulse Inhibition

Another way in which startle has been used in the investigation of social and personality psychology involves the application of prepulse inhibition (PPI) methodology (see Blumenthal, 1999; Graham, 1975). This technique, at its most fundamental, involves measuring startle reactivity to identical eliciting stimuli on two types of trials: Some trials have only the startle stimulus (control trials), whereas other trials have the same startle stimulus preceded by a prepulse (prepulse trials). The prepulse can be in the same modality as the startle stimulus or in a different modality; in fact, it can be any detectable change in the background present during the session. Prepulses usually cause some degree of inhibition of the response elicited by the later startle stimulus; this phenomenon is called PPI (see Figure 6.3). Depending on stimulus parameters, this inhibition can be weaker (e.g., decreasing the response to the startle stimulus by 10%) or stronger (e.g., completely blocking the response to the startle stimulus). PPI is maximal when the onset of the prepulse precedes the onset of the startle stimulus by 60–240 msec (Graham & Murray,

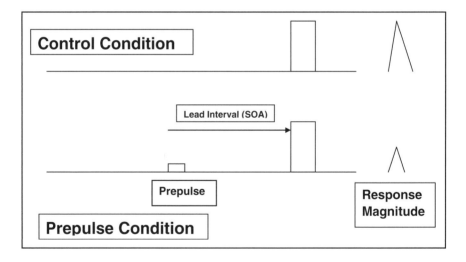

FIGURE 6.3. Schematic of the prepulse inhibition (PPI) method. Startle stimuli are identical in the control and prepulse conditions, with the only stimulus difference being the addition of a prepulse on some trials. Presence of the prepulse attenuates the response to the startle stimulus.

1977). The prepulse is often much less intense than the startle stimulus; indeed, the prepulse can be as weak as the detection threshold and still inhibit startle (Blumenthal & Gescheider, 1987; Reiter & Ison, 1977). Prepulses that are more intense, broadband, and longer result in greater PPI (Blumenthal, 1999). However, all that is required of a prepulse in order to inhibit startle is that it be a detectable change, with that detection occurring in the midbrain and not requiring conscious awareness of the presentation of the stimulus (Blumenthal, Burnett, & Swerdlow, 2001; Swerdlow et al., 2001). Paired pulse inhibition, in which two identical and intense startle stimuli are presented close together in time, can also result in PPI (Swerdlow et al., 2001).

PPI studies generally involve measuring the startle eyeblink reflex on control trials and prepulse trials, and then comparing the degree of PPI across groups or conditions. Some studies have failed to find expected PPI deficits, and this may be a function of symptom type, symptom severity, and medication history. In addition, three recently examined methodological factors have been shown to be important determinants of PPI. First, increased background noise has been found to decrease PPI, ostensibly due to increased sensory masking of the prepulse in the periphery (Blumenthal, Noto, Fox, & Franklin, 2006). Second, the related factor of signal-to-noise ratio (i.e., the ratio of the prepulse to background noise) has also been demonstrated to be an important determinant in PPI (Franklin, Moretti, & Blumenthal, 2007). These stimulus intensity relationships are important when investigating PPI, because when signal-to-noise ratio is too low (due to variations in either background noise or prepulse intensity settings), the effects of sensory masking are likely to introduce error variance into the study. Likewise, when the signal-to-noise ratio is too high, participants with "normal" PPI are likely to reach a ceiling of prepulse processing and allow participants who actually have sensorimotor gating deficits to approach similar PPI levels. Third, the way in which PPI is quantified can influence the outcome of PPI comparisons. Since baseline startle reactivity (i.e., startle reactivity in the control condition) varies greatly across individuals, this must be corrected for when PPI is quantified. Blumenthal and colleagues (2004) compared various methods for quantifying PPI, and concluded that the effects of baseline startle reactivity could be minimized by quantifying PPI as the proportion of difference; that is, (startle on prepulse trials – startle on control trials) / startle on control trials. However, since differences in baseline reactivity may exist as a function of personality/social traits or manipulations that may be of interest in the study, the researcher is advised to think about whether removing those baseline differences will remove the possibility of detecting such effects.

PPI is believed to reflect the extent to which the processing of the prepulse is protected from interruption by the startle stimulus (Graham, 1992). That is, the onset of the prepulse is believed to activate an inhibitory mechanism that decreases the subsequent impact of the startle stimulus, thereby decreasing the subsequent interruption caused by the startle response. Braff and colleagues (2001) describe PPI as an indicator of sensorimotor gating—an ability that is deficient in some clinical and preclinical groups, most notably in the schizophrenia spectrum (Braff, Grillon, & Geyer, 1992; Hazlett et al., 2007). For instance, PPI deficits have been found in patients with schizophrenia (Braff et al., 1978; Duncan et al., 2006), their first-degree asymptomatic relatives (Cadenhead, Swerdlow, Shafer, Diaz, & Braff, 2000; Kumari, Das, Zachariah, Ettinger, & Sharma, 2005), and asymptomatic individuals scoring high on schizotypal or psychosis-prone personality inventories (Cadenhead, Geyer, & Braff, 1993; Hazlett et al., 2003; Schell, Dawson, Hazlett, & Filion, 1995; Swerdlow, Filion, Geyer, & Braff, 1995). PPI has also been used to investigate state and trait anxiety, panic disorder, and social phobia (Duly, Hillman, & Coombes, 2007; Grillon & Baas, 2003; Larsen et al., 2002). Other research has demonstrated that PPI may be a useful measure of social processes, as studies have indicated that social isolation (Weiss & Feldon, 2001) and maternal separation (Zhang et al., 2005) in rats decrease PPI. Despite these promising findings, there has been little research concerning the effects of social factors and processes on PPI in humans. Nevertheless, further supporting the feasibility of this research, the proposed neural circuits for social information processing (Insel & Fernald, 2004; Nelson, Leibenluft, McClure, & Pine, 2005) overlap substantially with the neurological circuit for PPI (Swerdlow & Geyer, 1999). In addition, participants who display social information-processing deficits, such as those found in schizophrenia (Pinkham, Penn, Perkins, & Lieberman, 2003), also display PPI deficits (Hazlett et al., 2007). Indeed, Wynn and colleagues (2005) found a correlation between social cognition and PPI in a sample of patients with schizophrenia. Accordingly, this relationship should be examined in nonclinical participants and in other clinical groups. Moreover, PPI may be able to elucidate much about the psychophysiology of social processes if it is measured before, during, or after social interactions, or in relation to such things as social problem solving.

Attention-Modulated PPI

Researchers have also investigated the effects of attention on PPI, using approaches based primarily on the method described by Filion, Dawson, and Schell (1993). This method involves presenting tone prepulses at two or more frequencies, with these tones lasting several seconds. At some time after tone onset (e.g., 60–240 msec), the startle stimulus is presented. Participants are told to count the tones of one frequency that are longer than the other tones of that frequency—a task called the "discrimination-and-counting task." This makes tones of one frequency targets and tones of the other frequency nontargets, with the trials containing the latter often referred to as "ignore" trials. Several studies have shown that PPI is more pronounced on trials with target prepulses than on those with nontarget prepulses (e.g., Dawson, Hazlett, Filion, Nuechterlein, & Schell, 1993; Jennings, Schell, Filion, & Dawson, 1996; Thorne, Dawson, & Schell, 2005). This attentional modulation of PPI has been shown to be absent in patients with schizophrenia (Hazlett et al., 2007), suggesting an attentional deficit in these patients.

Not all studies in this area report such an attentional modulation of PPI, and the detection of an attention effect may be dependent upon a specific combination of methodological decisions. For example, Hawk, Redford, and Baschnagel (2002) found that only participants who were promised that they would be paid according to their accuracy on the attention task displayed attentional modulation of PPI. Other researchers have failed to find attentional modulation when background noise is presented throughout the session (background noise is used in many studies of PPI, with a 70-dB broadband noise often being presented throughout the entire session; Franklin, Fox, & Blumenthal, 2006). It may also be the case that the discrimination-and-counting task is required for the attentional modulation of PPI, since the effect is less reliably seen with other tasks (Heekeren, Meincke, Geyer, & Gouzoulis-Mayfrank, 2004). In sum, it appears that PPI can be used to investigate the effects of attention if this particular methodological combination (paid participants, no background noise, discrimination-and-counting task) is used. In addition, because attentional effects are only detected under specific methodological conditions, researchers need not worry that undirected attention will influence their results whenever this particular methodological combination is not used.

Although to date attention-modulated PPI has rarely been utilized in social and personality research, this paradigm does have the potential to provide insight in these areas. As mentioned earlier, the passive PPI paradigm may be able to index the functioning of the neural circuits of social information processing at rest; however, because it specifically assesses the ability to direct attention to a stimulus, attention-modulated PPI may be a more sensitive measure of processes that rely on the integrity of executive functioning, such as social problem solving. Similarly, attention-modulated PPI may be a more sensitive index of executive functioning deficits related to Cluster B personality disorder constructs.

Experimental Design Considerations

Overview

Many experimental design conditions have been described in the preceding sections of this chapter. In this section, we reiterate some of those and mention a few other things that the researcher should consider or keep in mind. These suggestions have to do with aspects of the experimental setting, the preparation of the participant, the collection of data, and the processing of those data. Most of these have to do with the fact that startle is sensitive to many things, and a failure to control as many of those things as possible will allow them to become influential in the data—either inducing real effects of uncontrolled variables (confounds), or simply adding to the error in the data set. Some of these suggestions have been empirically investigated, whereas others are based simply on our experience of measuring startle in many participants while investigating a variety of research questions.

Effect Size

One issue to consider is the effect size of the personality variable of interest. Differential startle reactivity as a function of a personality construct may not be evident if a relatively small group of participants is studied and a median split based on personality scale responses is conducted (Blumenthal, 2001). If the personality effect is weak, the researcher may decide instead to screen a large group of potential participants and select those scoring in the extreme high and low ranges of the questionnaire. The point is that a failure to find an effect of the personality variable on startle may be due to an absence of a difference between personality subgroups, or to a small effect size. Of course, this point is not unique to startle, but applies to any study of personality differences. As an alternative to comparing startle reactivity in people who score high or low on a personality questionnaire, a researcher may be able to get a more sensitive look at the relationship between startle and the personality construct by assessing the correlation between startle reactivity and scores on the personality questionnaire (Bowker, Franklin, & Blumenthal, 2007). To the extent that a significant correlation is found, the two measures—brainstem reflex and personality—may reflect an underlying relationship.

Experimental Setting

With regard to the experimental setting, researchers should put themselves in the place of the participant and try to take as fresh a look as possible at the testing environment. Is there anything potentially intimidating or anxiety-provoking in the testing room that does not need to be there? For example, some researchers inject conducting paste into their recording electrodes with a syringe, an effective way of filling the electrode cup with paste. If that syringe is left on a table or shelf in the testing room, within sight of a participant (or, worse, if the paste is injected into the cup within sight of the participant), the presence of the syringe may increase anxiety, which may increase startle reactivity. This would constitute an accidental manipulation of anxiety, with subsequent impact on startle. Are there pictures or decorations in the lab that the participants could consider either unpleasant (which may increase startle reactivity) or interesting and attention-getting (which may decrease startle reactivity)? Being observed by others may make some participants anxious, so the presence of an observation window or even a closed-circuit camera may cause a problem (Cacioppo, Rourke, Marshall-Goodell, Tassinary, & Baron, 1990). Of course, being able to see the participant is often important, and is sometimes required by the local human subjects committee. Also, the extent to which a participant hears external sounds such as other people talking or walking down the hall can be distracting (attention) or sensitizing (anxiety); testing in a sound-attenuated room will decrease this problem. If sound attenuation is not possible, the researcher may consider presenting a background noise throughout the session, to mask extraneous noises that are less intense than this background noise (a noise of 70 dB(A) is typically used). However, this background noise can influence both startle reactivity and startle PPI (Blumenthal et al., 2006; Franklin et al., 2007).

Data Collection

When researchers are measuring startle eyeblink reflexes, the way in which the recording electrodes are placed on the skin below the eye is an important consideration (see Blumenthal et al., 2005). The goal of electrode placement is to obtain a reliable EMG signal from the orbicularis oculi muscle under the skin just below the eye. Some researchers, in order to get as pure and strong a signal as possible, use abrasive pads to remove surface oil, makeup, dirt, and often epidermis; such abrasion can be quite uncomfortable for some participants. Given the sensitivity of startle to unpleasantness, this abrasion procedure may influence the data. Also, considering the fact that most participants know very little about psychophysiological measurements, and also know very little about the electrochemical signals that their bodies produce, referring to the recording electrodes as "electrodes" may heighten anxiety and/ or arousal in some participants. They may have the impression that the presence of "electrodes" will mean that they will receive electric shocks, and participants have heard enough about both electric shock and deception in "psychology experiments" for this false belief to increase anxiety in some cases. Researchers might rather refer to these electrodes instead as "sensors"—a distinction that may not seem important to the researchers, but may be important to naive participants. Again, such a seemingly minor point may have a more pronounced influence on participants at some level of a personality construct (e.g., trait anxiety) than on those at another level of that same construct, and this confound may be impossible to extract from the data.

Another consideration is the fact that the shape of the orbit, and its relation to the cheek, vary across participants: Some people have eyes that are further forward; some have eyes that are deeper in the orbital sockets; some have cheeks that are higher or wider; and so forth. The goal is to place the electrodes in as nearly the same place as possible on each participant. This is especially important when data are collected from the same participant at two points in time, or from both sides of the face at the same time.

The way in which a researcher interacts with a participant also may have an impact on the data. It is often a good idea to make participants as comfortable as possible, and this will be facilitated by experienced, well-trained, and polite researchers. This may seem to the reader both obvious and not worth mentioning—but again, the sensitivity of startle to a variety of factors suggests that variations in the participants' state, which can be influenced by their evaluation of the testing situation, can influence the data. Something that is considered a threat to one person may be irrelevant to another person; also, something that one person attends to may escape the notice of another person. In both cases, startle reactivity may be influenced more in one person than in the other. An extreme example of the extent to which what a participant believes, thinks, or expects has an influence on the data can be seen in research in which placebo responses are evident in startle data. Specifically, caffeine increases startle reactivity, but so does the presentation of decaffeinated coffee when a participant believes that the coffee is caffeinated (Flaten & Blumenthal, 1999). Another example involves increased startle when participants are told that a puff of air is directed "toward the eye" versus "toward the ear," when in fact the air puff delivery tube was directed to the same point between the eye and the ear in all cases (Haerich, 1994). This issue also highlights the fact that it may be necessary to deceive the participants in some cases, depending on the experimental question under study. Of course, such deception must be justifiable to the local human subjects committee.

Interpretation of Results

When designing a study and when interpreting the data from that study, a researcher must pay special attention to the possibility of uncontrolled factors. Since startle varies as a function of several factors, the more the researcher knows about the participants, the better. Knowledge of which medications they use; whether they use tobacco, caffeine, or other psychoactive substances; whether they are withdrawn from any of these substances at the time of testing; whether they have normal sensory sensitivity—all of these factors may be as influential as the personality or social construct under study. That is, something as simple as the fact that some participants use tobacco and others do not may have a larger effect size than whether the participants are introverted or extraverted, for example. This does not mean that startle is not useful in personality and social psychology research; it just means that startle must be used carefully.

Conclusions

Startle is affected by many events and qualities in the environment (stimulus parameters, background noise, multisensory input, etc.). It is also affected by numerous characteristics of the individual (personality, clinical conditions, pharmacological composition, sensory sensitivity, etc.), as well as by many processes of the individual (emotion, attention, arousal, etc.). The dividing lines among these three categories are not perfectly defined, and a good deal of interaction occurs. With these cautions in mind, there is a very high likelihood that the use of startle measures in social and personality research will continue to contribute information that is based on established physiological systems, leading to a fuller understanding of the mechanisms that determine many of the constructs underlying social and personality psychology.

References

Alheid, G., deOlmos, J. S., & Beltramino, C. A. (1995). Amygdala and extended amygdala. In G. Paxinos (Ed.), *The rat nervous system* (2nd ed., pp. 495–578). San Diego, CA: Academic Press.

Amodio, D. M., Harmon-Jones, E., & Devine, P. G. (2003) Individual differences in the activation and control of affective race bias as assed by startle eyeblink response and self-report. *Journal of Personality and Social Psychology, 84*, 738–753.

Benning, S. D., Patrick, C. J., & Iacono, W. M. (2005). Psychopathy, startle blink modulation, and electrodermal reactivity in twin men. *Psychophysiology, 42*, 753–762.

Berg, W. K., & Balaban, M. T. (1999). Startle elicitation: Stimulus parameters, recording techniques, and quantification. In M. E. Dawson, A. M. Schell, & A. H. Böhmelt (Eds.), *Startle modification: Implications for neuroscience, cognitive science, and clinical science* (pp. 21–50). Cambridge, UK: Cambridge University Press.

Blumenthal, T. D. (1999). Short lead interval modification. In M. E. Dawson, A. M. Schell, & A. H. Böhmelt (Eds.), *Startle modification: Implications for neuroscience, cognitive science, and clinical science* (pp. 51–71). Cambridge, UK: Cambridge University Press.

Blumenthal, T. D. (2001). Extraversion, attention, and startle response reactivity. *Personality and Individual Differences, 30*, 495–503.

Blumenthal, T. D., Avendano, A., & Berg, W. K. (1987). The startle response and auditory temporal summation in neonates. *Journal of Experimental Child Psychology, 44*, 64–79.

Blumenthal, T. D., Burnett, T. T., & Swerdlow, C. (2001). Prepulses reduce the pain of cutaneous electrical shocks. *Psychosomatic Medicine, 63*, 275–281.

Blumenthal, T. D., Cuthbert, B. N., Filion, D. L., Hackley, S., Lipp, O. V., & van Boxtel, A. (2005). Committee report: Guidelines for human startle eyeblink electromyographic studies. *Psychophysiology, 42*, 1–15.

Blumenthal, T. D., Elden, A., & Flaten, M. A. (2004). A comparison of several methods used to quantify prepulse inhibition of eyeblink responding. *Psychophysiology, 41*, 326–332.

Blumenthal, T. D., & Gescheider, G. A. (1987). Modification of the acoustic startle response by a tactile prepulse: Effects of stimulus onset asynchrony and prepulse intensity. *Psychophysiology, 24*, 320–327.

Blumenthal, T. D., Noto, J. V., Fox, M. A., & Franklin, J. C. (2006). Background noise decreases both prepulse elicitation and inhibition of acoustic startle blink responding. *Biological Psychology, 72*, 173–179.

Bowker, K. B., Franklin, J. C., & Blumenthal, T. D. (2007). Deficits in prepulse inhibition of startle with increased bulimic symptomology in a normative sample. *Psychophysiology, 44*, S24.

Bradley, M. M., Codispoti, M., & Lang, P. J. (2006). A multi-process account of startle modulation during affective perception. *Psychophysiology, 43*, 486–497.

Braff, D. L., Geyer, M. A., & Swerdlow, N. R. (2001). Human studies of prepulse inhibition of startle: Normal subjects, patient groups, and pharmacological studies. *Psychopharmacology, 156*, 234–258.

Braff, D. L., Grillon, C., & Geyer, M. A. (1992). Gating and habituation of the startle reflex in schizophrenic patients. *Archives of General Psychiatry, 49*, 206–215.

Braff, D. L., Stone, C., Callaway, E., Geyer, M., Glick, I., & Bali, L. (1978). Prestimulus effects on human startle reflex in normals and schizophrenics. *Psychophysiology, 15*, 339–343.

Britt, T. W., & Blumenthal, T. D. (1991). Motoneuronal insensitivity in extraverts as revealed by the startle response paradigm. *Personality and Individual Differences, 12*, 387–393.

Britt, T. W., & Blumenthal, T. D. (1992). The effects of anxiety on motoric expression of the startle response. *Personality and Individual Differences, 13*, 91–97.

Britt, T. W., & Blumenthal, T. D. (1993). Social anxiety and latency of response to startle stimuli. *Journal of Research in Personality, 27*, 1–14.

Brown, J. S., Kalish, H. I., & Farber, I. E. (1951). Conditioned fear as revealed by the magnitude of startle response to an auditory stimulus. *Journal of Experimental Psychology, 41*, 317–327.

Cacioppo, J. T., Rourke, P. A., Marshall-Goodell, B. S., Tassinary, L. G., & Baron, R. S. (1990). Rudimentary physiological effects of mere observation. *Psychophysiology, 27*, 177–186.

Cadenhead, K. S., Geyer, M. A., & Braff, D. L. (1993). Impaired startle prepulse inhibition and habituation in patients with schizotypal personality disorder. *American Journal of Psychiatry, 150*, 1862–1867.

Cadenhead, K. S., Swerdlow, N. R., Shafer, K. M., Diaz, M., & Braff, D. L. (2000). Modulation of the startle response and startle laterality in relatives of schizophrenia patients and in subjects with schizotypal personality disorder: Evidence of inhibitory deficits. *American Journal of Psychiatry, 157*, 1660–1668.

Cloninger, C. R. (1988). *The Tridimensional Personality Questionnaire*. St. Louis, MO: Department of Psychiatry and Genetics, Washington University School of Medicine.

Cornwell, B. R., Johnson, L., Berardi, L., & Grillon, C. (2006). Anticipation of public speaking in virtual reality reveals a relationship between trait social anxiety and startle reactivity. *Biological Psychiatry, 59*, 664–666.

Corr, P. J., Tynan, A., & Kumari, V. (2002). Personality correlates of prepulse inhibition of the startle reflex at three lead intervals. *Journal of Psychophysiology, 16*, 82–91.

Corr, P. J., Wilson, G., Fotiadou, M., Kumari, V., Gray, N., Checkley, S., et al. (1995). Personality and affective modulation of the startle reflex. *Personality and Individual Differences, 19*, 543–553.

Cuthbert, B. N., Bradley, M. M., & Lang, P. J. (1996). Probing picture perception: Activation and emotion. *Psychophysiology, 33*, 103–111.

Davis, M. (2006). Neural systems involved in fear and anxiety measured with fear-potentiated startle. *American Psychologist, 61*, 741–756.

Dawson, M. E., Hazlett, E. A., Filion, D. L., Nuechterlein, K. H., & Schell, A. M. (1993). Attention and schizophrenia: Impaired modulation of the startle reflex. *Journal of Abnormal Psychology, 102*, 633–641.

Dawson, M. E., Schell, A. M., & Böhmelt, A. H. (Eds.). (1999). *Startle modification: Implications for neuroscience, cognitive science, and clinical science*. Cambridge, UK: Cambridge University Press.

de Jong, P. J., Visser, S., & Merckelbach, H. (1996). Startle and spider phobia: Unilateral probes and the prediction of treatment effects. *Journal of Psychophysiology, 10*, 150–160.

Dillon, D. G., & LaBar, K. S. (2005). Startle modulation during conscious emotion regulation is arousal-dependent. *Behavioral Neuroscience, 119*, 1118–1124.

Downey, G., Mougios, V., Ayduk, O., London, B. E., & Shoda, Y. (2004). Rejection sensitivity and the defensive motivational system. *Psychological Science, 15*, 668–673.

Duly, A. R., Hillman, C. H., & Coombes, S. (2007). Sensorimotor gating and anxiety: Prepulse inhibition following acute exercise. *International Journal of Psychophysiology, 64*, 157–164.

Duncan, E. J., Bollini, A. M., Lewison, B., Keyes, M., Jovanovic, T., Gaytan, O., et al. (2006). Medication status affects the relationship of symptoms to prepulse inhibition of acoustic startle in schizophrenia. *Psychiatry Research, 145*, 137–145.

Eysenck, H. J., & Eysenck, M. W. (1985). *Personality and Individual Differences*. New York: Plenum Press.

Filion, D. L., Dawson, M. E., & Schell, A. M. (1993). Modification of the acoustic startle-reflex eyeblink: A tool for investigating early and late attentional processes. *Biological Psychology, 35*, 185–200.

Flaten, M. A., & Blumenthal, T. D. (1999). Caffeine-associated stimuli elicit conditioned responses: An experimental model of the placebo effect. *Psychopharmacology, 145*, 105–112.

Franklin, J. C., Fox, M. A., & Blumenthal, T. D. (2006). Effects of background noise and attention on startle reactivity and PPI. *Psychophysiology, 43*, S39.

Franklin, J. C., Moretti, N. A., & Blumenthal, T. D. (2007). Impact of stimulus signal-to-noise ratio on prepulse inhibition of acoustic startle. *Psychophysiology, 44*, 339–342.

Graham, F. K. (1975). The more or less startling effects of weak prestimulation. *Psychophysiology, 12*, 238–248.

Graham, F. K. (1992). Attention: The heartbeat, the blink, and the brain. In B. A. Campbell, H. Hayne, & R. Richardson (Eds.), *Attention and information processing in infants and adults: Perspectives from human and animal research* (pp. 3–29). Hillsdale, NJ: Erlbaum.

Graham, F. K., & Murray, G. M. (1977). Discordant effects of weak prestimulation on magnitude and latency of the reflex blink. *Physiological Psychology, 5*, 108–114.

Grillon, C. (2002). Startle reactivity and anxiety disorders: Aversive conditioning, context, and neurobiology. *Biological Psychiatry, 52*, 958–975.

Grillon, C., Ameli, R., Foot, M., & Davis, M. (1993). Fear-potentiated startle: Relationship to the level of state/trait anxiety in healthy subjects. *Biological Psychiatry, 34*, 566–574.

Grillon, C., Ameli, R., Woods, S. W., Merikangas, K., & Davis, M. (1991). Fear-potentiated startle in humans: Effects of anticipatory anxiety on the acoustic blink reflex. *Psychophysiology, 28*, 588–595.

Grillon, C., & Baas, J. M. (2003). A review of the modulation of startle by affective states and its application to psychiatry. *Clinical Neurophysiology, 114*, 1557–1579.

Grillon, C., & Davis, M. (1997). Fear-potentiated startle conditioning in humans: Explicit and contextual cue conditioning following paired vs. unpaired training. *Psychophysiology, 34*, 451–458.

Grillon, C., & Morgan, C. A., III. (1999). Fear-potentiated startle conditioning to explicit and contextual cues in Gulf War veterans with posttraumatic stress disorder. *Journal of Abnormal Psychology, 108*, 134–142.

Grillon, C., Morgan, C. A., III, Davis, M., & Southwick, S. M. (1998). Effect of darkness on acoustic startle in Vietnam veterans with PTSD. *American Journal of Psychiatry, 155*, 812–817.

Haerich, P. (1994). Startle reflex modification: Effects of attention vary with emotional valence. *Psychological Science, 5*, 407–410.

Hamm, A. O., Weike, A. I., & Schupp, H. T. (2001). The effect of neuroleptic medication on prepulse inhibition in schizophrenia patients: Current status and future issues. *Psychopharmacology, 156*, 259–265.

Hawk, L. W., Redford, J. S., & Baschnagel, J. S. (2002). Influence of a monetary incentive upon attentional modification of short-lead prepulse inhibition and long-lead prepulse facilitation of acoustic startle. *Psychophysiology, 39*, 674–677.

Hazlett, E. A., Levine, J., Buchsbaum, M. S., Silverman, J. M., New, A., Sevin, E. M., et al. (2003). Deficient attentional modulation of the startle response in patients with schizotypal personality disorder. *American Journal of Psychiatry, 160*, 1621–1626.

Hazlett, E. A., Romero, M. J., Haznedar, M. M., New, A. S., Goldstein, K. E., Newmark, R. E., et al. (2007). Deficient attentional modulation of startle eyeblink is associated with symptoms severity in the schizophrenia spectrum. *Schizophrenia Research, 93*, 288–295.

Heekeren, K., Meincke, U., Geyer, M. A., & Gouzoulis-Mayfrank, E. (2004). Attentional modulation of prepulse inhibition: A new startle paradigm. *Neuropsychobiology, 49*, 88–93.

Hutchison, K. E., Wood, M. D., & Swift, R. (1999). Personality factors moderate subjective and psychophysiological response to d-amphetamine in humans. *Experimental and Clinical Psychopharmacology, 4*, 493–501.

Insel, T. R., & Fernald, R. D. (2004). How the brain processes social information: Searching for the social brain. *Annual Review of Neuroscience, 27*, 697–722.

Jennings, P. D., Schell, A. M., Filion, D. L., & Dawson, M. E. (1996). Tracking early and late stages of information processing: Contributions of startle eyeblink reflex modification. *Psychophysiology, 33*, 148–155.

Kumari, V., Das, M., Zachariah, E., Ettinger, U., & Sharma, T. (2005). Reduced prepulse inhibition in unaffected siblings of schizophrenia patients. *Psychophysiology, 42*, 588–594.

Lang, P. J. (1995). The emotion probe: Studies of motivation and attention. *American Psychologist, 50,* 371–385.

Lang, P. J., Bradley, M. M., & Cuthbert, B. (1997). Motivated attention: Affect, activation, and action. In P. J. Lang, R. F. Simons, & M. Balaban (Eds.), *Attention and orienting* (pp. 97–136). Mahwah, NJ: Erlbaum.

Lang, P. J., Bradley, M. M., & Cuthbert, B. N. (2005). *International affective picture system (IAPS): Affective ratings of pictures and instruction manual* (Tech. Rep. No. A-6). Gainesville: University of Florida.

LaRowe, S. D., Patrick, C. J., Curtin, J. J., & Kline, J. P. (2006). Personality correlates of startle habituation. *Biological Psychology, 72,* 257–264.

Larsen, D. K., Norton, G., Walker, J. R., & Stein, M. B. (2002). Analysis of startle responses in patients with panic disorder and social phobia. *Cognitive Behaviour Therapy, 31,* 156–169.

Lee, Y., Lopez, D., Meloni, E., & Davis, M. (1996). A primary acoustic startle pathway: Obligatory role of cochlear root neurons and the nucleus reticularis pontis caudalis. *Journal of Neuroscience, 16,* 3775–3789.

Mahaffey, A. L., Bryan, A., & Hutchinson, K. E. (2005). Using startle eye blink to measure the affective component of antigay bias. *Basic and Applied Social Psychology, 27,* 37–45.

Marcin, M. S., & Nemeroff, C. B. (2003). The neurobiology of social anxiety disorder: The relevance of fear and anxiety. *Acta Psychiatrica Scandinavica, 108,* 51–64.

Nelson, E. E., Leibenluft, E., McClure, E. B., & Pine, D. S. (2005). The social reorientation of adolescence: A neuroscience perspective on the process and its relation to psychopathology. *Psychological Medicine, 35,* 163–174.

Neumann, D. L., Lipp, O. V., & McHugh, M. J. (2004). The effect of stimulus modality and task difficulty on attentional modulation of blink startle. *Psychophysiology, 41,* 407–416.

Panayiotou, G., & Vrana, S. R. (1998). Effect of self-focused attention on the startle reflex, heart rate, and memory performance among socially anxious and nonanxious individuals. *Psychophysiology, 35,* 328–336.

Patrick, C. J., Bradley, M. M., & Lang, P. J. (1993). Emotion in the criminal psychopath: Startle reflex modulation. *Journal of Abnormal Psychology, 102,* 82–92.

Pinkham, A., Penn, D. L., Perkins, D., & Lieberman, J. (2003). Implications of the neural basis of social cognition for the study of schizophrenia. *American Journal of Psychiatry, 160,* 815–824.

Reiter, L. A., & Ison, J. R. (1977). Inhibition of the human eyeblink reflex: An evaluation of the sensitivity of the Wendt–Yerkes method for threshold detection. *Journal of Experimental Psychology: Human Perception and Performance, 3,* 325–336.

Schell, A. M., Dawson, M. E., Hazlett, E. A., & Filion, D. L. (1995). Attentional modulation of startle in psychosis-prone college students. *Psychophysiology, 32,* 266–273.

Spielberger, C. D., Gorsuch, R. L., Lushene, R. E., Vagg, P. R., & Jacobs, G. A. (1983). *State–Trait Anxiety Inventory for Adults.* Palo Alto, CA: Mind Garden.

Swerdlow, N. R., Filion, D. L., Geyer, M. A., & Braff, D. L. (1995). "Normal" personality correlates of sensorimotor, cognitive, and visuospatial gating. *Biological Psychiatry, 37,* 286–299.

Swerdlow, N. R., & Geyer, M. A. (1999). Neurophysiology and neuropharmacology of short lead interval startle modification. In M. E. Dawson, A. M. Schell, & A. H. Böhmelt (Eds.), *Startle modification: Implications for neuroscience, cognitive science, and clinical science* (pp. 114–133). Cambridge, UK: Cambridge University Press.

Swerdlow, N. R., Geyer, M. A., & Braff, D. L. (2001). Neural circuit regulation of prepulse inhibition in the rat: Current knowledge and future challenges. *Psychopharmacology, 156,* 194–215.

Thorne, G. L., Dawson, M. E., & Schell, A. M. (2005). Attention and prepulse inhibition: The effects of task-relevant, irrelevant, and no-task conditions. *International Journal of Psychophysiology, 56,* 121–128.

Vrana, S. R., Constantine, J. A., & Westman, J. S. (1992). Startle reflex modification as an outcome measure in the treatment of phobia: Two case studies. *Behavioral Assessment, 14,* 279–291.

Vrana, S. R., Spence, E. L., & Lang, P. L. (1988). The startle probe response: A new measure of emotion? *Journal of Abnormal Psychology, 97,* 487–491.

Walker, D., & Davis, M. (1997). Double dissociation between the involvement of the bed nucleus of the stria terminalis and the central nucleus of the amygdala in startle increases produced by conditioned versus unconditioned fear. *Journal of Neuroscience, 17,* 9375–9383.

Weiss, I. C., & Feldon, J. (2001). Environmental animal models for sensorimotor gating deficiencies in schizophrenia: A review. *Psychopharmacology, 156,* 305–326.

Wynn, J. K., Sergi, M. J., Dawson, M. E., Schell, A. M., & Green, M. F. (2005). Sensorimotor gating, orienting, and social perception in schizophrenia. *Schizophrenia Research, 73,* 319–325.

Yeomans, J. S., Li, L., Scott, B. W., & Frankland, P. W. (2002). Tactile, acoustic, and vestibular systems sum to elicit the startle reflex. *Neuroscience and Biobehavioral Reviews, 26,* 1–11.

Zhang, T. Y., Chretien, P., Meany, M. J., & Gratton, A. (2005). Influence of naturally occurring variations in maternal care on prepulse inhibition of acoustic startle and the medial prefrontal cortical dopamine response to stress in adult rats. *Journal of Neuroscience, 25,* 1493–1502.

Zuckerman, M. (1994). *Behavioral expressions and biosocial bases of sensation seeking.* New York: Cambridge University Press.

7

Assessing Autonomic Nervous System Activity

Wendy Berry Mendes

C hanges in autonomic nervous system (ANS) activity can result from a variety of factors, including physical movement, postural changes, sleeping, disease, and aging. For social and personality psychologists, the value of examining the ANS may be that in many situations ANS responses can indicate shifts in emotion, motivation, attention, and preferences. Several obvious advantages of using ANS responses have been well established. For example, ANS responses are not susceptible to the self-report biases often engendered in sensitive contexts, in which individuals may be unwilling to report their unexpurgated feelings (Gardner, Gabriel, & Deikman, 2000; Guglielmi, 1999). In addition, obtaining data "online" allows for a dynamic analysis of moment-to-moment reactions that does not require introspective responses from participants. Other advantages are less obvious, however. ANS responses can temporally precede conscious awareness, revealing emotional responses or preferences that participants cannot yet report (Bechara, Damasio, Tranel, & Damasio, 1997). Finally, some patterns of ANS responding may be linked to mental and physical health vulnerabilities; these links may allow social and personality psychologists, along with clinical and health psychologists, to identify connections between social contexts or dispositions and disease etiology or progression.

In this chapter, I first describe some of the primary techniques, for measuring ANS responses, together with methodological considerations and psychological inferences associated with each technique. Following these descriptions, I provide examples of some research programs that have effectively used the ANS to explore questions within social and personality psychology; I also speculate on some possible domains that have not been examined but may prove to be promising. In the third part, I describe some critical design features that are relevant when social and personality researchers are examining ANS responses. I conclude by describing future directions for the use of these types of measures in psychological research.

Primary Techniques for Measuring ANS Responses

The ANS is part of the peripheral nervous system, and primarily serves a regulatory function by helping the body adapt to internal and environmental demands, thereby maintaining homeostasis. Various measures can be used to assess changes in ANS activity. Here I review three broad, but related, categories—electrodermal activity; cardiovascular activity (e.g., heart rate variability, respiration, and cardiac output); and blood pressure responses—with a specific focus on measuring, scoring, editing, and interpreting these responses. In what follows, each measure is briefly described, and the general physiology of the measure is outlined; then measurement, scoring, and interpretative caveats are discussed.[1]

Electrodermal Activity

Electrodermal activity (EDA), also known by its outdated name "galvanic skin responses," is a fairly common measure of ANS activity and has a long history in psychological research. EDA measures responses in the eccrine sweat glands, which are found widely distributed across the body, but are densely distributed in the hands and soles of the feet. The sympathetic branch of the ANS system innervates these sweat glands, but a difference from most sympathetic responses is that the neurotransmitter involved in changes is acetylcholine rather than epinephrine.

EDA is commonly measured in one of two ways. The first method, skin conductance (SC), uses a small current passed through the skin

---

[1] Given the scope of this chapter, my descriptions of the underlying structure and function of the various systems are greatly oversimplified. References are provided to point the reader to reviews that are essential for a thorough understanding of the physiological responses reviewed here.

via a bipolar placement of sensors, and the resistance to that current is measured. The reciprocal of this resistance is SC. The second method, skin potential (SP), uses no external current and is collected with a unipolar placement of sensors. In addition to these methods of assessing EDA, there are two categories of data quantification that are based on how the EDA data are aggregated. When examining responses to a specific and identifiable stimulus, one looks at phasic activity, or the "response." When describing EDA that is not associated with a specific stimulus onset, but involves changes over longer periods of time (i.e., minutes rather than seconds), it is appropriate to examine tonic activity, or "level." Thus, with two methods of collection and two methods of quantifying changes, there are four categories of EDA data: SC response (SCR), SC level (SCL), SP response (SPR), and SP level (SPL). Choice of method and quantification should be determined by the specific questions under investigation, which are described in more detail below.

Preparation and Recording

To record SC, a bipolar placement of Ag/AgCl sensors are placed on the fingers, palms, or soles of the feet. If finger placement is used, it is recommended to put the sensors on adjacent fingers (second and third fingers, or fourth and fifth fingers), because they will be innervated by the same spinal nerve (Venables & Christie, 1973) (Figure 7.1). Unlike SC recording, SP recording requires a unipolar placement in which one electrode is placed on an active site (typically the palm of the hand) and the other sensor is placed on an inactive site (typically the forearm, though any inactive site would work).

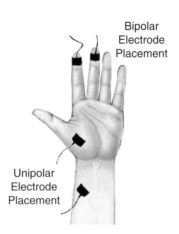

Bipolar
Electrode
Placement

Unipolar
Electrode
Placement

FIGURE 7.1. Placement of bipolar and unipolar leads for measurement of EDA.

Preparation of the skin should include a mild washing with water and a nonabrasive soap. Use of alcohol-based hand sanitizer or antibacterial soap prior to sensor placement is not recommended, because such products can excessively dry out the skin, resulting in lower levels of EDA and obscure sensitive changes. An electrolyte—either KCl, NaCl, or commercially available conductance cream—is then applied in a thin film on the two sensor sites, and also in the wells of the sensors. Once the sensors are attached, it is advised to wait several minutes (typically 5–15 min) before beginning the recording session. During this wait, one should check for sensor sensitivity. EDA responds to respiration, so the participant can be instructed to take a deep breath and hold the breath for a few seconds. A good EDA signal will show a change in response (an increase if SC is used, and a decrease if SP is used) within 2–3 sec once the breath is initiated.

Editing and Quantification

After data collection, waveforms should be inspected for movement artifact and electrical interference. Most scoring programs that are free or available for purchase will have options for editing waveforms that allow a coder to "spline," or interpolate, the area of the waveform that is affected by an artifact. This smoothing technique typically removes the influence of artifacts through interpolation by identifying the beginnings and ends of areas of the waveform that contain an artifact, and replacing them with estimates derived from adjacent areas.

When one is quantifying EDA to examine tonic levels (SCL or SPL), the decisions for averaging the waveform are time-based; that is, the waveform is averaged across a specified time period while a participant is at rest, and then over a similar time period when a participant is engaged in a task or activity. For example, reactivity values can be made in which 1 min of baseline data—typically the last minute or the minimum minute (when EDA reaches its nadir)—is subtracted from data quantified in 1-min intervals from a task. These new values then represent the change in EDA from resting to a task period. Alternatively, analysis of covariance or regression techniques can be used, in which baseline levels are added as covariates or repeated-measures analyses are used to examine changes over time.

A slightly more complicated approach related to quantification is required when one is examining responses linked to specific stimuli (SCR or SPR). In this case, an identifiable time-locked stimulus is presented to the participant, and a "trigger" or stimulus output is recorded online simultaneously with the EDA signal. A minimum threshold value of change needs to be determined so that a change in EDA can be identified as a "response" or not. Commonly, this threshold is set at 0.05

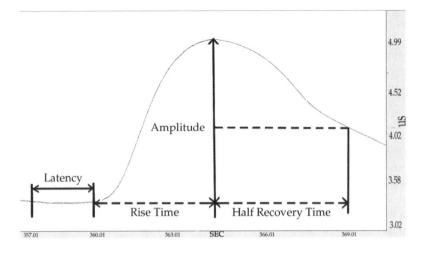

FIGURE 7.2. The SCR.

microsiemens (µS). Subsequent processing of data then allows for an estimate of the change in EDA linked to the specific stimulus. Several measures can be determined from this response: the latency from the stimulus to the initiation of rise time; the time from the initiation of rise time to the peak amplitude; the amplitude; and the time to reach "half-delta" (Figure 7.2). Half-delta is a time-based measure determined by examining the total magnitude of amplitude increase, dividing this by two, and then calculating the length of time from peak of amplitude to half of the magnitude of increase.

Levels versus Responses

The choice of collecting and scoring data based on either levels or responses should be dictated by the research questions and study design. For example, when experimental designs include presentations of specific stimuli in a time-locked, event-related design (e.g., affective pictures, pictures of members of different racial groups, etc.), it makes sense to score data as responses. When a study design includes events that unfold over time, and there are no specific time-locked events (e.g., social interactions, delivering speeches, nonscripted negotiations, etc.), then examining changes in EDA level from a baseline period to a task will be most appropriate. If the decision is made to examine changes in EDA level, one can still examine spontaneous responses, but the designation of these responses should be *nonspecific* SCRs. This measure is typically reported in number of nonspecific SCRs per minute, with resting or baseline averages ranging from 1 to 3 per minute. This measure can be used as a general index of anxiety or arousal resulting from some change in situational context, or linked to different dispositional factors.

Cardiovascular Measures

In simplest terms, the cardiovascular (CV) system consists of the heart and the pathways (vessels) through which oxygenated blood is delivered to the periphery of the body and deoxygenated blood returns to the heart. Psychologically, this system is responsive to affective states, motivation, attention, and reflexes. In addition, CV responses have been commonly linked to vulnerabilities in physical and mental illness. In this section, I review several methods that examine changes in the cardiac cycle: the electrocardiogram, measures of respiration, and impedance cardiography.

Electrocardiogram

The heart produces an electrical signal that can be measured with an electrocardiogram (ECG). A normal ECG recording is composed of various deflections referred to as P, Q, R, S, and T waves (Figure 7.3). Each heart cycle begins with an impulse from the sinoatrial node (not detected on the ECG wave), which results in a depolarization of the atria (P wave). The QRS complex represents the depolarization of the ventricles, and the T inflection indicates repolarization (or recovery) of the ventricles. These

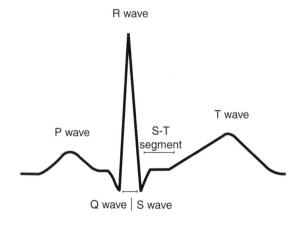

FIGURE 7.3. ECG waveform.

points in combination can be used to determine a variety of chronotropic (i.e., time-based) measures, such as the time of one complete heart cycle, known as the heart period (or interbeat interval). This measure is the inverse of heart rate (HR; beats per minute), though heart period is the preferred metric (see Berntson, Cacioppo, & Quigley, 1993).

PREPARATION AND RECORDING

ECG waveforms can be collected from several configurations of the limbs. Described below are three standard configurations in which placement results in an upward deflection of the Q-R complex:

Lead I: Electrodes are attached just above the right and left wrists on the inside of the arms. The left arm has the positively charged lead.

Lead II: Electrodes are attached on the right arm and left ankle. The ankle has the positively charged lead.

Lead III: Electrodes are attached on the left wrist and left ankle. The ankle has the positively charged lead.

Lead placements can be adjusted so that the sensors are placed on the torso rather than the limbs. For example, a modified Lead II configuration places the right lead below the sternum and the left lead on the left side of the torso below the ribcage. Torso placement may be deemed preferable over limb placement if there is anticipated movement of the limbs or if younger subjects (i.e., babies and toddlers) are being assessed.

Preparing the site for ECG placement can include gently abrading the skin and then applying a thin layer of conductance gel, but in many cases a clean signal can be obtained without any site preparation, given the strong electrical signal of the heart. Several factors that can interfere with an ECG recording should be anticipated, however. First, excessive hair on either the ankles or the chest can make recording difficult if adhesive disposable sensors are used. Shaving participants' ankles or chests may be possible, but could be problematic in some situations. Either adjusting the sensor location or using nonadhesive (i.e., band) electrodes may reduce the noise. Other potential problems include participants' skin type or changes in temperature during the course of the experiment. Skin that is especially oily or prone to sweat may require additional taping of disposable sensors, and even band electrodes may slip in extreme cases. Good lab practice includes taping the sensors with medical tape; this is especially true in summer months or for longer studies, when the risk of warmer skin temperature is greater.

EDITING AND QUANTIFICATION: ECG AND HRV

Editing an ECG waveform is typically done offline—that is, once the session is complete. The primary concerns in editing an ECG waveform are the proper identification of the R point and removal of artifacts that might appear to be an R point. Another critical point on the ECG waveform is the Q point, or the indication that the left ventricle is contracting. The Q point is critical for the calculation of the preejection period, which is considered to be one of the purest measures of sympathetic activation and is discussed below in the section on impedance cardiography.

Respiration can influence heart rate. For example, during inspiration, the influence of the vagus nerve on the heart is removed, and the HR accelerates; during expiration, the vagus nerve is applied, and HR decelerates. One way to examine cardiac changes from an ECG waveform, beyond HR/heart period, is to examine HR variability (HRV)—at its crudest level, $HR_{Max} - HR_{Min}$. HRV is influenced by a number of factors, but by deconstructing it one can isolate heart period changes due primarily to parasympathetic control, sympathetic control, or a combination of both. Of particular interest has been examining high-frequency HRV, because changes in variability in this range are believed to be due primarily to control of the vagus nerve and thus primarily indices of parasympathetic control. There are several measures of HRV estimates (time domain, frequency domain, and nonlinear measures), and a full committee report by the Society for Psychophysiological Research (SPR) is available for more details (Berntson, Bigger, & Eckberg, 1997). Here I briefly review some of the estimates and note what is needed to calculate these measures.

One of the simpler measures of HRV is based on time domain estimates—for example, root mean square of successive differences, which is calculated as the standard deviation of the beat-to-beat intervals. This measure is believed to reflect high-frequency HRV and respiratory sinus arrhythmia (RSA). A popular frequency domain technique to estimate HRV involves decomposing heart period variance into different frequency bands by using Fourier transformation. For example, the high-frequency band ranges from 0.15 to 0.4 Hz (cycles per second); it is thought to represent primarily vagal influence and, as such, parasympathetic activity. Lower-frequency bands (<0.15) have also been identified, and in these frequency domains the influence can be either sympathetic or parasympathetic.

Note that in the examples above, respiration rate is not factored into the analyses; instead, rate of breathing is assumed rather than measured. One commonly debated measurement issue in HRV research concerns the importance of controlling for respiration rate and depth in HRV analysis. For a thorough understanding of the complexities of this issue, see Denver, Reed, and Porges (2007) for justification that respiration frequency need not be included in estimates of RSA/HRV, and Grossman and Taylor (2007) for a discussion of why respiration frequencies are important.

Measures of Respiration

Respiration can be measured in a number of ways. One option is to use a strain gauge that measures pressure during inspiration and expiration, and rate and depth of breaths can be extracted. If a single strain gauge is used, the recommended placement is high on the torso immediately under the arms (and above the breasts). This placement will allow for measurement of upper respiration, but not lower abdominal respiration, which may be important if the research focuses on the type of deep breathing found in meditation or other focused breathing domains. In this case, two strain gauges can be used to provide both upper and lower respiration. Another option is to use impedance cardiography, which can extract respiration rate and amplitude.

Impedance Cardiography

Impedance cardiography is a noninvasive technique to estimate blood flow changes in the heart. This technique allows for estimates of how much blood is ejected during each heart cycle (stroke volume, or SV), and various changes in the cardiac cycle (e.g., the timing of the aortic valve's opening and closing). In combination with an ECG signal and blood pressure responses, a variety of cardiovascular changes can be assessed or derived.

Impedance cardiography requires the use of either spot or band electrodes[2] placed on the torso (Figure 7.4). Using an output of electrical current (ranging from 1 to 4 mA) to the two outer sensors, the inner sensors detect the resistance to the incoming current. This resistance to the current (or impedance) presents global blood flow in the thoracic cavity (typically referred to as Z_0, or basal impedance). As the blood volume increases, the impedance decreases. The first derivative of the

---

[2]The use of band versus spot electrodes is a topic of ongoing debate among psychophysiologists. For experimenter ease and participant comfort, spot electrodes may be preferable and appear to estimate SV reliably while subjects are at rest. However, band electrodes appear to more accurately reflect changes in cardiac output during stress/challenge conditions, because of detection of changes in the thoracic cavity that may be missed by spot electrodes (see Brownley, Hurwitz, & Schneiderman, 2000).

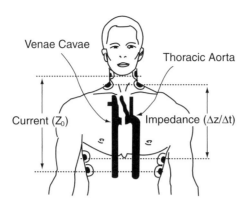

FIGURE 7.4. Impedance cardiography and placement of band sensors.

waveform—$\Delta z/\Delta t$, or the change in basal impedance over the change in time—provides a measure of the blood volume ejected from the heart on each beat.

As Figure 7.5 shows, the $\Delta z/\Delta t$ has several critical inflection and deflection points that are identified either with a software program or manually. Several of these points are critical to the identification of responses occurring in the cardiac cycle. For example, a chronotropic measure of ventricle contractile force is the preejection period (PEP). This is the time from the left ventricle contracting (Q point on the ECG wave) to the aortic valve opening (B point on the $\Delta z/\Delta t$ waveform). SV, the amount of blood ejected from the heart on any given cardiac cycle, is a measure that requires the identification of the B point and X point on the $\Delta z/\Delta t$ waveform to determine the time when blood is being emptied at the aorta, along with the maximum point of the $\Delta z/\Delta t$ waveform on the given cardiac cycle labeled Z^3 in Figure 7.5.

SV provides an estimate of the amount of blood ejected at each beat; however, in terms of an overall indication of how much blood is being pumped through the heart in any given minute, cardiac output (CO) is the preferred measure. CO is simply the product of SV and HR (SV × HR/1000). SV is reported in milliliters, so the product is divided by 1000 to report CO in liters per minute. Because CO is a combination of both heart speed and blood volume processed in the heart, it is believed to be a measure of cardiac efficiency.

When impedance cardiography is being used in a laboratory setting, it is important to tell participants to wear comfortable, two-piece cloth-

---

[3] The Z point is sometimes identified as the C point.

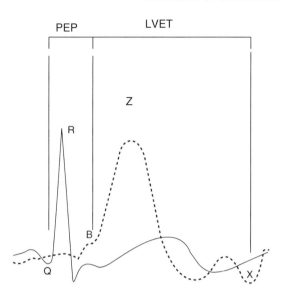

FIGURE 7.5. Dz/Dt and ECG waveforms needed to score PEP, LVET, and SV.

ing to the experiment. As the bands (or spots) require placement on the torso, directly on the skin, participants are required to lift their shirts to expose their torsos. In addition, placement of the neck sensors may be impeded by clothing that is snug on the neck. In my lab, we keep extra shirts and pants for participants who arrive in clothing that would make attachment of the bands difficult.

EDITING AND QUANTIFICATION

Probably among the greatest challenges for researchers interested in impedance cardiography are editing and summarizing the data. First, there are some important choices to be made regarding how the data are summarized for editing. One option uses ensembled waveform averages. This method determines the composite or average waveform across some specified time period (typically between 30 sec and 5 min). When the waveforms are "averaged" over time, random noise and movement are removed, and a more representative cardiac cycle can be obtained. Another option is to determine blood volume changes on a cycle-to-cycle basis (see an SPR committee guideline paper by Sherwood et al., 1990).

In addition to how the data are averaged, there are several different formulas that can be used to estimate SV. The Kubicek equation estimates SV from the derivative of the impedance signal and blood resistivity:

$$SV = \rho \times L2 / Z_0^2 \times \Delta Z/\Delta t_{max} \times LVET$$

where ρ = 135 (blood resistivity), L is the distance between electrodes, $\Delta Z/\Delta t_{max}$ is the peak amplitude of $\Delta Z/\Delta t$, and LVET is the left ventricle ejection time (time in milliseconds between B and X).

More recently, other equations have been offered that may be superior to Kubicek's. For example, the Sramek–Bernstein equation estimates SV from the volume of electrically participating tissue (VEPT), scaled according to body surface:

$$SV = \delta (VEPT) / Z_0 \times \Delta Z/\Delta t_{max} \times LVET$$

where $\delta (VEPT)$ = $weight_{max}$ /$weight_{ideal} \times (0.17H)^3$ / 4.25 (participant's height, weight, and ideal weight are needed).

Regardless of the equation used, one of the most critical decisions in scoring impedance data is accurately identifying the B point on the $\Delta z/\Delta t$ waveform. Though it is tremendously time- and labor-intensive, the technique that assures the greatest accuracy is manual detection of the B point. Specifically B should be placed at the beginning of the longest uphill slope before the Z point (Figure 7.5). Algorithms have been developed to assist in detecting the B point, such as placing the B point at 56% of the distance between Q and Z (see Berntson, Quigley, & Lozano, 2007), but in our own examination of this method, we have found that from 20% to 40% of the time the program does not mark the B point where we can visually confirm it (Mendes & Koslov, 2008). Importantly, the variability in accuracy changes, depending on whether the data are from a baseline period (where accuracy tends to be higher) or whether the participants are engaged in a stressful task (e.g., mental arithmetic in the presence of stoic evaluators).

Blood Pressure

Blood pressure (BP), measured in millimeters of mercury pressure (mm Hg), refers to the amount of pressure on the vessel walls during the cardiac cycle. Distinctions are made between systolic BP (SBP) and diastolic BP (DBP), which represent peak pressure and lowest pressure in the arteries, respectively. Though correlated, these measures may provide unique information and are thus typically both presented. For example, during stressful or emotionally provocative situations, increases in SBP compared to DBP have been identified as part of an adaptive defense patterning (see Brownley et al., 2000). SBP responses have also been linked specifically to effort expenditure (Wright & Kirby, 2001). Moreover, health consequences have been identified as resulting from increases in SBP and not necessarily DBP; for example, Chobanian and colleagues (2003) reported that elevated SBP, and not necessarily DBP, predicts the development of coronary heart disease.

Although SBP and DBP are often presented separately, one will also find instances in which researchers combine the two in some meaningful way. For example, pulse pressure (PP) is calculated by subtracting DBP from SBP (PP = SBP – DBP). At rest, average PP is approximately 40 mm Hg. During exercise, SBP typically increases more than DBP. Extremes in PP in both directions can indicate abnormalities. When PP is too high, this is likely due to artery stiffness, leaky aortic valves, or hyperthyroidism and has been linked to CV complications (Blacher et al., 2000). Low PP values, typically influenced by low SV, can indicate abnormalities such as congestive heart failure.

Another type of averaging is mean arterial pressure (MAP), which is calculated as a type of average (though not an exact mathematical average, because DBP is weighted more, given its longer time course within a given cardiac cycle): MAP ≈ [(2 × DBP) + SBP]/3. MAP is often used in combination with CO to determine total peripheral resistance (TPR), according to this formula: TPR = (MAP/CO) × 80. Changes in TPR can be construed as an estimate of the amount of constriction versus dilation occurring in the blood vessels—specifically, the arterioles. When the arterioles constrict, less blood can flow to the periphery, and this is indicated by an increase in TPR. In contrast, when arterioles expand, or vasodilate, this allows more blood flow and is indicated by decreases in TPR.

BP can be obtained from various places on the body, including the brachial artery (upper arm), the radial artery (wrist), or the finger. It is important to point out, however, that as the distance from the heart is increased, the accuracy of BP changes is reduced. BP measurements can be obtained via several techniques. One option is the auscultatory method, which consists of temporally stopping blood flow at the brachial artery and listening for Kortokoff sounds indicating blood flow in the arteries—the pressure when blood first begins to flow is SBP, and the pressure when blood flow sounds stop is DBP. A trained professional using this technique employs a sphygmomanometer and stethoscope to obtain BP.

However, in many cases psychologists want to obtain BP in a less labor-intensive way, and/or one that minimizes the self-consciousness that may arise from having BP measured. Digital BP machines are relatively inexpensive and fairly accurate measures of BP levels (though not as precise as a trained professional using a sphygmomanometer). Again, these BP machines typically require occluding the brachial artery every time a BP measurement is desired. This is not difficult, but could potentially distract participants from the experimental situation. A potential solution for obtaining BP responses over time, which is only minimally invasive, is with a continual or continuous BP monitor. *Continual* monitors are so designated because BP responses are estimated over some given number of cardiac cycles (e.g., BP over 15 cardiac cycles). *Continuous* BP machines have the additional advantage of obtaining BP responses on every cardiac cycle. Commercially available machines are manufactured by Colin Medical Instruments (San Antonio, TX) and Mindware Technologies (Gahanna, OH).

Many continual or continuous BP machines use either oscillometric or tonometric technology. Oscillometric technology initially inflates a cuff over the brachial artery, deflates until the point at which SBP can be measured, and then keeps a constant cuff pressure. The technology and algorithms used for these machines are proprietary, so there is some concern about comparing results across laboratories. Tonometric technology consists of BP measurement from the radial (wrist) artery, and uses a sweep technique, which applies a varying force on the artery. This technology can be very sensitive to movement and sensor positioning relative to the heart. Manufacturers recommend putting the arm in a sling so as to position the sensor at heart height and limit movement. For social and personality psychologists, who often aim for strong ecological validity, restraining the arm can be problematic. However, my lab's own use of this technology suggests that movement is the greater problem. Fashioning a cradle that will keep the arm and wrist stable throughout the experiment is imperative to obtaining good measurements. Some of the more expensive machines include an additional brachial cuff BP device to allow for online comparisons from the two sites; the wrist cuff can be signaled to reposition if the brachial BP responses differ from BP measured at the radial artery.

ANS Responses in Social and Personality Psychology

Social and personality research using ANS responses is plentiful. Here I review some selected studies; this review is not meant to be exhaustive and is influenced by my own research interests in emotion, stress, motivation, attitudes, and intergroup relations. For ease, I have based the organization of sections on the physiological measurements used rather than the psychological constructs under examination.

Electrodermal Responses

As previously described, changes in EDA can index general arousal; thus the use of these measures may at first seem limited. However, both classic and contemporary uses of these measures show that compelling information can be obtained by looking at EDA. Indeed, using peripheral measures in the domains of emotion, motivation, and attention has provided important empirical evidence for social and personality psychologists.

For example, SC has been used in the context of emotional disclosure. Pennebaker, Hughes, and O'Heeron (1987) examined changes in SCL while participants disclosed traumatic events from their lives. Talking about traumatic events decreased SCL in participants classified as high disclosers, relative to those classified as low disclosers. This finding has been used as a possible explanation of why there are physical and mental health benefits of confession: High disclosers showed lower sympathetic activation than low disclosers.

Whereas getting something traumatic off one's chest may be beneficial, forcing oneself to feel good may be detrimental. Wegner, Broome, and Blumberg (1997) instructed participants either to relax or not to relax while answering questions that were believed to index intelligence (a high-cognitive-load condition) or answering the same questions that were described as test items (a low-cognitive-load condition). For participants in the high-cognitive-load condition, the instruction to relax resulted in higher SCL than did the instruction not to relax. These findings nicely demonstrate the potentially ironic effects of *trying* to relax, which resulted in greater sympathetic activation.

Not surprisingly, ANS responses in general, and EDA measures in particular, are often used in research examining gender biases and race relations because of the difficulty in obtaining unexpurgated self-reported responses. In a recent study, changes in SCL were used to examine threatening gender environments, involving an imbalance of males to females (Murphy, Steele, & Gross, 2007). In this research, male and female participants viewed one of two videos that presented either a gender-balanced group of students or a gender-unbalanced group (mostly white males) in the domain of a math and engineering science camp. Changes in SCL from a baseline period to watching the videos were computed. The findings were that female participants showed greater increases in SCL when watching the gender-unbalanced video than watching the gender-balanced video, and male participants did not differ in their SCL responses as a function of the videos' gender composition. The authors concluded that the gender imbalance was especially threatening for women.

In these examples, EDA was used as a general measure of arousal or anxiety. However, by limiting the context, one can increase the inference of EDA changes. For example, in fear conditioning paradigms, an electric shock or other aversive stimulus is paired with some unconditioned stimulus while SCRs are measured. In learning phases, the shock or other aversive stimulus is repeatedly linked in time with the conditioned stimulus. Later the shock is removed and SCRs are examined upon exposure to the conditioned stimulus. The critical examination is the length of the extinction phase, or how long it takes for participants to cease showing SCRs to the conditioned stimulus once the aversive element is removed. An exceptionally creative adaptation of this design has been described in a *Science* article by Olsson, Ebert, Banaji, and Phelps (2005). In this study, the researchers paired electric shock with ingroup and outgroup male faces. They argued that individuals might be evolutionarily "prepared" to fear outgroup members and, because of this, that extinction of the fear response would take longer when the shock was paired with outgroup faces than when it was paired with ingroup faces. Indeed, when shocks were paired with outgroup faces compared to ingroup faces, SCRs persisted longer and were of greater magnitude in the extinction phase. In this example, SCRs could be interpreted as fear responses because the context was constrained to a fear-eliciting (shock) situation.

SC changes may index emotional responses even prior to the conscious awareness of those emotions. An elegant example of the possibility that physiology may provide information regarding emotional and motivational responses before conscious awareness is provided by Bechara and colleagues (1997). These investigators measured SC changes while participants (individuals with and without prefrontal brain damage) learned decision rules for a card task. Although self-reported indications related to "hunches" regarding decks that were associated with more gain than loss cards developed by the 50th trial for the control participants (i.e., those without brain damage), SC changes in anticipation to the loss decks occurred typically by the 10th trial, which preceded conscious awareness by approximately 40 trials. That is, SCRs suggested an intuition of an impending loss prior to the nondisabled participants' conscious awareness of the intuitions they were developing.

Heart Rate Variability

Of growing interest to social and personality psychologists are measures capitalizing on the variability of the cardiac cycle. Initially, HRV was believed to be a measurement artifact or nuisance, but further exploration into spontaneous changes in the timing of the heart cycle proved to be psychologically and physiologically meaningful. Though there are still disagreements on the specifics related to measurement, quantification, and psychological meaningfulness of vagal tone and cardiac vagal reactivity (see Chambers & Allen, 2007), these measures may prove to be especially important for social and personality psychologists interested in emotion and/or mental effort.

Though most work has focused on resting/baseline RSA (also known as cardiac vagal tone) and its links to dispositions and responses to social and emotional situations, there is also a growing literature on vagal reactivity and vagal rebound. Vagal rebound is the extent to which RSA responses return to or even overshoot baseline levels after some suppression of the vagal brake. Below I review some literature exploring these various components of HRV.

One theory that has received much attention in terms of the inferences one can draw from HRV is Porges's polyvagal theory (e.g., Porges, 2007). Porges (2007) argues that vagal regulation stemming from the nucleus ambiguus and enervation from cranial nerve X acts on the vagus nerve to modulate heart period. The polyvagal theory further specifies that primates uniquely have vagal nerve modulation (but see Grossman & Taylor, 2007), which has evolved as part of the social engagement system. One of the primary postulates of polyvagal theory is that social factors (affiliation, social engagement) or personality factors (bonding, compassion) can modulate vagal activity. Specifically, Porges argues that higher RSA (higher cardiac vagal tone) can be used as an index of adaptive emotional regulation and responsiveness to the social environment. Similarly, cardiac vagal reactivity may also index appropriate social engagement, in that increased vagal reactivity during a task may be associated with calmness, equanimity, and a lack of distress.

Adding some complexity to these effects, however, is the nature of the social context. In highly stressful situations or tasks that require some amount of mental attention or effort, then one should expect a withdrawal of the vagal brake (resulting in lower RSA) to indicate greater attentional control and effort. Indeed, cognitive psychophysiologists have used decreased RSA as an index of attention or mental effort (Tattersall & Hockey, 1995). In one study relying on this type of interpretation for HRV reactivity, Croizet, Després, and Gauzins (2004) examined changes in RSA during a stereotype threat paradigm. They found that participants assigned to receive a stereotype threat prime had a greater decrease in RSA and poorer performance than those in the control condition, and that RSA changes mediated the relationship from the condition to the performance effects.

Applications of cardiac vagal tone and vagal reactivity are increasing in personality and social psychology. Some applications have focused on the extent to which dispositional emotional styles are linked with cardiac vagal tone (Demaree & Everhart, 2004; Sloan, Bagiella, & Shapiro, 2001). For example, do individuals with greater hostile tendencies have lower cardiac vagal tone? In an examination of this question, researchers found that those higher in hostility tended to have lower cardiac vagal tone at baseline, during an emotional induction task, and at recovery than those lower in hostile tendencies did (Sloan et al., 2001; cf. Demaree & Everhart, 2004).

Recently, RSA has been examined as a possible mediator for why implicit goal setting may result in improved performance. In a previous study, participants who exaggerated reports of their grade point average (GPA) tended to improve their GPA more than those who did not exaggerate (Gramzow & Willard, 2006). Was exaggeration a form of implicit goal setting or simply a form of anxious repression? We examined RSA reactivity as a way to differentiate anxious orientation while exaggerating from motivated goal setting (Gramzow, Willard, & Mendes, 2008). In this study, participants first reported their GPA and course grades in private, and then met with an experimenter to review their academic history. During this interview, the participant's ECG and respiration were recorded, and RSA responses were then calculated. We found that the more participants exaggerated their GPA, the greater the increase in RSA from baseline to the interview, suggesting that participants who exaggerated their GPA were not necessarily anxious about their exaggerated standards. In addition, those who had greater increases in RSA when discussing their GPA tended to improve their GPA in a subsequent semester. Converging evidence from nonverbal behavior coded during the interview suggested that exaggerators appeared composed rather than anxious, supporting the interpretation that higher RSA while discussing one's GPA was associated with equanimity rather than anxiety.

Impedance Cardiography

CV responses have been used extensively in the areas of motivation, emotion, and stress. Interest in these measures is further fueled by the possibility that certain patterns or response profiles of CV responses repeatedly experienced over time may be linked to health outcomes. Early work linking Type A personality and coronary heart disease examined CV responses as one of the likely mechanisms through which physical health was affected. Specifically, it was theorized that excessive CV responses would create tears in the endothelial lining, resulting in greater calcifications and plaque buildup that could possibly initiate ischemic events or strokes. Primarily, CV responses in this context included HR (heart period) and BP responses.

A combination of CV and BP responses is used in research attempting to index challenge and threat states. Though not without its critics (Wright & Kirby, 2003; see also Blascovich, Mendes, Tomaka, Salomon, & Seery, 2003), this line of research attempts to differentiate motivational states by using various CV measures, such as PEP, CO, and TPR. The theory behind this research argues that in motivated performance situations (i.e., those that are active rather than passive and require some cognitive or behavioral responses), CV responses produce a distinct profile of reactions that can differentiate motivational states related to approach/activation from those related to defeat/inhibition (Mendes, Major, McCoy, & Blascovich, 2008). Early work on this theory showed that task appraisals that showed greater resources relative to demands were associated with greater CV responses: shorter PEP (indicating greater ventricle contractility), increased HR and CO, and decreases in vascular resistance (lower TPR). This pattern of CV reactivity was believed to be a marker of psychological states of challenge. In contrast, appraisals that showed greater perceived demands relative to resources to cope were associated with comparatively less CO and higher TPR (Tomaka, Blascovich, & Kelsey, 1993). These responses were thought to index threat states. To test for the possible bidirectionality of these responses, these physiological states were engendered with nonpsychological events—specifically, exercise (challenge) or cold pressor (threat)—to determine whether appraisals associated with challenge and threat would follow from the physiological responses (Tomaka, Blascovich, Kibler, & Ernst, 1997). Results showed that although appraisals preceded CV responses as described above, the relationship was not invariant. That is, physiological responses engendered in nonpsychological ways did not influence subsequent appraisals.

Challenge and threat theory has been used in a variety of social and personality domains. In the social domain, these indices have been explored to examine responses within a dyadic social interaction when one member of the dyad is stigmatized in some way. Stigmas were operationalized as physical stigmas (e.g., birthmarks), stigmas resulting from group membership (e.g., race/ethnicity), or socially constructed stigmas (e.g., accents, socioeconomic status). Across more than a dozen studies, participants who interacted with stigmatized partners were more likely to exhibit threat (i.e., lower CO and higher TPR) than were those interacting with nonstigmatized partners. If the results had been found only with physiological responses, they would have still been intriguing—but in many cases the physiological responses also correlated with other automatic or less consciously controlled responses, such as cognitive performance, emotional states, and various nonverbal behaviors (such as freezing, orientation away from the partner, and closed posture) (Mendes et al., 2008; Mendes, Blascovich, Hunter, Lickel, & Jost, 2007; Mendes, Blascovich, Lickel, & Hunter, 2002). Also of interest was the lack of correlations between participants' CV responses and their self-reported appraisals and partner ratings. In contrast with the CV responses, self-reported partner ratings showed a preference for stigmatized over nonstigmatized partners, suggesting that deliberate and consciously controlled measures may be more vulnerable to attempts to correct for racial bias (Blascovich, Mendes, & Seery, 2002; Mendes & Koslov, 2008).

In the personality domain, these measures have been used to assess individuals' reactions to stressful situations. For example, individuals who scored higher on scales assessing belief in a just world (e.g., the view that hard work is rewarded) tended to exhibit greater increases in cardiac and decreases in TPR during stressful tasks than those who scored lower on these scales, who exhibited lower CO and higher TPR—consistent with threat profiles (Tomaka & Blascovich, 1994). Self-perceptions in the form of level and stability of self-esteem have been explored with these methods as well (Seery, Blascovich, Weisbuch, & Vick, 2004). For participants with high and stable self-esteem, positive performance feedback resulted in more challenge responses than for those with high and unstable self-esteem.

Loneliness also appears to result in these patterns of CO and TPR (Cacioppo, Hawkley, & Crawford, 2002; Hawkley, Burleson, & Berntson, 2003). Cacioppo and colleagues (2002) have shown in various settings that individuals reporting higher levels of loneliness are likely to show lower CO and higher TPR than individuals reporting lower levels of loneliness. This effect has been found both in lab-based studies in response to social evaluation, and in field studies using ambulatory impedance and BP devices. In one field study, due to lack of ability to determine whether individuals were actually in motivated performance situations, the authors interpreted these profiles as indicating passive versus active coping styles (Sherwood et al., 1990), with lonely individuals adopting more passive coping styles within the context of their day.

Blood Pressure

Social psychologists have used BP to index several psychological states, including stress, threat, and effort. Much evidence has been accumulated by Wright and colleagues (see Wright & Kirby, 2001, for a review) supporting their theory of effort mobilization. In this extension of Brehm's motivational intensity analysis, it has been empirically demonstrated that participants' effort increases monotonically with difficulty until the task is perceived as too difficult, and then effort is withdrawn. Ability is also a critical factor; when individuals have lower levels of ability, effort is withdrawn at lower levels of difficulty. In this model, Wright's group typically uses SBP as a measure of effort. Although HR and DBP may also follow patterns similar to those for SBP, SBP is thought to be more closely aligned with effort, given its tighter relationship to the sympathetic component of the cardiac cycle (systole).

Experimental Design Considerations

Before incorporating ANS responses into the methodological toolbox, one should consider several important issues that are reviewed here. These considerations include the level of inference one can draw; the complex relationship between the sympathetic and parasympathetic nervous systems; the nature of the experimental context and task; the ways in which health and aging can influence responses; individual and situational stereotypy; the need for knowledge of biological systems; and guidelines for data editing.

Establishing Level of Inference

It is critical to begin with the first major obstacle to any psychophysiologist, which is determining the level of psychological inference that can be attributed to any physiological response. "Inference," in this context, refers to the extent to which an observed physiological response or constellation of responses indicates the presence, absence, or intensity of a psychological state. Here I summarize the main points of psychological inference, and suggest what social and personality psychologists should and should not expect from incorporating ANS responses into their methodological toolboxes.

When one is interpreting physiological responses in terms of what the changes might reflect psychologically, it is useful to evoke the taxonomy of physiological responses outlined by Cacioppo, Tassinary, and Berntson (2000). In this conceptualization, the level of inference is determined by (1) the generality of the context in which the response occurs, and (2) the specificity of the physiological response in relation to the psychological state. The context distinction focuses on whether the context is free and unconstrained (context-independent) or constrained (context-dependent). That is, does one expect that only in a specific context a psychological state would correlate with a physiological response (constrained), or that in any context the psychological–physiological relationship would emerge (unconstrained)?

The specificity dimension refers to the relationship between psychology and physiology. Do many psychological states relate to a physiological response, or do the psychology and physiology have a one-to-one relationship? For example, many psychological states are thought to bring about an increase in SC (e.g., arousal, attention, fear, anxiety); this would be an example of a many-to-one relationship. In contrast, the relationship between negative affect and potentiated startle responses is thought to reflect a one-to-one or invariant relationship. When individuals are experiencing negative emotions, either elicited incidentally or evoked via images, an auditory or visual probe is presented that potentiates the startle response, as evidenced by increased eyeblink magnitude and shortened latency to blink.

When these dimensions of context and specificity are combined, various levels of psychophysiological relationships emerge. When the context is constrained, many-to-one relationships are referred to as "outcomes," whereas one-to-one relationships are referred to as "markers." In an unconstrained context, many-to-one relationships are called "concomitants," and one-to-one relationships are referred to as "invariants." Knowledge of the level of inference is essential to interpreting the psychological meaning of any physiological response.

An additional question related to determining inference is this: What is the "gold standard" for evaluating whether a physiological response is indexing the psychological state of interest? In a somewhat tautological argument, the inferences of physiological responses are often determined by their relationship to a self-reported psychological state. Following the confirmation of the established relationship, some psychophysiologists then will conclude that their physiological responses are revealing responses that are closer to the true and valid experience of the respondents, ignoring the fact that self-reports are often used to establish inference in the first place. Determining psychophysiological inference should be a dynamic process that includes testing and validating relationships between psychology and physiology, and examining the predictive validity of physiological responses to behavior, performance, and health. Most importantly, however, one should not infer that physiological responses *are* the psychological constructs.

Autonomic Space

A second critical factor in examining ANS responses is an understanding of how the sympathetic and parasympathetic branches of the ANS interact and influence each other. In a seminal paper, Berntson, Cacioppo, and Quigley (1991) outline the importance of considering the complexity of the relationships between the two branches. The idea that the sympathetic and parasympathetic branches are reciprocally related (as sympathetic activation increases parasympathetic activity decreases) has been deemed overly simplistic. Instead, it is more accurate to construe these systems as complementary and complexly interactive. For example, increases in sympathetic activation can be associated with decreases in parasympathetic responses; however, this is not exclusively the case. Instead, the systems can be reciprocal, coactivated, or decoupled. An understanding of these relationships can protect against inaccurate conclusions when one system is being observed in the absence of the other. For example, increases in HR may be incorrectly interpreted as reflecting an increase in sympathetic activation, when instead HR increases are due to parasympathetic withdrawal or to a combination of activations in both branches.

Nature of the Experimental Context and Task

The characteristics of the experimental context and task play an important role in the choice of an ANS measure, as well as in how the data are collected, quantified, and (most critically) interpreted. When one is incorporating ANS measures in an experiment, among the first decisions to make is the context in which to collect ANS responses. As described earlier, many of the inferences that can be drawn from the physiological responses are context-bound. For example, although the SCRs that Olsson and colleagues (2005) used in their fear conditioning paradigm are broadly recognized as indexing a fear response, SCRs are by no means universally accepted as indexing fear responses. Indeed, SCRs can result from strong positive emotion, anxiety, deception, attention, and other psychological factors that are certainly distinct from fear. So it is important to know whether a physiological response is believed to be context-bound or context-free. As the context becomes more constrained, one can imagine that the inference level is likely to be increase, though little has been written on this topic.

One of the critical context distinctions in examining ANS responses is the extent to which the participant is engaged in an active versus a passive task (Obrist, 1981). Active tasks are ones in which some response is required from participants, as opposed to passive tasks, in which participants simply experience some event without necessarily having to respond in some instrumental way. This distinction is critical, because in many cases ANS changes are functional; that is, they are responses to the required needs of a task, rather than reflecting the psychological change brought on by the situation. For example, giving a speech requires modulation of respiration to produce vocal tones, and often postural changes are made to improve vocal projection; both of these can influence ANS responses that have nothing to do with stress, emotion, or motivation. In addition, many ANS patterns or profiles are thought to index psychological states stemming from active situations and not passive ones. Challenge and threat, for example, are thought to occur only in active situations and not passive ones. So either watching a scary movie or giving a talk to a room filled with people who disagreed with the speaker might be terrifying, but only in the latter case would the ANS responses yield a pattern associated with threat.

Health of Participants and Individual Response Stereotypy

Recruiting participants for psychophysiology studies poses some challenges. Depending on the response of interest, some health conditions may need to be considered and screened. Of course, when the interest is in HRV or other CV responses, people with heart conditions, pacemakers, or cardiac-altering prescriptions (e.g., beta-blockers) should be excluded. This is probably also true of doctor-diagnosed arrhythmias, though in the 10 years that I have been running participants (resulting in over 3,000 participants), my colleagues and I did not detect any abnormalities on the ECG waveform for the few participants who claimed to have an arrhythmia. Instead, in a small number of cases when participants have claimed *not* to have an arrhythmia, we have noted ECG abnormalities (e.g., bradycardia and premature ventricle contractions). What to do when an arrhythmia is detected is actually a matter of debate (see Stern, Ray, & Quigley, 2003). One perspective is that if a nonmedical professional informs a participant of possible ECG abnormalities and causes undue distress, only to be proven wrong when the person does have a medical screening, this would outweigh the risk of occasionally being correct. The other perspective is that abnormalities can be detected in ECG waveforms, and that an informed opinion about these could be beneficial to participants, so they should be told. Decisions to report should be guided by the policy of the local institutional review board, as well as by the quality of one's knowledge of ECG abnormalities. For several years, I received advice from a cardiovascular surgeon when I was concerned about possible cardiac abnormalities. Forging a relationship with a medical professional may be critical if the institutional review board or funding agency wants any detected abnormalities to be reported to participants. Importantly, though, undergraduate research assistants with limited experience and graduate students just starting their careers should not make these decisions, and each lab should have some plan for how to deal with these possible situations.

For social psychologists, another potential source of difficulties with participants is individual response stereotypy. That is, for some individuals' ANS responses will not be modulated by the experimental situation, no matter what it is. For example, some individuals are thought to be chronic vasoconstrictors and, regardless of the situation, will show constriction rather than dilation in their arteries and arterioles in any change from homeostasis. There is considerable disagreement in the literature regarding the percentage of individuals who respond without psychological modulation, but it is something that could add error and reduce the ability to detect differences based on the experimental manipulation. Certainly older participants are more likely to have sluggish responses and tend to have more individual response stereotypy than younger persons do. Overweight individuals may also show less psychological modulation.

Situational Stereotypy

Parallel with the idea that some individuals respond in stereotyped ways without the influence of the social setting, some situations are thought to bring about stereotyped responses without individual modulation. One of the most obvious situations is the startle reflex, in which sound or visual presentations occur at such high decibels or lumens that the eyeblink reflex occurs for everyone. At lower levels of sound, for example, psychological modulation can occur, so only at intense levels is the startle response universal.

The Need for Knowledge of Biological Systems

The most common question I hear from researchers considering incorporating psychophysiology into their methodological toolboxes is "How much physiology do I need to know?" There is really only answer to this question: "As much as possible." A good understanding of biological systems will inform research questions, choices of context, and (probably most importantly) interpretations of the data. The good news is that obtaining training in biological systems generally and the ANS specifically is easier than some readers may think. Biology departments often have terrific courses in anatomy and physiology. Auditing a medical school class on the CV system can provide invaluable information. Joining such organizations as the SPR and the American Psychosomatic Society, and attending their conferences, can immerse psychologists in a world that does not consider the ANS a mere tool for answering research questions related to social and personality questions; instead, this system *is* their research question. The ways in which the body responds to stress, emotion, temperature changes, age, and other factors differently or similarly are some of the critical issues. Indeed, one might not want to claim brazenly that one is merely interested in ANS measures as mere methods of obtaining answers to psychological research questions. Examining the ANS and the complexities of all its changes is a worthy pursuit in its own right and provides important foundational work for social and personality psychologists whose interest in the system may be merely methodological.

Guidelines for Data Editing

Though one can find many software programs that can edit, score, and ensemble data with a push of the button, I strongly advocate either designing one's own software or scoring the data manually whenever possible. Putting trust in any software program, even those designed by researchers at the top of the field, is a leap of trust that one might not want to make when considering the multiple problems that might arise during data collection. Also, there is nothing quite like editing data to make one appreciate how the system reacts to stimuli, stressors, or events. In addition, after reviewing over a dozen software programs to score impedance waveforms, for example, I have yet to see a program that can consistently detect one of the critical inflection points on the $\Delta z/\Delta t$ waveform—the B point. Under- or overestimating this point can dramatically change SV and CO measures.

We have established several guidelines in my lab to determine the quality of the data while scoring. One guiding rationale is "physiological plausibility." Each measure has a range of responses that are plausible, given the physiological marker. In addition to the plausibility of any single measure, there is the plausibility of a constellation of related measures. Table 7.1 shows plausible ranges of PEP, HR, and LVET (left ventricle ejection time—time from the aortic valve opening to its closing). These relationships demonstrate that when the heart is beating faster, decreases in PEP and LVET can be expected. These ranges are not presented as the only possible ranges that could occur, but rather general guidelines for determining whether the data are typical or not. When scoring or examining data, one should be aware of general ranges in which these measures are related to each other.

Future Directions

One of the greatest advantages of ANS recording is one that has probably been underexamined: testing the dynamic nature of changes in ANS responses as a result of moment-to-moment changes in experience. In many cases, psychophysiologists spend a great amount of time and effort reducing their data to a reasonable number of time epochs and critical responses. However, such statistical techniques as hierarchical linear modeling and time series analyses allow researchers to model tem-

TABLE 7.1. Plausibility of Physiological Ranges: HR, PEP, and LVET

HR (bpm)	PEP (msec)	LVET (msec)
40–60	100–140	300–450
60–80	90–130	250–400
80–120	80–120	250–350
100–120	70–100	200–300
120+	<80	180–300

poral changes in a more fine-grained fashion than ever before (Vallacher, Read, & Nowak, 2002). An additional benefit of these online responses is that they do not require a conscious assessment of what participants are thinking or feeling. Thus responses can be viewed as relatively automatic and less consciously controlled than online subjective reports obtained with rating dials.

Moreover, ANS responses are not limited to lab-based designs. Advances in ambulatory monitoring allow responses to be collected continually throughout a person's daily life and coordinated with experience-sampling techniques. Ambulatory monitoring of ANS responses presents infinite possibilities for social and personality psychologists, particularly those whose work intersects with public health, clinical science, and organizational behavior. The possibilities are endless and limited only by researchers' finances, imagination, and knowledge. I am hopeful that this chapter has offered at least some initial inspiration for expanding the latter two limits.

References

Bechara, A., Damasio, H., Tranel, D., & Damasio, A. R. (1997). Deciding advantageously before knowing the advantageous strategy. *Science, 275,* 1293–1294.

Berntson, G. G., Bigger, J. T., Jr., & Eckberg, D. L. (1997). Heart rate variability: Origins, methods, and interpretive caveats. *Psychophysiology, 34*(6), 623–648.

Berntson, G. G., Cacioppo, J. T., & Quigley, K. S. (1991). Autonomic determinism: The modes of autonomic control, the doctrine of autonomic space, and the laws of autonomic constraint. *Psychological Review, 98*(4), 459–487.

Berntson, G. G., Cacioppo, J. T., & Quigley, K. S. (1993). Cardiac psychophysiology and autonomic space in humans: Empirical perspectives and conceptual implications. *Psychological Bulletin, 114*(2), 296–322.

Berntson, G. G., Quigley, K. S., & Lozano, D. (2007). Cardiovascular psychophysiology. In J. T. Cacioppo, L. G. Tassinary, & G. G. Berntson (Eds.), *Handbook of psychophysiology* (3rd ed., pp. 182–210). New York: Cambridge University Press.

Blacher, J., Staessen, J. A., Girerd, X., Gasowske, J., Thijs, L., Liu, L., et al. (2000). Pulse pressure not mean pressure determines cardiovascular risk in older hypertensive patients. *Archives of Internal Medicine, 160,* 1085–1089.

Blascovich, J., Mendes, W. B., & Seery, M. D. (2002). Intergroup threat: A multi-method approach. In D. M. Mackie & E. R. Smith (Eds.), *From prejudice to intergroup emotions: Differentiated reactions to social groups* (pp. 89–109). New York: Psychology Press.

Blascovich, J., Mendes, W. B., Tomaka, J., Salomon, K., & Seery, M. D. (2003). The robust nature of the biopsychosocial model of challenge and threat: A reply to Wright and Kirby. *Personality and Social Psychology Review, 7(3),* 234–243.

Brownley, K. A., Hurwitz, B. E., & Schneiderman, N. (2000). Cardiovascular psychophysiology. In J. T. Cacioppo, L. G. Tassinary, & G. G. Berntson (Eds.), *Handbook of psychophysiology* (2nd ed., pp. 224–264). New York: Cambridge University Press.

Cacioppo, J. T., Hawkley, L. C., & Crawford, E. (2002). Loneliness and health: Potential mechanisms. *Psychosomatic Medicine, 64*(3), 407–417.

Cacioppo, J. T., Tassinary, L. G., & Berntson, G. G. (Eds.). (2000). *Handbook of psychophysiology* (2nd ed.). New York: Cambridge University Press.

Chambers, A. S., & Allen, J. J. B. (2007). Cardiac vagal control, emotion, psychopathology, and health. *Biological Psychology, 74,* 113–115.

Chobanian, A. V., Bakris, G. L., Black, H. R., Cushman, W. C., Green, L. A., Izzo, J. L., Jr., et al. (2003). Seventh report of the Joint National Committee on Prevention, Detection, Evaluation, and Treatment of High Blood Pressure. *Hypertension, 42*(6), 1206–1252.

Croizet, J., Després, G., & Gauzins, M. (2004). Stereotype threat undermines intellectual performance by triggering a disruptive mental load. *Personality and Social Psychology Bulletin, 30,* 721–731.

Demaree, H. A., & Everhart, D. E. (2004). Healthy high-hostiles: Reduced parasympathetic activity and decreased sympathovagal flexibility during negative emotional processing. *Personality and Individual Differences, 36*(2), 457–469.

Denver, J. W., Reed, S. F., & Porges, S. W. (2007). Methodological issues in the quantification of respiratory sinus arrhythmia. *Biological Psychology, 74*(2), 286–294.

Gardner, W. L., Gabriel, S., & Diekman, A. B. (2000). Interpersonal processes. In J. T. Cacioppo, L. G. Tassinary, & G. G. Berntson (Eds.), *Handbook of psychophysiology* (2nd ed., pp. 643–664). New York: Cambridge University Press.

Gramzow, R. H., & Willard, G. B. (2006). Exaggerating current and past performance: Motivated self-enhancement versus reconstructive memory. *Personality and Social Psychology Bulletin, 32*(8), 1114–1125.

Gramzow, R. H., Willard, G. B., & Mendes, W. B. (2008). Big tales and cool heads: GPA exaggeration is related to increased parasympathetic activation. *Emotion, 8*(1), 138–144.

Grossman, P., & Taylor, E. W. (2007). Toward understanding respiratory sinus arrhythmia: Relations to cardiac vagal tone, evolution and biobehavioral functions. *Biological Psychology, 74*(2), 263–285.

Guglielmi, R. S. (1999). Psychophysiological assessment of prejudice: Past research, current status, and future directions. *Personality and Social Psychology Review, 3*(2), 123–157.

Hawkley, L. C., Burleson, M. H., & Berntson, G. G. (2003). Loneliness in everyday life: Cardiovascular activity, psychosocial context, and health behaviors. *Journal of Personality and Social Psychology, 85*(1), 105–120.

Mendes, W. B., Blascovich, J., Hunter, S., Lickel, B., & Jost, J. (2007). Threatened by the unexpected: Challenge and threat during inter-ethnic interactions. *Journal of Personality and Social Psychology, 92*(4), 698–716.

Mendes, W. B., Blascovich, J., Lickel, B., & Hunter, S. (2002). Cardiovascular reactivity during social interactions with white and black men. *Personality and Social Psychology Bulletin, 28*, 939–952.

Mendes, W. B., & Koslov, K. (2008). *Over-correction*. Manuscript under review.

Mendes, W. B., Major, B., McCoy, S., & Blascovich, J. (2008). How attributional ambiguity shapes physiological and emotional responses to social rejection and acceptance. *Journal of Personality and Social Psychology, 94*(2), 278–291.

Murphy, M. C., Steele, C. M., & Gross, J. J. (2007). Signaling threat: How situational cues affect women in math, science, and engineering settings. *Psychological Science, 18*(10), 879–885.

Obrist, P. A. (1981). *Cardiovascular psychophysiology: A perspective.* New York: Plenum Press.

Olsson, A., Ebert, J. P., Banaji, M. R., & Phelps, E. A. (2005). The role of social groups in the persistence of learned fear. *Science, 309*, 785–787.

Pennebaker, J. W., Hughes, C. F., & O'Heeron, R. C. (1987). The psychophysiology of confession: Linking inhibitory and psychosomatic processes. *Journal of Personality and Social Psychology, 52*(4), 781–793.

Porges, S. W. (2007). The polyvagal perspective. *Biological Psychology, 74*(2), 116–143.

Seery, M. D., Blascovich, J., Weisbuch, M., & Vick, S. B. (2004). The relationship between self-esteem level, self-esteem stability, and cardiovascular reactions to performance feedback. *Journal of Personality and Social Psychology, 87*(1), 133–145.

Sherwood, A., Allen, M. T., Fahrenberg, J., Kelsey, R. M., Lovallo, W. R., & van Doormen, L. J. P. (1990). Methodological guidelines for impedance cardiography. *Psychophysiology, 27*, 1–23.

Sherwood, A., Dolan, C. A., & Light, K. C. (1990). Hemodynamics of blood pressure responses during active and passive coping. *Psychophysiology, 27*, 656–668.

Sherwood, A., Royal, S. A., & Hutcheson, J. S. (1992). Comparison of impedance cardiographic measurements using band and spot electrodes. *Psychophysiology, 29*(6), 734–741.

Sloan, R. P., Bagiella, E., & Shapiro, P. A. (2001). Hostility, gender, and cardiac autonomic control. *Psychosomatic Medicine, 63*(3), 434–440.

Stern, R. M., Ray, W. J., & Quigley, K. S. (2003). Psychophysiological recording. *Psychophysiology, 40*(2), 314–315.

Tattersall, A. J., & Hockey, G. R. (1995). Level of operator control and changes in heart rate variability during simulated flight maintenance, *Human Factors, 37,* 682–698.

Tomaka, J., & Blascovich, J. (1994). Effects of justice beliefs on cognitive appraisal of and subjective physiological, and behavioral responses to potential stress. *Journal of Personality and Social Psychology, 67*(4), 732–740.

Tomaka, J., Blascovich, J., & Kelsey, R. M. (1993). Subjective, physiological, and behavioral effects of threat and challenge appraisal. *Journal of Personality and Social Psychology, 65*(2), 248–260.

Tomaka, J., Blascovich, J., Kibler, J., & Ernst, J. M. (1997). Cognitive and physiological antecedents of threat and challenge appraisal. *Journal of Personality and Social Psychology, 73*(1), 63–72.

Vallacher, R. R., Read, S. J., & Nowak, A. (2002). The dynamical perspective in personality and social psychology. *Personality and Social Psychology Review, 6*(4), 264–273.

Venables, P. H., & Christie, M. J. (1973). Mechanisms, instrumentation, recording techniques, and quantification of responses. In W. F. Prokasy & D. C. Raskin (Eds.), *Electrodermal activity in psychological research* (pp. 1–124). New York: Academic Press.

Wegner, D. M., Broome, A., & Blumberg, S. J. (1997). Ironic effects of trying to relax under stress. *Behaviour Research and Therapy, 35*(1), 11–21.

Wright, R. A., & Kirby, L. D. (2001). Effort determination of cardiovascular response: An integrative analysis with applications in social psychology. *Advances in Experimental Social Psychology, 33,* 255–307.

Wright, R. A., & Kirby, L. D. (2003). Cardiovascular correlates of challenge and threat appraisals: A critical examination of the biopsychosocial analysis. *Personality and Social Psychology Review, 7*(3), 216–233.

8

Patient Methodologies for the Study of Personality and Social Processes

Jennifer S. Beer

There may be a reason why "patience" and "patients" sound so similar. Although they can be time-consuming, patient studies are a less expensive and potentially more accessible methodology than the neuroimaging techniques so often used by social and personality psychologists interested in the brain's implications for psychological processes (see Table 8.1; see also Beer & Lombardo, 2007). Patient studies offer a number of advantages over neuroimaging techniques, such as functional magnetic resonance imaging (fMRI) or event-related potentials (ERPs). Conducting a patient study is much more similar to conducting a typical social or personality psychology experiment than to conducting one that involves neuroimaging techniques. It is often possible to adapt a social or personality paradigm to use with patients with little modification. In addition, a wider range of paradigms is possible, because patient studies do not require the large number of trials, timing restrictions, or physical restraint associated with most neuroimaging techniques. For example, experimental paradigms that involve social interaction are much easier to conduct with patients in a laboratory than with healthy controls in a scanner. Studies with patients also do not require expensive equipment

TABLE 8.1. Advantages and Disadvantages of Patient Methods in Comparison to Neuroimaging Techniques

Advantages

- Lower cost: Payment is often limited to cost of materials and compensation to participants.
- The procedures used are more similar to the behavioral experiments typically conducted by social–personality psychologists.
- A wider range of paradigms is possible.
- Patient studies do not require special equipment, such as a magnetic resonance scanner or electrophysiology hookup.

Disadvantages

- Success depends on the availability of patient populations and appropriate control participants.
- Even if patients of interest are available, it may take years to complete the study with a reasonable sample size.
- Measures of patient condition may require clinical expertise.

or in-depth knowledge of topics that are far afield from traditional social and personality psychology training (e.g., the physics underlying fMRI and electrophysiology).

The study of patient populations is a classic methodology for understanding the relation between brain and behavior (Kolb & Whishaw, 2003; Rorden & Karnath, 2004). In contrast to neuroimaging techniques that examine function, the patient methodology is deficit-focused. Patients with brain damage resulting from trauma or disorders are studied to understand how underlying neural deficits relate to behavioral function and impairment. This chapter discusses general issues for researchers to keep in mind when planning a patient study, and then illustrates these issues in patient populations that are often studied by social and personality psychologists: patients with brain injury resulting from trauma, stroke, or dementia; patients with depression; and patients with autism spectrum disorders. The goals of this chapter are to (1) provide guidelines for designing a scientifically rigorous patient study, and (2) help social and personality psychologists become informed consumers of research using patient methodologies.

General Issues to Consider in Designing a Study with Patients

When it comes to designing a research study, social and personality psychologists are no strangers to the usual concerns about statistical power, experimental control, and measurement reliability and validity. The addition of a patient population to a research study does not suddenly change the principles of the scientific method; however, a new layer of concerns must be addressed to execute a study that utilizes the scientific method to the fullest extent. Specifically, researchers who are planning a study that involves one or more patient populations will need to consider issues of *categorization, capability, comorbidity, availability,* and *control* in their study design (see Table 8.2). In short, how will they measure the difference between the patient and control populations (categorization); what modifications are needed to ensure that the patient population can complete the experiment (capability), are there possible confounding conditions associated with the patient population (comorbidity); what types of sample sizes should be expected for particular patient populations (availability); and what types of control populations are needed for the study (control)?

Categorization

How will researchers measure whether a participant belongs in the patient population of interest? First, they need to familiarize themselves with the "gold standard" assessment of that particular patient population. Just as social and personality psychologists use experimental manipulations or questionnaire data to establish experimental groups, patient studies require a criterion for categorizing a participant as part of the patient population of interest. For example, researchers interested in group relations may measure ingroup and outgroup status by assessing racial identity or using an experimental manipulation to create group identities (e.g., the "minimal group" paradigm; Tajfel, Billig, Bundy, & Flament, 1971). If researchers want to study participants with particular kinds of brain damage, dementia, depression, or autism spectrum disorders, what is the best way to measure those variables? What measures are considered valid and reliable? Do they require a trained professional to administer and score? Unlike the experimental manipulations and questionnaires used in social and personality psychology research, many of these evaluations are lengthy. Therefore, it is also important to consider whether these measures can be administered in the same session as the experimental paradigms.

Capability

In addition to considering whether potential referral sources will permit the kind of experimental procedure of interest, it is important to understand the capability of the patient population. Particular patient populations may involve children or older adults, or patients whose deficits

TABLE 8.2. Summary of Considerations for Patient Studies

	Brain injury resulting from trauma, stroke, or dementia	Depression	Autism spectrum disorders
Categorization	Standardized measurement requires clinical expertise and may require a separate session than the experimental session.		
	Neuropsychological batteries are helpful for establishing specificity of disorder.		
	Measures of subclinical levels do not require clinical expertise.		
Capability	Experimental sessions should be kept short.		
	Extra instruction and task practice may be necessary.		Extra instruction and task practice may be necessary.
Comorbidity	Patients may take medications that interfere with deficits and neural impairments of interest.		
	Depression, other psychiatric disorders, substance abuse	Dementia, other psychiatric disorders, substance abuse	Psychiatric disorders, mental retardation
Availability	Selective damage from trauma is rare; stroke and dementia are more common.	Availability depends on local patient referral source rather than incidence or prevalence.	
	Patient referral sources may restrict the frequency of referrals and experimental paradigms.		
Control	Patients with a different type of selective damage; patients with a different type of dementia	Patients with mania or manic symptoms	Patients with a different pervasive developmental disorder

make it difficult to use particular experimental paradigms that might be of interest to social and personality psychologists. Can the instructions and measurement tools be administered in a way that is understandable to the patient population of interest? In comparison to studies with healthy individuals, patient populations may require simpler or repeated instructions and more practice of the experimental procedure. Asking patients to verbalize their understanding of the task instructions may be necessary to confirm that they understand the task. Patient studies may also require different measurement tools. If the patients are likely to be children or to have compromised IQ because of their condition, they may have difficulty with Likert scales and questionnaires that exceed their reading level. Measures that use pictures or verbal questions and responses may be more appropriate; therefore, it is important to consider whether alternative measures are available. In addition to needing more time and special task measures, patient populations often get tired easily. Depending on the population, sessions lasting more than 1–2 hours are likely to have confounding effects of fatigue in paradigms administered near the end of the session. Although it can be more time-consuming and require more resources, it is advisable to conduct multiple sessions that are shorter in length, rather than one long session.

Comorbidity and Medication Confounds

If the goal is to study a particular patient population because of specific neural deficits, then potential comorbidities need to be identified and evaluated for possible confounding effects on brain function. Just as there are correlations among personality traits that are important to consider in studies of individual differences, many patient populations are characterized by two or more correlated diagnoses. In other words, certain disorders may co-occur with other conditions and/or require medication. The comorbid conditions and/or medication may change the underlying neural deficits in a confounding manner. Comorbid conditions may be associated with generalized brain dysfunction, making it difficult to test strongly whether deficits are associated with specific neural systems. Medications may bolster function and reduce the deficits that make the patient population of interest. If there is a possible confound, then it will be necessary to exclude participants on the basis of comorbidity. The measurement of comorbid conditions will be subject to all of the same considerations mentioned for measuring the condition of interest.

Availability

Other important issues to consider in planning a patient study are the number of potential participants and the frequency with which patients become available to participate in research. Access to particular patient populations may be restricted for a variety of reasons. Some patient populations may be difficult to access without a collaborator who has clinical or medical expertise. Even with such a collaborator, some conditions that lead to selective brain damage are rare, and it may be difficult to find more than a few participants. For example, research on amygdala damage is often conducted with patients who have Urbach–Wiethe disease. This disease affects only about 200,000 people in the U.S. population; amygdala calcification only occurs in about 50% of these people; and the calcification often extends beyond the amygdala (e.g., Anderson & Phelps, 2000; Siebert, Markowitsch, & Bartel, 2003). Even if a local patient referral source had information on these patients already, the low prevalence of this disease as well as the even lower prevalence of selective amygdala damage guarantees a small sample size. It is important to anticipate a small sample size, so that researchers can focus on paradigms that will yield effect sizes detectable in small samples.

Established patient cohorts that are sampled by a large number of researchers may be also subject to certain restrictions. Coordinators of patient referrals often put restrictions on how frequently they will provide information on potential study participants, to ensure that the participants are not overwhelmed with requests for testing. Scientists who have used the patient cohort in previous studies will be a valuable source of information about expected sample sizes and time investment for completing a study. This information will be important for deciding whether it is feasible to have access to the necessary testing facility and study funding for that time period (often more than a year for one study with rare patients). In addition, coordinators of established patient cohorts may restrict the types of experimental paradigms that can be used with their population. In order to retain patients' participation in the recruitment pool, coordinators may not allow them to take part in experimental procedures that may be upsetting. For example, deception is used in a number of social psychology procedures; patient coordinators may be concerned that patients will have a negative response to the debriefing and will refuse to participate in any further research studies.

Control

In patient studies, control procedures and populations may be more extensive than in studies that only include healthy participants. Patients are likely to have a wide variety of deficits, and therefore control tasks are needed to test whether patients' deficits are really specific to the social or personality process of interest. For example, if patients do not accurately identify emotional states or personality traits from pictures of people, is it because they have trouble representing the mental states of other people? Or is it because they have impaired perception of faces, because they perform more poorly on any abstract task, and/or because they perform poorly on all tasks? Most studies include neuropsychological batteries that measure the cognitive capabilities of the patient population. However, the neuropsychological battery may not address all of the relevant abilities. For example, a study of emotional or personality facial judgment might also include a test of general facial judgment, such as the Benton Facial Recognition Test (BFRT: Benton, Sivan, Hamsher, Varney, & Spreen, 1983). The BFRT will assess participants' level of facial perception abilities, such as whether they can match faces on the basis of physical features.

In addition to control tasks that may not be included in the categorization measurement, it is important to identify meaningful control populations. It is optimal to include a healthy control population as well as a relevant control patient population. The inclusion of a control patient population ensures that any significant deficits are specific to the patient population of interest and not to any patient population. In addition, it is often necessary to match control participants to the patient populations on age, gender, and education level. Healthy control participants who are willing to take part in experiments tend to be adults with at least a college education. In contrast, some patient populations tend to be children, older adults, or adults with a high school education or less. Therefore, it is important to anticipate the recruitment of appropriate control participants.

Unlike participants from university recruitment pools, patients and healthy control participants are unfamiliar with experimental procedures and may try to engage in conversation with the experimenter. Often these participants are uncomfortable in the unfamiliar experimental setting, so every effort should be made to reduce their anxiety. However, it is also important to remember that the content of conversation should be kept standardized and focused on the experiment as much as possible, so as not to introduce any confounding factors. For example, studies with patients that examine social interaction skills such as teasing (e.g., Beer, Heerey, Keltner, Scabini, & Knight, 2003; Heerey, Capps, Keltner, & Kring, 2005) could be confounded if the experimenters were to make personal small talk with either the patient population or the control participant population. The personal nature of side conversations could result in a greater feeling of intimacy, which could affect participants' comfort levels with different types of teasing. If the patients expressed teasing behaviors that is not appropriate between strangers, it might not be because of their condition, but because the experimenter was accurately perceived as less of a stranger by the group that engaged in personal conversation.

Finally, another important control issue is the lack of random assignment in all patient research. Often researchers will get referrals from a clinician who works with the patient population of interest. It is important to think through the role of the patient referral source. If the person who refers the patients for study is aware of the study hypothesis and also conducts the experimental sessions, he or she may inadvertently select patients from the patient pool who are likely to confirm the hypothesis, or may create experimental demand when conducting the experimental session. Lack of random assignment also needs to be considered in the interpretation of the data. In contrast to patients with selective brain injury, patients who have psychiatric disorders or develop progressive neurological disorders may have different developmental neural trajectories. Therefore, there are potential differences in general brain function within these latter two groups, not just in the areas typically implicated by a particular condition.

Issues to Consider in Planning Studies with Specific Patient Populations

Social and personality psychologists interested in investigating brain–behavior relationships usually have one of two reasons for studying patient populations. First, they may want to understand commonalities between psychological processes by investigating whether they are governed by the same neural systems. Second, the brain dysfunction associated with some conditions results in selective deficits in a social or personality process. In this case, the comparison of the patient population with a healthy control population is a proxy for manipulating the psychological process and understanding its downstream effects on other processes. This may be particularly helpful for investigating psychological processes that are difficult to elicit in a laboratory setting. Therefore, the selection of a patient population should focus on the specificity of brain damage and/or the specificity of psychological impairment. Patients with *specific lesions* provide the strongest avenue for understanding how damage to specific brain regions affects one or more personality and social processes. Patients with *specific social or personality impairments* provide the strongest avenue for understanding how that behavioral impairment affects subsequent behavior. Drawing on these principles and the general considerations outlined above, social and personality psychologists often study patient populations that have (1) fairly specific brain injuries resulting from either trauma, stroke, or early-stage frontotemporal dementia; or (2) mood and/or social impairments such as depression and autism spectrum disorders.

Patients with Brain Injury Resulting from Trauma, Stroke, or Dementia

Studying patients with selective brain damage is one way to understand how psychological processes are related to one another. For example, research with patients who have amygdala lesions shows that these patients may have difficulty recognizing facial expressions of emotion, but they do not have trouble posing facial expressions of emotion (Adolphs et al., 1999; Anderson & Phelps, 2000). This research suggests that the ability to recognize an emotional expression does not depend on being able to pose that expression. Patients with selective damage can also be helpful for manipulating psychological processes that are otherwise difficult to manipulate in the lab. For example, patients with orbitofrontal cortex damage have poor self-regulation skills and frequently make social mistakes such as disclosing too much personal information, assuming that others share their perspective, and making poor decisions about how to resolve interpersonal dilemmas (e.g., Beer et al., 2003; Beer, Knight, & D'Esposito, 2006; Beer, Shimamura, & Knight, 2004; Kaczmarek, 1984; Saver & Damasio, 1991). Although social mistakes do occur in everyday life, they are few and far between because of socialization processes. Participants may be particularly self-conscious in a lab setting and exert extra effort to avoid social mistakes. Therefore, comparing patients with orbitofrontal damage to healthy controls is one way to test the relation between self-regulatory ability and dependent social–personality processes. For example, the self-regulation deficits of patients with orbitofrontal damage are associated with impaired self-conscious emotions, not with other kinds of emotions (Beer et al., 2003, 2006). These studies provide support for the theory that self-conscious emotions are important for regulating social behavior (e.g., Keltner & Beer, 2005; Tangney, 2003).

Researchers desiring specificity of brain damage will benefit most from studies of patients with brain injury from trauma, stroke, and (to a lesser degree) early-stage frontotemporal dementia. Focal lesions are most often the results of trauma from accidents, although strokes and the early stages of dementia can also affect brain function in fairly selective ways (e.g., Gazzaniga, Ivry, & Mangun, 2009; Kolb & Whishaw, 2003; Perry et al., 2001). Furthermore, trauma, stroke, and dementia often impair brain regions that are most likely to interest social and personality psychologists. For example, the jagged ridges that hold the eye orbits in place often selectively damage the orbitofrontal cortex. In a high-speed collision, the brain may bounce against the back of the skull and then shoot forward against the jagged ridges, causing damage to the orbitofrontal region. Strokes of the anterior communicating artery may also affect orbitofrontal tissue in a relatively selective manner (e.g., Bechara, Damasio, Tranel, & Damasio, 1997). In the early stages, patients with frontotemporal lobe dementia may experience relatively pronounced atrophy in specific brain regions, including the orbitofrontal cortex, amygdala, or temporal lobe (e.g., Perry et al., 2001).

Categorization

Categorizing patients with brain injury from trauma, stroke, or dementia can be fairly straightforward but may require neurological expertise. Most patient studies include information about each patient's specific brain damage (location and volume); the cause of injury, whether it be trauma, stroke, or disease; and the length of time since the injury or onset of disease. This information requires some expertise with identifying damage from a brain scan, as well as permission to access patients' medical records. The extent and regional specificity of damage will not be exactly the same for all participants, even if they all sustained their damage in the same way. If the volume of the damage differs dramatically among patients, it might be necessary to test lesion volume as a predictor for the experimental effects of interest. The length of time since the injury is also important, because the brain may swell after sustaining injury, and function may be affected outside the primary area of injury for 6 months to 1 year afterward.

Capability

Patient studies should include assessments of IQ and basic cognitive functioning to understand whether experimental effects are accounted for by a general impairment. Many standardized measures of IQ and basic cognitive functioning require some neuropsychological training to administer and score properly. These tests are often included in neuropsychological batteries in medical facilities, and the source for patient referrals may have access to patients' scores. The Mini-Mental State Exam (Folstein, Folstein, & McHugh, 1975) takes about 10 min and is widely used to measure basic cognitive functioning. Measures of IQ may include the Barona Demographic Index (Barona, Reynolds. & Chastain, 1984); the National Adult Reading Test (NART; Nelson, 1982); and the Wechsler Abbreviated Scale of Intelligence (WASI; Wechsler, 1999). The Barona Demographic Index and NART are typically used to estimate preinjury IQ, and the WASI measures current IQ. Memory and cognitive flexibility may be measured with the Wechsler Memory Scale—Third Edition (Wechsler, 1997); the California Verbal Learning Test (Delis, Kramer, Kaplan, & Ober, 1987); the Rey–Osterrieth Complex Figure (Meyers & Meyers, 1995) and the Wisconsin Card Sorting Test (Heaton, Chelune, Talley, Kay, & Curtiss, 1993). Extensive guides to neuropsychological assessment are also available (Kolb & Whishaw, 2003; Lezak, 1995).

Patients with brain injury, particularly those stemming from stroke or dementia, tend to be elderly, and it is usually important for researchers to allow extra time and practice when providing experimental instructions. Such patients may also tire easily, so experimental sessions should be kept short. Researchers will understandably want to include as many measures as possible once they have managed to recruit a patient for the study. However, it cannot be stressed enough that the best way to get reliable data in patient populations that are vulnerable to fatigue is to conduct multiple shorter sessions, rather than one long session.

Comorbidity

Although patients with brain injury resulting from trauma, stroke and early-stage frontotemporal dementia may be the best bets for studying the psychological consequences of fairly specific brain damage, comorbidity issues still need to be considered. Nonrandom assignment may be a particular concern for scientists interested in individual differences. If focal lesions result from trauma or stroke, it is important to consider whether these patients differed prospectively on personality dimensions (e.g., risk taking or chronic stress) or psychopathology, which may have made them more likely to incur their brain injury. Patients from any of these groups may also suffer from depression, which may extend their deficits past the effect of their selective lesions. Furthermore, antidepressant medications and medications such as Aricept that bolster cognitive and memory functioning (often prescribed for dementia) may diminish the brain deficits that are of interest. Finally, because many of the regions selectively damaged by traumatic brain injury, stroke, and frontotemporal dementia result in disinhibited behavior, these patients may abuse drugs and alcohol. Therefore, it is important to screen for possible substance and alcohol dependence (see, e.g., Neary, 1999).

Availability

The frequency of patients with specific kinds of brain damage differs, depending on whether the brain damage resulted from traumatic injury, stroke, or frontotemporal dementia. Focal lesions that arise from traumatic injury (e.g., a car accident) are rare, and it is not the case that all parts of the brain are affected. For example, even though patients with orbitofrontal damage are rare, it is even rarer to find patients with selective damage to other brain regions of interest to social and personality psychologists. Selective damage to regions such as the medial prefrontal cortex, caudate, or anterior cingulate is not very likely to occur. These regions are deep within the brain and are either buffered in traumatic accidents or damaged in addition to surface areas. Patients sustaining brain damage from strokes are more frequent than patients with focal lesions caused by trauma. Like traumatic lesions, strokes tend to affect particular brain regions more than others. Strokes are mostly attributed to burst aneurysms in the circle of Willis at the base of the brain, or occur in "watershed" areas (i.e., the brain regions that are the most distal to major arteries). Therefore, patients with strokes that affect regions outside these areas are fairly rare; patients with specific stroke-related damage to the orbitofrontal cortex or dorsolateral prefrontal cortex may be of the most interest to social and personality psychologists. Patients with frontotemporal dementia are rarer than patients with Alzheimer dementia (e.g., Neary, 1999), but are potentially easier to find than patients with very selective damage from traumatic injury. Patients with early-stage frontotemporal dementia may have a large percentage of atrophy concentrated in the frontal lobes, the amygdala, or the temporal lobes (e.g., Perry et al., 2001). It is important to remember that dementias are progressive diseases. Although atrophy may appear concentrated to a particular region, it is likely that atrophy has begun in other regions, even though it may not be detectable in a brain scan at the early stages. The limited availability of these patients makes it important to focus on experimental paradigms that yield reliable and robust effects in small numbers of healthy comparison subjects.

Control

Studies that include patients with brain injury resulting from trauma, stroke, or early-stage frontotemporal dementia should ideally include healthy comparison participants as well as a patient control population. The patient control population rules out the possibility that experimental effects are accounted for by any kind of brain damage. In other words, it is important to test whether experimental effects are seen in any patient population or are significant in the patient population of interest. For example, patients with orbitofrontal lesions caused by trauma or stroke are often compared to healthy control participants and participants with selective damage to a different region in the frontal cortex (e.g., Beer et al., 2006; Berlin, Rolls, & Kischka, 2004). The inclusion of patients with different kinds of frontal lobe damage is an especially strong design, because the frontal lobes are involved in a number of executive functions. Significant effects in one group suggest that the deficits are associated not only with a particular brain region, but with a specific kind of executive function as well. Studies of patients with frontotemporal dementia often include a patient control population that has a different kind of dementia (such as Alzheimer dementia), or a psychiatric disorder that involves the frontal lobes (such as depression) (e.g., Elderkin-Thompson, Boone, Hwang, & Kumar, 2004; Mioshi et al., 2007).

The inclusion of specific, a priori patient populations is important, because studies of patients with diffuse brain damage begin to lose utility as a measure of the neurobiology underlying social and personality processes. For example, one study compared the pretrauma and post-trauma measures of the "Big Five" dimensions of personality between patients with head injuries and patients with non-head injuries (Lannoo, de Deyne, Colardyn, de Soete, & Jannes, 1997). Peer reports from relatives were collected for almost all of the patients with head injuries. The researchers found that both patient groups reported significant changes in their personalities following their traumas, but did not differ from one another. Specifically, patients reported increased neuroticism, decreased extraversion, and decreased conscientiousness after their traumas. In comparison to their relatives, patients with head injuries reported a smaller reduction in extraversion and conscientiousness. However, it is difficult to draw any conclusions from this study, because the area and extent of head injury for each patient were not reported. If patients had been classified as to type and area of brain damage, the results might have suggested whether particular personality traits change more as a function of damage to areas associated with specific functions.

Patients with Social and Personality Deficits Resulting from Depression and Autism Spectrum Disorders

Although the study of patients with selective brain damage provides the strongest avenue for understanding how one or more psychological processes share a common neural basis, another possible methodology is to patients who have mood and/or social deficits because of a condition that affects multiple brain regions, such as depression or autism spectrum disorders. One particular advantage is that it may be easier to access patients with such conditions. Generally, studying psychiatric populations is most beneficial for understanding how behavioral impairments relate to other behavioral impairments.

Patients with Depression

Depression is associated with dysfunction in limbic areas of the brain (e.g., frontal lobes, temporal lobes, anterior cingulate), which presumably gives rise to the chronic negative mood of patients with this condition (Ressler & Mayberg, 2007). Comparisons of patients with depression and healthy controls are one approach to understanding the effects of negative mood on a variety of social and personality processes. For example, research from studies of patients with depression provides support for theories that cognitions are often influenced in a mood-congruent manner (e.g., Bower, 1981); it may be that the dysphoric mood of these patients especially influences effortful information processing (Hartlage, Alloy, Vazquez, & Dykman, 1993). In comparison to healthy control participants, patients with depression interpret facial expressions of emotion with a negative bias. Sad and angry faces are most easily recognized; neutral faces are perceived as sad; and happy faces are perceived as neutral (e.g., Gur et al., 1992; Mandel & Battacharya, 1985).

Categorization

There are several standardized measures of depression; some require administration by a trained clinician, and others do not. Some of the most common measurements are the Structured Clinical Interview for DSM-IV (SCID-II; First, Spitzer, Gibbon, & Williams, 1997); the Modified Hamilton Rating Scale for Depression (Miller, Bishop, Norman, & Maddever, 1985); and the Beck Depression Inventory (Beck, Ward, Mendelson, Mock, & Erbaugh, 1961). The administration of the SCID-II can be quite a lengthy process, because it is an interview rather than a questionnaire, unlike the other measures. If the SCID-II is used, it may be a good idea to plan two sessions, so that patients begin the experimental portion without having just completed the lengthy interview. As mentioned above, often the referral source for patients with depression may have access to scores on these measures that were acquired when the patients were initially accepted for treatment.

Capability

It is unlikely that depressed patients will struggle with task instructions because of their depression. However, if the patients are elderly, it is important to include repeated task instructions, to provide extra practice for the experimental tasks, and to keep the length of the experimental session reasonable. A neuropsychological battery will be essential for testing the extent of deficits.

Comorbidity

Clinical levels of depression may commonly co-occur with any number of other psychiatric disorders (e.g., somatization disorder, schizophrenia), Axis II (personality) disorders, dementia, and substance abuse. In addition, many patients with depression take medications to change the deficits that make them of interest to social and personality researchers. Screening for clinical levels of depression and the possible comorbid conditions requires a big time investment, and thorough measurement requires clinical training. For social and personality researchers, it is ideal to have a collaborator refer patients who have already had expert assessments. Another possibility is for social and personality researchers to measure subclinical levels or proneness to depressive symptoms. For example, the General Behavior Inventory (Depue, Krauss, Spoont, & Arbisi, 1989) measures how prone individuals are to developing mania or depression and is easily administered without a clinician.

Availability

Patients with clinical or subclinical levels of depression are relatively prevalent, in comparison to the other patient populations mentioned in this chapter. The main restriction may be access to a collaborator who can refer patients for research. University participant pools may be characterized by meaningful individual differences in dysphoric mood states (rather than severe depression). Therefore, studies of patients with depression or participants with dysphoria are likely to involve larger samples than many of the patient populations discussed in this chapter. Researchers interested in studying psychological phenomena with smaller effect sizes may find that they are able to get sufficient statistical power from a population with depression.

Control

In addition to healthy control participants, studies of depression might include patient populations with a different mood disorder, in order to rule out general patient effects. Comparisons between patients with unipolar depression and patients with either a manic or a depressive state are one way of studying the effects of chronic negative and positive moods. For example, one study found that patients with bipolar disorder show mood-congruent effects on perception of emotional facial expressions (less sensitivity to happy faces and increased attention to negative emotional faces) when they exhibited depressed symptoms but not manic symptoms (Gray et al., 2006).

Patients with Autism Spectrum Disorders

Autism spectrum disorders are interesting examples of disorders that affect limbic structures (e.g., Bachevalier & Loveland, 2006; Kennedy, Redcay, & Courchesne, 2006) and primarily have consequences for social and personality processes (e.g., Bryson, Rogers, & Fombonne, 2003). Comparing patients with autism, high-functioning autism, and

Asperger syndrome to healthy control children is one way to understand how one social deficit may be related to another. In addition, the comparisons of these patients and healthy controls are one avenue for manipulating psychological processes that may be difficult to manipulate experimentally. "Theory of mind"—that is, the ability to understand that other people have mental states that differ from one's own mental states—is typically impaired in patients with autism spectrum disorders (e.g., Capps & Sigman, 1996; Flavell, 1999). Therefore, comparisons of patients with autism and healthy participants can be considered to be a proxy manipulation of theory-of-mind ability. One study showed that patients with high-functioning autism and Asperger syndrome had difficulty recognizing facial expressions of self-conscious emotions, and that this deficit was mediated by their theory-of-mind deficits (Heerey, Keltner, & Capps, 2003).

Categorization

Standardized measures of autism and Asperger syndrome often involve interviews with one or both parents of a patient. For example, the Autism Diagnostic Interview—Revised (Lord, Rutter, & Le Couteur, 1994) and the Pervasive Developmental Disorders Screening Test (Siegel, 1986) are often used to confirm diagnoses. Many of the neuropsychological measures mentioned in the section on patients with brain injury are also administered in studies of autism spectrum disorders, in order to understand the depth of deficits in the experimental sample.

Capability

The high comorbidity of autism and mental retardation (Bregman & Volkmar, 1988; Ghaziuddin, Tsai, & Ghaziuddin, 1992; Zafeiriou, Ververi, & Vargiami, 2007) makes administration of a thorough neuropsychological battery essential with this patient population. It will be necessary to report IQ scores and other measures of basic cognitive functioning, in order to test whether deficits are related to general impairment.

Most studies of autism spectrum disorders include children; therefore, it is essential to consider the developmental appropriateness of the measurement used in experimental sessions. For example, many theory-of-mind measures require the experimenter to read vignettes aloud to the participants and often have accompanying pictures (Baron-Cohen, Leslie, & Frith, 1985; Happé, 1994; Wimmer & Perner, 1983). Another option is to act out social scenarios with standardized puppet shows (Measelle, Ablow, Cowan, & Cowan, 1998).

In addition, it is important to consider the capabilities of the healthy children who will be studied in comparison. For example, certain emotions and emotion regulation processes develop across the lifespan. Therefore, if the children with autism spectrum disorders are studied to examine impaired emotion regulation processes or complex emotion, it will be important to consider whether the comparison healthy children will really be capable of the processes in question. For example, in the study of facial expressions of emotion conducted mentioned above (Heerey et al., 2003), the youngest participants were 8 years old; healthy children who were younger may have shown the same recognition deficits as the patient population.

Comorbidity

Autism spectrum disorders are comorbid with a large number of other conditions. Patients with autism may also be diagnosed with other types of psychiatric disorders, such as bipolar disorder and possibly depression (e.g., Matson & Nebel-Schwalm, 2007). Patients with autism may also have various forms of mental retardation, such as those associated with Down syndrome and fragile X syndrome (e.g., Bregman & Volkmar, 1988; Ghaziuddin et al., 1992; Zafeiriou et al., 2007). Therefore, it is essential to collaborate with a clinician or medical facility that can evaluate possible comorbidities in patients with autism.

Availability

The availability of patients with autism spectrum disorders may not be a problem, particularly if there is a local medical facility devoted to their treatment. It is important to note that autism spectrum disorders affect boys more often than girls (Capps & Sigman, 1996); therefore, there may be some difficulty in recruiting equal numbers of male and female patients. Researchers studying psychological processes that may be related to significant gender differences may find that autism is not well suited for their interests, or that more time will need to be spent in order to get equal numbers of patients of both genders.

Control

Patient studies of autism spectrum disorders most often include children, and therefore it is important to consider where healthy comparison participants will be recruited. The comparison participants need to be screened for autism spectrum disorders, other pervasive developmental disorders, and psychiatric history. The groups are typically matched on a number of demographic and ability characteristics, such as verbal IQ, chronological age (as opposed to developmental age), and gender (see Ozonoff, Rogers, & Pennington, 1991).

Conclusion

Patient studies are a useful approach for examining the implications of neural function for social and personality processes. Studies with patients may require some modification of experimental measures and greater time investment than studies that only include healthy participants. However, they lend themselves to a wider range of experimental paradigms in comparison to most neuroimaging techniques. Although this chapter has focused on brain injury resulting from trauma, stroke, and dementia, as well as on depression and autism spectrum disorders, all of the information here can be applied to any patient population of interest. With a little attention to issues of categorization, capability, comorbidity, availability, and control, social and personality psychologists will find that patient studies are useful tools to add to their current repertoire and may provide new insight into their psychological phenomena of interest.

References

Adolphs, R., Tranel, D., Hamann, S., Young, A. W., Calder, A. J., Phelps, E. A., et al. (1999). Recognition of facial emotion in nine individuals with bilateral amygdala damage. *Neuropsychologia, 37*, 1111–1117.

Anderson, A., & Phelps, E. (2000). Expression without recognition: Contributions of the amygdala to emotional communication. *Psychological Science, 11*, 106–111.

Bachevalier, J., & Loveland, K. A. (2006). The orbitofrontal–amygdala circuit and self-regulation of social-emotional behavior in autism. *Neuroscience and Biobehavioral Reviews, 30*, 97–117.

Barona, A., Reynolds, C. R., & Chastain, R. (1984). A demographically based index of premorbid intelligence for the WAIS-R. *Journal of Consulting and Clinical Psychology, 52*, 885–887.

Baron-Cohen, S., Leslie, A., & Frith, U. (1985). Does the autistic child have a "theory of mind"? *Cognition, 21*, 37–46.

Bechara, A., Damasio, H., Tranel, D., & Damasio, A. R. (1997). Deciding advantageously before knowing the advantageous strategy. *Science, 275*, 1293–1295.

Beck, A. T., Ward, C. H., Mendelson, M., Mock, J., & Erbaugh, J. (1961). An inventory for measuring depression. *Archives of General Psychiatry, 4*, 561–571.

Beer, J. S., Heerey, E. H., Keltner, D., Scabini, D., & Knight, R. T. (2003). The regulatory function of self-conscious emotion: Insights from patients with orbitofrontal damage. *Journal of Personality and Social Psychology, 85,* 594–604.

Beer, J. S., Knight, R. T., & D'Esposito, M. (2006). Integrating emotion and cognition: The role of the frontal lobes in distinguishing between helpful and hurtful emotion. *Psychological Science, 17,* 448–453.

Beer, J. S., & Lombardo, M. V. (2007). Patient and neuroimaging methodologies. In R. W. Robins, R. C. Fraley, & R. F. Krueger (Eds.), *Handbook of research methods in personality psychology* (pp. 360–369). New York: Guilford Press.

Beer, J. S., Shimamura, A. P., & Knight, R. T. (2004). Frontal lobe contributions to executive control of cognitive and social behavior. In M. S. Gazzaniga (Ed.), *The cognitive neurosciences III* (pp. 1091–1104). Cambridge, MA: MIT Press.

Benton, A. L., Sivan, A. B., Hamsher, K. de S., Varney, N. R., & Spreen, O. (1983). *Facial recognition: Stimulus and multiple choice pictures.* New York: Oxford University Press.

Berlin, H. A., Rolls, E. T., & Kischka, U. (2004). Impulsivity, time perception, emotion and reinforcement sensitivity in patients with orbitofrontal cortex lesions. *Brain, 127,* 1108–1126.

Bower, G. H. (1981). Mood and memory. *American Psychologist, 36,* 129–148.

Bregman, J. D., & Volkmar, F. R. (1988). Autistic social dysfunction and Down's syndrome. *Journal of the American Academy of Child and Adolescent Psychiatry, 27,* 440–441.

Bryson, S. E., Rogers, S. J., & Fombonne, E. (2003). Autism spectrum disorders: Early detection and intervention, education, and psychopharmacological management. *Canadian Journal of Psychiatry, 48,* 506–516.

Capps, L., & Sigman, M. (1996). Autistic aloneness. In R. D. Kavanaugh, B. Zimmerberg, & S. Fein (Eds.), *Emotion: Interdisciplinary perspectives* (pp. 273–296). Mahwah, NJ: Erlbaum.

Delis, D. C., Kramer, J. H., Kaplan, E., & Ober, B. A. (1987). *California Verbal Learning Test: Adult Version manual.* San Antonio, TX: Psychological Corporation.

Depue, R. A., Krauss, S., Spoont, M. R., & Arbisi, P. (1989). General Behavior Inventory identification of unipolar and bipolar affective conditions in a nonclinical university population. *Journal of Abnormal Psychology, 98,* 117–126.

Elderkin-Thompson, V., Boone, K. B., Hwang, S., & Kumar, A. (2004). Neurocognitive profiles in elderly patients with frontotemporal dementia or major depressive disorder. *Journal of the International Neuropsychological Society, 10,* 753–771.

First, M. B., Spitzer, R. L., Gibbon, M., & Williams, J B. W. (1997). *Structured Clinical Interview for DSM-IV Personality Disorders (SCID-II).* Washington, DC: American Psychiatric Press.

Flavell, J. H. (1999). Cognitive development: Children's knowledge about the mind. *Annual Review of Psychology, 50,* 21–45.

Folstein, M. F., Folstein, S. E., & McHugh, P. R. (1975). Mini-Mental State: A practical method for grading the cognitive state of patients for the clinician. *Journal of Psychiatric Research, 12,* 189–198.

Gazzaniga, M. S., Ivry, R. I., & Mangun, G. M. (2009). *Cognitive neuroscience: The biology of the mind* (3rd ed.). New York: Norton.

Ghaziuddin, M., Tsai, L., & Ghaziuddin, N. (1992). Autism in Down's syndrome: Presentation and diagnosis. *Journal of Intellectual Disability Research, 36,* 449–456.

Gray, J., Venn, H., Montagne, B., Murray, L., Burt, M., Frigerio, E., et al. (2006). Bipolar patients show mood-congruent biases in sensitivity to facial expressions of emotion when exhibiting depressed symptoms but not when exhibiting manic symptoms. *Cognitive Neuropsychiatry, 11,* 505–520.

Gur, R. C., Erwin, R. J., Gur, R. E., Zwil, A. S., Heimberg, C., & Kraemer, H. C. (1992). Facial emotion discrimination: II. Behavioural findings in depression. *Psychiatry Research, 42,* 241–251.

Happé, F. G. E. (1994). An advanced test of theory of mind: Understanding of story characters' thoughts and feelings by able autistic, mentally handicapped, and normal children and adults. *Journal of Autism and Developmental Disorders, 24,* 129–154.

Hartlage, S., Alloy, L. B., Vazquez, C., & Dykman, B. (1993). Automatic and effortful processing in depression. *Psychological Bulletin, 113,* 247–278.

Heaton, R. K., Chelune, G. J., Talley, J. L., Kay, G. G., & Curtiss, G. (1993). *Wisconsin Card Sorting Test manual.* Odessa, FL: Psychological Assessment Resources.

Heerey, E. A., Capps, L. M., Keltner, D., & Kring, A. M. (2005). Understanding teasing: Lessons from children with autism. *Journal of Abnormal Child Psychology, 33,* 55–68.

Heerey, E. A., Keltner, D., & Capps, L. (2003). Making sense of self-conscious emotion: Linking theory of mind and emotion in children with autism. *Emotion, 3,* 394–400.

Kaczmarek, B. L. J. (1984). Neurolinguistic analysis of verbal utterances in patients with focal lesions of frontal lobes. *Brain and Language, 21,* 52–58.

Keltner, D., & Beer, J. S. (2005). Self-conscious emotion and self-regulation. In A. Tesser, J. V. Wood, & D. A. Stapel (Eds.), *On building, defending and regulating the self* (pp. 197–216). New York: Psychology Press.

Kennedy, D. P., Redcay, E., & Courchesne, E. (2006). Failing to deactivate: Resting functional abnormalities in autism. *Proceedings of the National Academy of Sciences USA, 103,* 8275–8280.

Kolb, B., & Whishaw, I. Q. (2003). *Fundamentals of human neuropsychology.* New York: Worth.

Lannoo, E., de Deyne, C., Colardyn, F., de Soete, G., & Jannes, C. (1997). Personality change following head injury: Assessment with the NEO Five-Factor Inventory. *Journal of Psychosomatic Research, 43,* 505–511.

Lezak, M. (1995). *Neuropsychological assessment* (3rd ed.). New York: Oxford University Press.

Lord, C., Rutter, M., & Le Couteur, A. (1994). Autism Diagnostic Interview— Revised: A revised version of the diagnostic interview for caregivers of individuals with possible pervasive developmental disorders. *Journal of Autism and Developmental Disorders, 31,* 367–376.

Mandel, M. K., & Bhattacharya, B. B. (1985). Recognition of facial affect in depression. *Perceptual and Motor Skills, 61,* 13–14.

Matson, J. L., & Nebel-Schwalm, M. S. (2007). Comorbid psychopathology with autism spectrum disorder in children: An overview. *Research on Developmental Disorders, 28,* 341–352.

Measelle, J. R., Ablow, J. C., Cowan, P. A., & Cowan, C. P. (1998). Assessing young children's self-perceptions of their academic, social and emotional lives: An evaluation of the Berkeley Puppet Interview. *Child Development, 69,* 1556–1576.

Meyers, J., & Meyers, K. (1995). *The Meyers Scoring System for the Rey Complex Figure and the Recognition Trial: Professional manual.* Odessa, FL: Psychological Assessment Resources.

Miller, I. W., Bishop, S., Norman, W. H., & Maddever, H. (1985). The modified Hamilton Rating Scale for Depression: Reliability and validity. *Psychiatry Research, 14,* 131–142.

Mioshi, E., Kipps, C. M., Dawson, K., Mitchell, J., Graham, A., & Hodges, J. R. (2007). Activities of daily living in frontotemporal dementia and Alzheimer disease. *Neurology, 68,* 2077–2084.

Neary, D. (1999). Overview of frontotemporal dementias and the consensus applied. *Dementia, Geriatric and Cognitive Disorders, 10*(Suppl. 1), 6–9.

Nelson, H. E. (1982). *The National Adult Reading Test (NART).* Windsor, Ontario, Canada: Nelson.

Ozonoff, S., Rogers, S. J., & Pennington, B. F. (1991). Asperger's syndrome: Evidence of an empirical distinction from high-functioning autism. *Journal of Child Psychology and Psychiatry, 32,* 1107–1122.

Perry, R. J., Rosen, H. R., Kramer, J. H., Beer, J. S., Levenson, R. L., & Miller, B. L. (2001). Hemispheric dominance for emotions, empathy and social behaviour: Evidence from right and left handers with frontotemporal dementia. *Neurocase, 7,* 145–160.

Ressler, K. J., & Mayberg, H. S. (2007). Targeting abnormal neural circuits in mood and anxiety disorders: Drom the laboratory to the clinic. *Nature Neuroscience, 10,* 1116–1124.

Rorden, C., & Karnath, H. O. (2004). Using human brain lesions to infer function: A relic from a past era in the fMRI age? *Nature Reviews Neuroscience, 5,* 813–819.

Saver, J. L., & Damasio, A. R. (1991). Preserved access and processing of social knowledge in a patient with acquired sociopathy due to ventromedial frontal damage. *Neuropsychologia, 29,* 1241–1249.

Siebert, M., Markowitsch, H. J., & Bartel, P. (2003). Amygdala, affect and cognition: Evidence from 10 patients with Urbach–Wiethe disease. *Brain, 12,* 2627–2637.

Siegel, B. (1986). Empirically derived subclassification of the autistic syndrome. *Journal of Autism and Developmental Disorders, 16*, 275–293.

Tajfel, H., Billig, M. G., Bundy, R. F., & Flament, C. (1971). Social categorization and intergroup behavior. *European Journal of Social Psychology, 1*, 149–177.

Tangney, J. P. (2003). Self-relevant emotions. In M. R. Leary & J. P. Tangney (Eds.), *Handbook of self and identity* (pp. 384–400). New York: Guilford Press.

Wechsler, D. (1997). *Wechsler Memory Scale—Third Edition*. San Antonio, TX: Psychological Corporation.

Wechsler, D. (1999). *Wechsler Abbreviated Scale of Intelligence*. San Antonio, TX: Psychological Corporation.

Wimmer, H., & Perner, J. (1983). Beliefs about beliefs: Representation and constraining function of wrong beliefs in young children's understanding of deception. *Cognition, 13*, 103–128.

Zafeiriou, D. I., Ververi, A., & Vargiami, E. (2007). Childhood autism and associated comorbidities. *Brain Development, 29*, 257–272.

9

Electroencephalographic Methods in Social and Personality Psychology

Eddie Harmon-Jones
Carly K. Peterson

Physiology Underlying Electroencephalography

The recording of electrical brain activity from the human scalp is referred to as electroencephalography (EEG). It was discovered by Hans Berger in the late 1920s (see Berger, 1929), and since then has been used as a measure of brain function in studies on basic psychological and motor processes, as well as in studies of psychological and motor dysfunction.

The observed EEG at the human scalp is the result of electrical voltages generated inside the brain. Electrical activity associated with neurons comes from "action potentials" and "postsynaptic potentials" (see Figure 9.1 for an illustration of a neuron). An action potential is a discrete voltage spike that runs from the beginning of the axon at the cell body to the axon terminals where neurotransmitters are released. A postsynaptic potential is a voltage that occurs when the neurotransmitters bind to receptors on the membrane of the postsynaptic cell. This

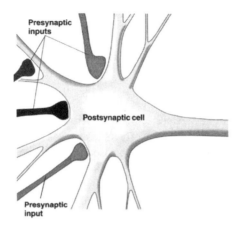

FIGURE 9.1. Illustration of a neuron.

binding causes ion channels to open or close, and it leads to a graded
change in the electrical potential across the cell membrane. In contrast
to EEG measurements, when electrical activity is measured by placing
an electrode in the intercellular space, action potentials are more easily measured than postsynaptic potentials, because of the difficulty of
isolating a single neuron's postsynaptic potentials in extracellular space.
Thus recording of individual neurons or single-unit recordings measure
action potentials and not postsynaptic potentials.

Scalp-recorded EEG does not measure action potentials because of
the timing of action potentials and the physical arrangement of axons.
That is, unless the neurons fire within microseconds of each other,
action potentials in different axons will typically cancel each other out.
If one neuron fires shortly after another one, then current at a given
location will be flowing into one axon at the same time that it is flowing
out of another one, and thus they cancel each other out and produce a
much smaller signal at the electrode. Whereas the duration of an action
potential is approximately 1 msec, the duration of postsynaptic potentials is much longer, often tens or hundreds of milliseconds. Postsynaptic
potentials are also mostly confined to dendrites and cell bodies, and
occur instantaneously rather than traveling down axons at a fixed rate.
These factors allow postsynaptic potentials to summate rather than cancel each other out, and thus make it possible to record them at the scalp.
Because of the need for summation of electrical potentials, EEG activity
is most likely the result of postsynaptic potentials, which have a slower
time course and are more likely to be synchronous and summate than
presynaptic potentials.

Thus scalp-recorded electrical activity is the result of activity of populations of neurons. The activity can be recorded on the scalp surface, because the tissue between the neurons and the scalp acts as a volume conductor. Because the activity generated by one neuron is small, it is thought that the activity recorded at the scalp is the integrated, synchronous activity of numerous neurons. Moreover, for activity to be recorded at the scalp, the electric fields generated by each neuron must be oriented in such a way that their effects accumulate. That is, the neurons must be arranged in an open as opposed to a closed field. In an open field, the neurons' dendrites are all oriented on one side of the structure, while their axons all depart from the other side. Open fields are present where neurons are organized in layers, as in most of the cortex, parts of the thalamus, the cerebellum, and other structures.

The raw EEG signal is a complex waveform that can be analyzed in the temporal domain or frequency domain. Processing of the temporal aspect is typically done with event-related potential designs and analyses, and is discussed by Bartholow and Amodio (Chapter 10, this volume). In the present chapter, we focus on frequency analyses of EEG, where frequency is specified in hertz or cycles per second.

Recording

In contemporary social and personality research, EEG is recorded from 32, 64, 128, or more electrodes that are mounted in a stretch Lycra electrode cap. The cap is relatively easy to position and has electrodes positioned over the entire scalp surface. Electrodes are often made of tin (Sn) or silver/silver chloride (Ag/AgCl); the latter are nonpolarizable, but are typically much more expensive. Because most modern EEG amplifiers with high input impedance use very low electrode currents, polarizable electrodes (Sn) can often be used to record slow potentials without distortion. However, for frequencies less than 0.1 Hz, nonpolarizable electrodes are recommended.

The electrode placements are typically based on the original 10–20 system (Jasper, 1958), which has been extended to a 10% electrode system (Chatrian, Lettich, & Nelson, 1985) and beyond. The naming convention for electrode positions is as follows. The first letter of the name of the electrode refers to the brain region over which the electrode sits; thus Fp refers to the frontal pole, F refers to the frontal region, C to the central region, P to the parietal region, T to the temporal region, and O to the occipital region. Electrodes in between these regions are often designated by using two letters, such as FC for frontal–central. After the letter is a number, as in F3, or another letter, as in Cz. Odd numbers are used to designate sites on the left side of the head, and even numbers are used to designate sites on the right side of the head. Numbers increase as distance from the middle of the head increases, so F7 is farther from the midline than F3. The letter z is used to designate the midline, which runs from front to back of the head. Caps often contain a ground electrode, which is connected to the isoground of the amplifier and assists in reducing electrical noise. Recording of eye movements (electro-oculography, or EOG) is also carried out, to facilitate artifact scoring of the EEG. EOG can be recorded from the supra- and suborbit of the eyes to assess vertical eye movements, and from the left and right outer canthus to assess horizontal eye movements. Additional electrodes are often placed on earlobes, so that offline digitally derived references can be computed. See below for a more complete discussion of reference electrodes. See Figure 9.2 for an example of the original 10–20 layout, and Figure 9.3 for a 64-channel layout.

Sites where electrodes will be placed must be abraded to reduce electrode impedances, typically under 5000 ohms. Conductive gel is used as a medium between the scalp and electrodes. EEG, EOG, and other signals are then amplified with bioamplifiers. For EEG frequency analyses, the raw signals are often bandpass-filtered online (e.g., from 0.1 to 100 Hz), because the frequencies of interest fall between 1 and 40 Hz. Online notch filters (60 Hz in the United States, 50 Hz in Europe) are also often used to reduce electrical noise further. From the amplifiers, the raw signals are then digitized onto a computer at a sampling rate greater than twice the highest frequency of interest. For example, if one is only interested in frequencies below 40 Hz, then 80 samples per second would be collected. This sampling rate is necessary because of the Nyquist theorem, which states that exact reconstruction of a continuous signal from its samples is possible if the signal is of limited bands

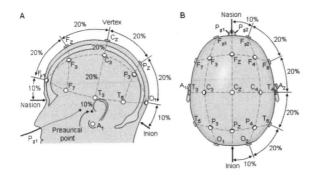

FIGURE 9.2. Illustration of original 10–20 electrode system.

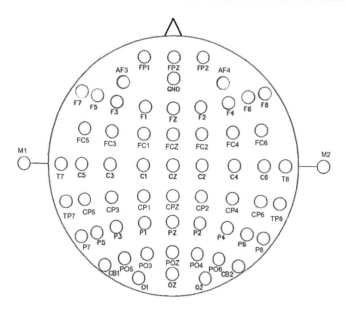

FIGURE 9.3. Illustration of 64-channel EEG cap layout.

and is sampled at least twice as great as the actual signal bandwidth. If this sampling condition is not met, then frequencies will overlap; that is, frequencies above half the sampling rate will be reconstructed as, and appear as, frequencies below half the sampling rate. This distortion is called "aliasing," because the reconstructed signal is said to be an alias of the original signal.

Preparing the Participant

We recommend that the EEG equipment be calibrated prior to running each participant, by running a sine wave of known characteristics through the amplifiers to ensure that everything is working appropriately. Many commercial systems have calibration routines that can be used.

Because most EEG protocols require the researcher to spend almost 1 hour preparing the participant for EEG data collection, we feel it important to offer a few comments regarding the researcher's behavior. When talking with our participants, we avoid referring to electricity, electrodes, needles, or anything that sounds painful. "I am going to be putting a cap on you to measure brain activity," is a nice, calming thing to say. We also train all individuals who apply EEG equipment to participants to adopt the mindset of a person who has done this *very routine procedure* many times. We work with them so that they appear confident and do not cause participants to worry about the procedure. We explain to our research assistants that they may make mistakes, but there is no need to announce these, since they can correct them easily. We also encourage research assistants to avoid being too friendly or displaying too much empathy, as doing so could drastically alter the mood of the participants. In general, research assistants should be encouraged to adopt a professional mindset and wear lab coats.

Once the equipment is calibrated, and all of the materials needed for the attachment of the EEG electrodes are ready (e.g., adhesive collars, conductive gel), the participant is brought into the experiment room. With most EEG systems, electrical impedance of the scalp will need to be brought under 5000 ohms. To assist in reducing impedance, we ask participants to "brush your hair vigorously about 5 min. Make sure to press the brush hard against your scalp as you brush. It helps with the hookup process. I will tell you when you can stop."

Once they are finished brushing their scalps, participants are told that we are going to use an exfoliant to clean some areas of their skin and use rubbing alcohol to remove the exfoliant. We clean their foreheads, earlobes, temples, and areas above/below the eyes with a mildly abrasive cleaning solution (e.g., Green Prep) and gauze pad. We follow the cleaning by wiping the areas with alcohol.

As most labs now use EEG caps instead of single electrodes to collect EEG data, we describe the capping procedure in some detail. We first use a metric tape to measure the length from the nasion (a point just below the eyebrows where there is an indentation at the top of the nose) to the inion (the bump on the occipital lobe at the back of the head). Then 10% of this total distance (in centimeters) is calculated and is measured up from the nasion. We mark this spot on a participant's forehead with a wax pencil and explain this by saying, "I am going to make a mark on your forehead with a wax pencil. It will wipe right off." Cap size is determined by measuring the distance around the participant's head, crossing the marks on the forehead and the inion. Caps often come in small, medium, and large sizes. Then two adhesive, cushioned collars are placed on cap sites Fp1 and Fp2 (if the cap has high-profile plastic housing enclosures around the electrodes). These collars are then adhered to the forehead, in line with the wax pencil marks, and centered over the nose. The cap is then stretched toward the back of the head and down. Having the participant hold the cap in place on the forehead helps with getting the cap over the head. After the cap is straightened so that the midline electrodes actually go down the midline of the head, we remeasure from the naison to the inion and ensure that Cz is halfway between these sites. If it is not, we adjust the cap so that it is. Ensuring that Cz is centered horizontally is accomplished by measuring from the preauricular indention in front of each ear (we locate the indention by having the participant open his or her mouth and feeling for the indention).

After attaching the cap's connectors to the preamp, we place electrodes on each earlobe by placing an adhesive collar on the flat side and sticking it on the ear; additional adhesive collars can be placed on top of the electrode, to ensure that the electrode remains attached. We then fill the sensors with gel but do not overfill; that is, we avoid having gel run between two sensors or outside the adhesive collar, because this will cause measurement problems. Then we abrade the ground site with the blunt tip of a wooden Q-tip or blunt tip of a needle, and apply gel with a syringe. To the participant, we say, "I am going to put gel into each sensor," and we demonstrate how we will do this by making a motion with the syringe and blunt tip on the participant's hand so that he or she will know what to expect. Impedances should be below 5000 ohms. Then we attach the chin strap to the cap and position it under the participant's chin. Some systems permit measuring EEG with higher impedances, but some have questioned the reliability and validity of such data under certain recording conditions (Kappenman & Luck, 2007).

Eye movements are often measured in EEG research, so that procedures can later be taken to remove eye movements from the EEG or to correct the EEG from these movements (see below). As noted earlier, eye movement measurement is referred to as EOG. Electrodes are affixed to the face with double-sided adhesive collars. For measuring vertical eye movements, one electrode is placed 10% of the inion–nasion distance above the pupil, whereas another is placed 10% of the inion–nasion distance below the pupil. These two electrodes are referenced to each other, rather than to the EEG reference electrode. For measuring horizontal eye movements, one electrode is placed on the right temple, and another is placed on the left temple. These electrodes are also referenced to each other. Because the EOG is relatively large, we attempt to reduce EOG impedance to only 10,000 ohms, so as to avoid overabrading the face.

Now the participant is ready. In addition to making sure that the EEG equipment is properly attached, it is equally important to ensure that the participant is in the state of mind desired for the research question. For instance, if a researcher is interested in personality characteristics or individual differences, it is important that characteristics of the situation not be too intense to overwhelm potential individual differences of interest. Along these lines, we avoid making participants more self-conscious by covering the computer monitor until it is ready to be used, as a black screened computer monitor serves as a mirror. Similarly, video cameras are best hidden, so as to avoid the arousal of excessive self-consciousness.

Artifacts

Artifacts, whether of biological or nonbiological origin, are much easier to deal with if they are prevented from occurring. However, if artifacts are recorded in the EEG, procedures exist to handle them.

Muscle Artifact

Muscle artifact (electromyography, or EMG) is typically of higher frequencies than EEG. Most EEG signals of interest are less than 40 Hz, whereas EMG is typically greater than 40 Hz. However, some EMG blends in with the EEG frequencies, so it is advisable to limit muscle artifact by training the participants to limit muscle movements. If muscle artifacts do appear in studies in which muscle movements should not occur, the artifacts can be removed during the data-processing stage. Often this is done by hand, after training from an EEG expert.

In some experiments, particularly those that evoke emotion, muscle artifacts cannot be avoided. That is, if an intense amount of disgust is evoked, the facial muscles of the participant will move and create muscle artifact in the EEG, particularly in frontal and temporal regions. Removing these muscle movements is not advisable, as emotions are occurring during these movements. One way to handle the EMG that may contaminate the EEG is to measure facial EMG and then use the facial EMG responses (in EMG frequency ranges, such as 50–250 Hz) in covariance analyses, to assess whether statistically adjusting the EEG data for several possible covariates has eliminated the effects on EEG of interest. Similarly, one could obtain EMG frequencies from the EEG sites and use these EMG frequencies in covariance analyses. Another way to address this concern is to assess the EEG frequency of interest in the facial EMG sites, and test whether this covariate would account for the EEG effects (see Coan, Allen, & Harmon-Jones, 2001, for examples).

Eye Movement Artifacts

Eye movement artifacts are also often best dealt with in advance of EEG recording. That is, training participants to limit eye movements during EEG recording is recommended. However, researchers must not encourage participants to control their blinking, because blinks and spontaneous eye movements are controlled by several brain systems in a highly automatic fashion (e.g. Brodal, 1992), and the instruction to suppress these systems may act as a secondary task (see Verleger, 1991, for a discussion).

Participants do blink, and these blinks will influence the EEG data (particularly data obtained from frontal electrodes), so epochs containing blinks should be removed from the EEG or corrected via a computer algorithm (Gratton, Coles, & Donchin, 1983; Semlitsch, Anderer, Schuster, & Presslich, 1986). These algorithms rely on regression techniques. In general, the actual EEG time series is regressed on the EOG time series, and the resulting residual time series represents a new EEG from which the influence of the ocular activity is statistically removed. Then EOG-corrected EEG data may be processed as would EEG data without EOG artifact. The latter has the advantage of not losing data, as the eye movement rejection procedure does. Some disadvantages of eye movement artifact correction have been discussed (Hagemann & Naumann, 2001), but evidence suggests that it does not cause a distortion of frontal EEG asymmetry (Hagemann, 2004)—a measure of interest in contemporary social and personality psychology that is discussed in detail later.

Nonbiological Artifacts

Nonbiological artifacts are those that typically involve external electrical noise (coming from elevator motors, electric lights, computers, etc.). Most of these problems can be dealt with through filtering of the signal; that is, 60-Hz activity can be removed with an online filter or after the data are collected. High electrode impedances or a faulty ground connection can increase 60-Hz noise. Electrodes need to be carefully washed after each use, to prevent corrosion and thus to assist in prevention of artifacts.

Offline Data Processing

Referencing

After the data are scored for artifacts, EEG signals are often re-referenced. The issue of referencing is the subject of some debate (Allen, Coan, & Nazarian, 2004; Davidson, Jackson, & Larson, 2000; Hagemann, 2004; Nunez & Srinivasan, 2006). All bioelectrical measurements must reflect the difference in activity between at least two sites. In EEG research, one site is typically placed on the scalp, whereas the other site could also be on the scalp or on a nonscalp area, such as an earlobe or nose tip.

Because researchers strive for obtaining measures that reflect activity in particular brain regions, they often search for a relatively inactive reference, such as the earlobe. However, there are no "inactive sites," and all sites near the scalp reflect some EEG because of volume conduction. To address this issue, some researchers suggest using an average reference consisting of the average of activity at all recorded EEG sites. The average reference should approximate an inactive reference if a sufficiently large array of electrodes is placed in a spherical arrangement around the head. That is, activity generated from dipoles will be positive at one site and negative at a site 180° opposite this site, and thus the sum across sites should approach zero with a representative sample of the sphere. Because electrodes are not placed under the head, though, the assumption is rarely met. Moreover, use of smaller montages of electrodes causes more residual activity in the average reference.

Other researchers have recommended the use of linked ears as a reference, because of the ears' relatively low activity and because the linking of the ears should theoretically center the reference on the head, making the determination of lateralized activity more accurate. However, the physical linking of the ears into one reference electrode has been questioned (Katznelson, 1981), because it was thought that the linking of the ears could produce a low-resistive shunt between the two sides of the head and thus reduce any asymmetries observed at the scalp. Research, however, has determined that physically linking the ears does not alter the observed EEG asymmetries (Gonzalez Andino et al., 1990). Some suggested that the original idea was ill conceived, because the electrode impedances would be higher than the internal resistance within the head, and thus would not be able to provide a shunt lower in resistance than what is present inside the head (Davidson et al., 2000). However, physically linking the ears is inappropriate for another reason. When the ears are linked prior to being input to the amplifier, variations in the impedances of the left and right electrodes will change the spatial location of the reference, and thus will potentially alter the magnitude and direction of any observed differences in left versus right EEG activity.

Such does not happen when a linked-ears reference is created offline, after the data have been collected. This is because most contemporary amplifiers have very high input impedances (about 100 k-ohms), and variations in electrode impedances of several thousand ohms will have a tiny effect on the observed voltage. To create an offline linked- or averaged-ears reference, the collected EEG data need to be referenced online to one of the ears or some other location (e.g., Cz). Then the other ear (if the reference is one ear) or both ears (if the reference is Cz) will need to be collected with the EEG. Offline, the data will be re-referenced to the average of the two ears.

So which reference should be used? From the perspective of psychological construct validity, use and comparison of different reference schemes in each study may be advisable (see Coan & Allen, 2003, for an example). A significant interaction involving the reference factor would indicate that the relationship between the EEG and the psychological variable is moderated by the reference. If such research is conducted over several years, EEG researchers may establish good psychological construct validity of the particular EEG measure.

However, from the perspective of neurophysiological construct validity, selecting a particular reference in advance may be advisable, and such a selection may consider the advantages and disadvantages of each method for the EEG measurement construct. For example, in research on asymmetrical frontal cortical activity and emotion/motivation, Hagemann (2004) has recommended against use of the average reference if only limited head coverage is used, as in the 10–20 system. He indicates that the average reference may cause increased anterior alpha activity, because anterior regions have much lower alpha power than posterior regions, and the averaging of the whole head would thus inflate anterior alpha. On the other hand, the offline average of earlobes may be more appropriate. Although this reference shows some alpha activity and thus is not "inactive," it may yield greater signal-to-noise ratios for anterior sites that are better than the average reference.

Obtaining the Frequencies of the EEG Signal

Several steps are involved in transforming EEG signals into indices used in data analyses. First, a signal is collected in the time domain; it is then converted to a frequency domain representation, usually in the form of a power spectrum. The spectrum, which collapses data across time, summarizes which frequencies are present. Spectral analysis involves examining the frequency composition of short windows of time (epochs), often 1 or 2 sec each. The spectra are averaged across many epochs. Epochs of 1 or 2 sec in length are used to meet an assumption underlying the Fourier transform, which is the method used to derive power spectra. The Fourier transform assumes a periodic signal, or one that is repeated at uniformly spaced intervals. Any periodic signal can be decomposed into a series of sine and cosine functions of various frequencies, with the function for each frequency beginning at its own particular phase. EEG signals are not exactly periodic, because the repetition of features is not precisely spaced at uniform intervals. However, the use of short epochs allows one to analyze small segments of data with features that are repeated in a highly similar fashion at other points in the waveform.

Often in EEG research, the epochs are overlapped, so that the weighting functions applied in the process of "windowing" cause the central portion of the epoch to receive the most weight, and distal portions to receive less weight. When the epochs are overlapped, all data points receive maximum weighting in some epoch. Windowing, such as a Hamming window, is used to avoid creating artifactual frequencies in the resultant power spectra. Windowing reduces the ends of the epoch to near-zero values, so that discontinuities will not occur if copies of the epochs are placed immediately before or after the epoch. This assists in meeting the Fourier assumption regarding periodic signals—that is, the assumption that the epoch will be repeated infinitely both forward and backward in time. Fourier methods will introduce spurious frequencies if windowing is not used to prevent discontinuities in the signal. Windowing prevents discontinuity, but also prevents data near the ends of the epoch from being fully represented in the power spectrum. Overlapping the epochs provides a solution to this problem, because data minimally weighted at the end of one epoch will be weighted more heavily in subsequent epochs.

Most signal-processing programs use a fast Fourier transform (FFT). The FFT requires that the epochs to be analyzed have data points that are a power of 2 (e.g., 128, 256, 512, or 1048 data points). The FFT produces two spectra, a power spectrum and a phase spectrum. The power spectrum reflects the power in the signal at each frequency from direct current to the Nyquist frequency, with a spectral value every $1/T$ points, where T is the length of the epoch analyzed. The phase spectrum presents the phase of the waveform at each interval $1/T$. Often analyses focus only on the power spectrum.

The FFT of each epoch produces many power spectra results, and the average of these power spectra is used in analyses. Further reduction is accomplished by summarizing data within conventionally defined frequency bands.

Frequency Bands of Interest

Previous discussions of EEG frequency bands suggested that there are five bands with relationships to psychological and behavioral outcomes. These bands are delta (1–4 Hz), theta (4–8 Hz), alpha (8–13 Hz), beta (13–20 Hz), and gamma (>20 Hz). Many of the psychological and behavioral correlates of these frequency bands mentioned in past reviews were based on visual inspection of the frequency bands and not on mathematical derivations of the frequencies of interest, as is now commonly done with spectral analyses. Recent research with these more precise and accurate methods of measuring EEG frequencies has questioned some of the earlier conclusions, though much of this recent work has not been incorporated into social and personality psychology as yet. Moreover, the extent to which these bands are discrete from each other or differ as a function of scalp region has not been examined in a rigorous statistical fashion. Finally, research has suggested that the frequency bands below 20 Hz are highly and positively correlated (Davidson, Chapman, Chapman, & Henriques, 1990; Harmon-Jones & Allen, 1998). Consequently, we review research focusing on alpha power, as this has attracted most of the attention of social and personality psychologists.

Research Examples

Much social and personality research has examined differences in left and right frontal cortical activity in relationship to emotional and motivational processes. In this research, alpha power has been used, because alpha power has been found to be inversely related to cortical activity assessed with a variety of methods, such as positron emission tomography (PET) (Cook, O'Hara, Uijtdehaage, Mandelkern, & Leuchter, 1998) and functional magnetic resonance imaging (fMRI) (Goldman, Stern, Engel, & Cohen, 2002). Moreover, behavioral tasks presumed to activate one brain region lead to alpha power suppression in that region (e.g., Davidson et al., 1990).

Power within the alpha frequency range is obtained by using the methods described in the preceding section. These alpha power values are often log-transformed for all sites, to normalize the distributions. Then, in the research to be described, asymmetry indices (natural log right minus natural log left alpha power) are computed for all homologous sites, such as F3 and F4 or P3 and P4. Because alpha power is inversely related to cortical activity, higher scores on the asymmetry indices indicate greater relative left-hemisphere activity.

Frontal Alpha Power Asymmetry at the Trait Level

A large portion of the frontal EEG alpha power asymmetry literature on individual differences has examined relationships of personality with resting baseline asymmetry. In these studies, resting asymmetry is utilized as a stable index of an individual's dispositional style across situations. For example, resting EEG asymmetry has been found to relate to social behavior. In one study, EEG data recorded from infants at age

9 months were used to predict social wariness at age 4 years (Henderson, Fox, & Rubin, 2001). It was found that negative emotionality, as reported by the infants' mothers, predicted social wariness in infants who displayed a pattern of right frontal EEG. However, this relationship was not found in infants with a pattern of left frontal EEG asymmetry (Henderson et al., 2001). Another study found that socially anxious preschool children exhibited greater right frontal EEG activation than their peers did (Fox et al., 1995).

The largest body of literature examining relationships with resting EEG asymmetry stems from the research on emotion. Greater relative left and greater relative right frontal EEG activity have been found to relate to individual differences in dispositional positive and negative affect, respectively (Tomarken, Davidson, Wheeler, & Doss, 1992). Individuals with stable relative left frontal activity report greater positive affect to positive films, while individuals with stable relative right frontal activity report greater negative affect to negative films (Wheeler, Davidson, & Tomarken, 1993). This notion of positive affect/left frontal versus negative affect/right frontal asymmetry has been referred to as the "affective valence hypothesis" of frontal EEG asymmetry.

However, more recent research has suggested that affective valence may not explain the relationship of emotive traits with asymmetrical frontal activity, and that motivational direction may provide a more accurate explanation of this relationship (Harmon-Jones, 2003). For example, Harmon-Jones and Allen (1997) compared resting frontal EEG asymmetry to behavioral withdrawal–approach sensitivities, as measured by the Behavioral Inhibition System/Behavioral Activation System (BIS/BAS) Scales (Carver & White, 1994). They found that higher left frontal cortical activity during resting baseline was related to higher trait approach motivation scores. Sutton and Davidson (1997) replicated this effect and found that asymmetrical frontal activity was more strongly related to approach–withdrawal motivation than was positive and negative affect (as measured by the Positive and Negative Affect Schedule; Watson, Clark, & Tellegen, 1988).

Other research examining relationships between resting frontal EEG asymmetry and psychopathology has also supported the role of motivational direction. Depression, for example, has been characterized by a general lack of approach motivation and decreased positive affect. Research has shown that higher scores on the Beck Depression Inventory (Beck, Ward, Mendelson, Mock, & Erbaugh, 1961) relate to greater relative right frontal cortical activity at resting baseline (Schaffer, Davidson, & Saron, 1983). Further studies support the relationship, showing that depression relates to trait-level increased right frontal activity and/or reduced left frontal activity (Allen, Iacono, Depue, & Arbisi,

1993; Henriques & Davidson, 1990, 1991). Other examples come from research on bipolar disorder. Increased relative right frontal EEG activity at resting baseline has been observed in bipolar depression (Allen et al., 1993), whereas increased relative left frontal activity at resting baseline has been observed in mania (Kano, Nakamura, Matsuoka, Iida, & Nakajima, 1992).

The evidence that most strongly challenges the affective valence hypothesis lies within the research on anger. Most research examining relationships with frontal asymmetry and emotion confound valence and motivational direction, since, for example, most negative affects examined are withdrawal-oriented (e.g., fear, disgust). Anger, however, is an approach-oriented negative emotion, and has been shown to relate to relatively greater left frontal resting cortical activity rather than relatively greater right frontal cortical activity (Harmon-Jones, 2004). For example, Harmon-Jones and Allen (1998) assessed dispositional anger with the Buss and Perry (1992) Aggression Questionnaire, and then measured resting alpha power asymmetries over the whole head. Results indicated that trait anger correlated positively with left frontal activity and negatively with right frontal activity (Harmon-Jones & Allen, 1998). These findings support the "motivational direction model" of frontal asymmetry, which proposes that approach motivation relates to relatively greater left than right frontal activity, whereas withdrawal motivation relates to relatively greater right than left frontal activity (Harmon-Jones, 2004).

Frontal Asymmetry and State Manipulations

Although resting baseline frontal asymmetries have been found to predict certain dispositional styles and psychopathologies, there have been failures to replicate some of the findings of relationships between resting baseline asymmetry and affective traits (see Coan & Allen, 2004, for a review). This may be because asymmetrical frontal cortical activity is also sensitive to state manipulations (e.g., Hagemann, Naumann, Becker, Maier, & Bartussek, 1998; Reid, Duke, & Allen, 1998). In fact, approximately half of the variance in baseline resting measurements is state rather than trait variance (Hagemann, Naumann, Thayer, & Bartussek, 2002). Variance in resting EEG may even be caused by the time of day and time of year the measurement is taken; for example, relative right frontal activity is greatest during fall mornings (Peterson & Harmon-Jones, 2008a). This latter finding fits with other work suggesting (1) that seasonal variations influence mood, such that the fall is associated with more depression than other seasons; and (2) that circadian variations influence release of the stress hormone cortisol, such that mornings are associated with higher cortisol levels. These factors need to be considered in EEG asymmetry research.

Failures in replicating some findings may also lie within the context in which the data were collected. Some researchers believe that simply using resting baseline EEG to predict personality is not enough, given that personality is best evident when elicited in particular states or situations (Wallace, 1966). Such an idea prompted Coan, Allen, and McKnight (2006) to propose the "capability model" of frontal EEG asymmetry and personality. This model hypothesizes that there are meaningful individual differences in frontal EEG asymmetry, but that individuals have different capabilities, depending on the demands of the specific situation.

One early study investigating frontal asymmetry in response to state manipulations of emotion and motivation used water, sugar, and citric acid to elicit facial expressions of interest and disgust in newborn infants (Fox & Davidson, 1986). Disgust expressions during the water stimulus were associated with increased right frontal activation, whereas interest expressions during the sugar stimulus were associated with increased left frontal activation (Fox & Davidson, 1986). Coan and colleagues (2001) also examined the effect of facial expressions on frontal asymmetry. Participants made expressions of disgust, fear, anger, joy, and sadness while brain activity was recorded. Relatively less left than right frontal activity was found during facial expressions of withdrawal-oriented emotions (disgust, fear), compared to expressions of approach-oriented emotions (joy, anger) and to a control condition (Coan et al., 2001).

To further compare the affective valence (positive–negative) model with the motivational direction (approach–withdrawal) model of asymmetrical frontal cortical activity, experiments were conducted in which anger was manipulated. For example, Harmon-Jones and Sigelman (2001) manipulated state anger by leading participants to believe another participant (ostensibly in the next room) had insulted them on an essay they wrote on an important social issue. EEG activity recorded immediately following the insult revealed an increase in left frontal activation, compared to individuals in the no-insult condition. This increase in left frontal activation was found to relate to an increase in self-reported anger and aggressive behavior, which was not the case in the no-insult condition (Harmon-Jones & Sigelman, 2001). Additional research has found that manipulating sympathy prior to an angering event reduces left frontal activation caused by anger (Harmon-Jones, Vaughn-Scott, Mohr, Sigelman, & Harmon-Jones, 2004). Moreover, other research has revealed that it is specifically the approach motivational character of anger that increases relative left frontal activation (Harmon-Jones,

Lueck, Fearn, & Harmon-Jones, 2006; Harmon-Jones, Sigelman, Bohlig, & Harmon-Jones, 2003). In these latter studies, anger and approach motivation were manipulated, and EEG was assessed.

To more firmly establish the causal role of relative left frontal activity in aggressive motivation, a study was conducted in which asymmetrical frontal cortical activity was manipulated, and the effects of this manipulation on aggression were measured (Peterson, Shackman, & Harmon-Jones, 2008). In this experiment, participants made either left-hand or right-hand contractions for four periods of 45 sec each. The contractions caused contralateral activation of the motor cortex and prefrontal cortex (i.e., right-hand contractions caused greater relative left activation, and vice versa) (see also Harmon-Jones, 2006). Participants were then insulted by another ostensible participant. Following the insult, participants played a reaction time game against the insulting participant. Participants were told that they would be able to administer a blast of white noise (of which the level and length would be up to them) to the other participant if they were fastest to respond to the stimulus on the screen. Individuals who made right-hand contractions were significantly more aggressive during the game than individuals who made left-hand contractions, and the degree of relative left frontal activation correlated with aggression within the right-hand contraction condition (Peterson et al., 2008).

The motivational direction model can also be compared with the affective valence model by examining positive affects that differ in motivational intensity. Some positive affects are more strongly associated than others with approach motivation. According to the motivational direction model, positive affects higher in approach motivational intensity should evoke greater relative left frontal activation than should positive affects lower in approach motivational intensity. To test these ideas, participants were asked to recall and write about one of three things: (1) a neutral day; (2) a time when something positive happened to them that they did not cause, such as a surprise gift from a friend; or (3) a goal they were committed to achieving. The second condition was designed to manipulate positive affect that was lower in approach motivation. The third condition was designed to manipulate positive affect that was higher in approach motivation. Past research suggested that this third condition increases positive affect (Harmon-Jones & Harmon-Jones, 2002; Taylor & Gollwitzer, 1995). Results from the experiment revealed that the two positive affect conditions caused greater self-reported positive affect than the neutral condition did. More importantly, the approach-oriented positive affect condition caused greater relative left frontal cortical activity than either the neutral condition or the low-approach positive affect condition did (Harmon-Jones, Harmon-Jones, Fearn, Sigelman, & Johnson, 2008).

*The Role of Individual Differences in Asymmetry
during State Manipulations*

Research has also examined the role of individual differences in responses to state manipulations. For example, the BAS dysregulation theory posits that individuals with bipolar disorder are extremely sensitive to cues of reward and failure, so that they show "an excessive increase in BAS activity in response to BAS activation-relevant events (e.g., reward incentives, goal striving) and an excessive decrease in BAS activity in response to BAS deactivation-relevant events (e.g., definite failure)" (Nusslock, Abramson, Harmon-Jones, Alloy, & Hogan, 2007, p. 105). Given that the left frontal cortical region is associated with approach motivation, it was predicted and confirmed that individuals with bipolar disorder would show increased left frontal activation in response to goal striving (Harmon-Jones, Abramson, et al., 2008).

Another study examined how hypomanic and depressive traits affected frontal asymmetry in response to an anger-inducing event (Harmon-Jones et al., 2002). Research on hypomania has suggested the involvement of increased BAS activity, whereas depression may be associated with decreased BAS activity. In support of these ideas, it was found that proneness toward hypomania related to an increase in left frontal activation, and proneness toward depression related to a decrease in left frontal activation, in response to the anger-inducing event (Harmon-Jones et al., 2002).

Research has also been conducted on populations without mood disorder traits. Gable and Harmon-Jones (2008) examined individual differences in response to appetitive stimuli. They found that self-reported time since last eaten and liking for dessert related to greater relative left frontal activation during viewing of desirable food pictures (Gable & Harmon-Jones, 2008).

The research on asymmetrical frontal cortical activity has shed light on several questions of interest to social and personality psychologists. Indeed, it accounts for the largest share of the EEG frequency research to date within social and personality psychology. Other EEG frequency research has recently occurred that is of interest to social and personality psychologists, and we briefly review some of this exciting work below.

Other Analyses of Interest

Relationships among Frequency Bands

Recent research has suggested that the ratio between resting state frontal theta and beta activity may shed light on important processes related to social and personality psychology. For example, increased theta–beta ratio has been observed in children with attention-deficit/ hyperactivity disorder (Barry, Clarke, & Johnstone, 2003). Other research has revealed that increased theta–beta ratios are associated with disadvantageous decision-making strategies on the Iowa gambling task (Schutter & van Honk, 2005). Scientists have suggested that slower-frequency waves (such as delta and theta) are associated with subcortical brain regions involved in affective processes (Knyazev & Slobodskaya, 2003), whereas faster-frequency waves (such as beta) are associated with thalamocortical and corticocortical level activations that may be involved in cognitive control processes (Pfurtscheller & Lopes da Silva, 1999).

Event-Related Desynchronization

Event-related desynchronization (ERD) is a measurement of the time-locked average power associated with the desynchronization of alpha rhythms. It is measured via event-related potential designs, which are described by Bartholow and Amodio (Chapter 10, this volume). That is, across multiple experimental events, an average is taken within the same stimulus condition. The time window is usually 1 sec in length, and the amount of desynchronization is examined over 100-msec bins within the 1-sec window. Gable and Harmon-Jones (2008) recently examined alpha ERD in an experiment in which participants viewed photographs of attractive desserts or neutral items. Results indicated that relatively greater left frontal activity, as measured by ERD, occurred during the first second of viewing of the photograph. Moreover, this effect appeared to peak at 400 msec.

Coherence

Coherence measures the degree to which EEG signals (within a given frequency band) measured at two distinct scalp locations are linearly related to one another. High coherence implies that amplitudes at a given frequency are correlated across EEG samples. Moreover, there tends to be a constant phase angle (or time lag) between the two signals. Research has suggested that high EEG coherence occurs between scalp regions connected by known white matter tracts (Thatcher, Krause, & Hrybyk, 1986). In an extension of this work, we found that during right-hand contractions, individuals with greater trait approach motivational tendencies showed greater EEG alpha power coherence between the left motor cortex and left frontal region (Peterson & Harmon-Jones, 2008b). Perhaps the appetitive behaviors associated with trait approach motivation and activation of the left frontal cortical region, such as goal striving and reward responsiveness, require close connectivity with the motor cortex. Greater coherence between these regions may facilitate activation of approach "motor-vational" behaviors.

Source Localization

EEG frequency analyses, as described above, do not provide direct information about the anatomical origins of the observed signals. With high-density EEG arrays, it is possible to conduct source localization techniques to estimate intracerebral electrical sources underlying EEG activity recorded at the scalp. These methods thus provide information regarding the neural generators of the observed signals. These techniques use mathematical models to represent the location, orientation, and strength of a hypothetical dipolar current source.

A number of source localization methods have been proposed. One that has generated much interest is low-resolution brain electromagnetic tomography (LORETA) (Pascual-Marqui et al., 1999). It computes current density (i.e., the amount of electrical current flowing through a solid) without assuming any number of active sources. The LORETA solution space (i.e., the locations in which sources can be found) is composed of 2394 cubic elements (voxels, $7 \times 7 \times 7$ mm) and is limited to cortical gray matter and hippocampi, as defined by a digitized MRI available from the Montréal Neurological Institute and Hospital (Montréal, Québec, Canada).

LORETA solutions have been cross-modally validated with studies combining LORETA and fMRI (Mulert et al., 2004; Vitacco, Brandeis, Pascual-Marqui, & Martin, 2002), structural MRI (Worrell et al., 2000), PET (Pizzagalli et al., 2004), and intracranial recordings (Seecka et al., 1998). The core assumptions of LORETA, its mathematical implementation, and additional technical details, including relations between scalp-recorded EEG and LORETA data, are described in detail elsewhere (Pascual-Marqui et al., 1999; Pizzagalli et al., 2002, 2004).

Advantages and Disadvantages of EEG Methods

We hope we have conveyed some advantages of using EEG methods in our brief review of such research in social and personality psychology. In addition to these advantages, EEG methods are relatively inexpensive, compared to other neuroimaging methods. For instance, time on an fMRI scanner averages $500 per hour (as of August 2008), and that assumes the presence of a scanner, which costs about $5 million to purchase and set up. The hourly rate charged to researchers assists in covering the maintenance contracts and salaries of the support personnel. In contrast, most EEG researchers have their own equipment, which costs less than $100,000. In this situation, no hourly fees are charged and maintenance contracts rarely exceed $3000 per year. EEG caps need to be replaced approximately once per year (depending on use), and they cost between $300 and $2000, depending on number of electrodes and type of electrode used. There are also other regular expenses for conducting gel, adhesive collars, and sterilizing solution, but these costs are relatively minimal.

In relation to PET and fMRI, EEG provides better temporal resolution but poorer spatial resolution. EEG measures electrical activations instantaneously, at submillisecond resolution, but is less able to give precise information regarding the anatomical origin of the electrical signal. In contrast, PET and fMRI have better spatial resolution but poorer temporal resolution. Ultimately, both PET and fMRI rely on metabolism and blood flow to brain areas recently involved in neuronal activity, though other changes also affect fMRI, such as oxygen consumption and blood volume changes. Because both PET and fMRI measure blood flow rather than neuronal activity, the activations are not in real time with neuronal activations, but are blood responses to neuronal responses. Thus there is a biological limit on the time resolution of the response, such that even in the best measurement systems, the peak blood flow response occurs 6–9 sec after stimulus onset (Reiman, Lane, van Petten, & Bandettini, 2000). However, there are suggestions that experimental methods can be designed to detect stimulus condition differences as early as 2 sec (Bellgowan, Saad, & Bandettini, 2003). Finally, PET and EEG permit measurement of tonic (e.g., resting, baseline) activity as well as phasic (e.g., in response to a state manipulation) activity, whereas fMRI permits measurement of phasic but not tonic activity.

Spatial and temporal resolution comparisons are often made between EEG and fMRI/PET, but rarely do researchers consider that EEG and PET/fMRI may provide different information about neural activity. For instance, correlations between EEG alpha power and fMRI/PET measures are only of moderate magnitude, suggesting that the two types of measures are not measuring exactly the same signals or activations. Moreover, EEG measures are very selective measures of current source activity, often corresponding to small subsets of total synaptic action in tissue volumes and largely independent of action potentials, as discussed earlier. By contrast, hemodynamic and metabolic measures are believed to increase with action potential firing rates (Nunez & Silberstein, 2000). Consider cortical stellate cells. They occupy roughly spherical volumes, and as such their associated synaptic sources provide a "closed-field" structure. Thus these stellate cells are electrically invisible to EEG sensors. But stellate cells constitute only about 15% of the neural population of the neocortex (Braitenberg & Schuz, 1991; Wilson, O'Scalaidhe, & Goldman-Rakic, 1994). However, they contribute disproportionately to cortical metabolic activity, because of their higher firing frequencies of action potentials (Connors & Gutnick, 1990). Thus they would show up as large signals in fMRI and PET. On the other hand, there are cases where strong EEG signals appear while weak metabolic activity occurs. EEG can be large if only a few percent of neurons in each cortical column are "synchronously active," provided that a large-scale synchrony among different columns produces a large dipole in which individual columns tend to be phase-locked in particular frequencies. Because, in this scenario, the majority of neurons in each intracolumn population are relatively inactive, minimal metabolic activity is produced. Very consequential dissociations between electrical and metabolic measures have been found in studies of epilepsy (e.g., Olson, Chugani, Shewmon, Phelps, & Peacock, 1990). For example, in one study of children with lateralized epileptic spikes (measured with EEG), regional glucose metabolism measured with PET was not lateralized, suggesting that "metabolic changes associated with interictal spiking cannot be demonstrated with PET with 18F-flurodeoxyglucose" (Van Bogaert, Wikler, Damhaut, Szliwowski, & Goldman, 1998).

Conclusion

As we have conveyed, EEG frequency measures are useful, and recent advances in EEG measures suggest even more important uses in testing theories and hypotheses of social and personality psychologists. Among the most exciting new developments in EEG awaiting applications in social and personality psychological studies is the examination of distributed patterns of activation. Many psychological processes likely involve widely distributed networks of brain dynamics, and most past work in EEG, fMRI, and PET has failed to examine the dynamics of brain activations as they unfold on the order of milliseconds. Given the exquisite temporal resolution of EEG, it will be the method of choice in addressing these questions. When brain operations are viewed as a "combination of quasi-local processes allowed by functional segregation and global processes facilitated by functional integration" (Nunez & Silberstein, 2000, p. 93), the importance of EEG methods in conjunction with other neurobiological methods at addressing important psychological questions is obvious.

References

Allen, J. J. B., Coan, J. A., & Nazarian, M. (2004). Issues and assumptions on the road from raw signals to metrics of frontal EEG asymmetry in emotion. *Biological Psychology, 67*, 183–218.

Allen, J. J., Iacono, W. G., Depue, R. A., & Arbisi, P. (1993). Regional electroencephalographic asymmetries in bipolar seasonal affective disorder before and after exposure to bright light. *Biological Psychiatry, 33*, 642–646.

Barry, R. J., Clarke, A. R., & Johnstone, S. J. (2003). A review of electrophysiology in attention-deficit/hyperactivity disorder: I. Qualitative and quantitative electroencephalography. *Clinical Neurophysiology, 114*(2), 171–183.

Beck, A. T., Ward, C. H., Mendelson, M., Mock, J., & Erbaugh, J. (1961). An inventory for measuring depression. *Archives of General Psychiatry, 4*, 561–571.

Bellgowan, P. S., Saad, Z. S., & Bandettini, P. A. (2003). Understanding neural system dynamics through task modulation and measurement of functional MRI amplitude, latency, and width. *Proceedings of the National Academy of Sciences USA, 100*(3), 1415–1419.

Berger, H. (1929). Über das Elektrenkephalogramm das Menschen. *Archiv für Psychiatrie und Nervenkrankheiten, 87*, 527–570.

Braitenberg, V., & Schuz, A. (1991). *Anatomy of the cortex: Statistics and geometry.* New York: Springer-Verlag.

Brodal, P. (1992). *The central nervous system.* New York: Oxford University Press.

Buss, A. H., & Perry, M. (1992). The Aggression Questionnaire. *Journal of Personality and Social Psychology, 63*, 452–459.

Carver, C. S., & White, T. L., (1994). Behavioral inhibition, behavioral activation, and affective responses to impending reward and punishment: The BIS/BAS Scales. *Journal of Personality and Social Psychology, 22*, 319–333.

Chatrian, G. E., Lettich, E., & Nelson, P. L. (1988). Modified nomenclature for the 10–percent electrode system. *Journal of Clinical Neurophysiology, 5*(2), 183–186.

Coan, J. A., & Allen, J. J. B. (2003). Frontal EEG asymmetry and the behavioral activation and inhibition systems. *Psychophysiology, 40*(1), 106–114.

Coan, J. A., & Allen, J. J. B. (2004). Frontal EEG asymmetry as a moderator and mediator of emotion. *Biological Psychology, 67*(1–2), 7–49.

Coan, J. A., Allen, J. J. B., & Harmon-Jones, E. (2001). Voluntary facial expression and hemispheric asymmetry over the frontal cortex. *Psychophysiology, 38*(6), 912–925.

Coan, J. A., Allen, J. J. B., & McKnight, P. E. (2006). A capability model of individual differences in frontal EEG asymmetry. *Biological Psychology, 72*(2), 198–207.

Connors, B. W., & Gutnick, M. J. (1990). Intrinsic firing patterns of diverse neocortical neurons. *Trends in Neurosciences, 13*, 99–104.

Cook, I. A., O'Hara, R., Uijtdehaage, S. H. J., Mandelkern, M., & Leuchter, A.

F. (1998). Assessing the accuracy of topographic EEG mapping for determining local brain function. *Electroencephalography and Clinical Neurophysiology, 107*(6), 408–414.

Davidson, R. J., Chapman, J. P., Chapman, L. J., & Henriques, J. B. (1990). Asymmetrical brain electrical activity discriminates between psychometrically-matched verbal and spatial cognitive tasks. *Psychophysiology, 27*(5), 528–543.

Davidson, R. J., Jackson, D. C., & Larson, C. L. (2000). Human electroencephalography. In J. T. Cacioppo, L. G. Tassinary, & G. G. Berntson (Eds.), *Handbook of psychophysiology* (2nd ed., pp. 27–52). New York: Cambridge University Press.

Fox, N. A., & Davidson, R. J. (1986). Taste-elicited changes in facial signs of emotion and the asymmetry of brain electrical activity in human newborns. *Neuropsychologia, 24*, 417–422.

Fox, N. A., Rubin, K. H., Calkins, S. D., Marshall, T. R., Coplain, R. J., Porges, S. W., et al. (1995). Frontal activation asymmetry and social competence at four years of age. *Child Development, 66*, 1770–1784.

Gable, P. A., & Harmon-Jones, E. (2008). Relative left frontal activation to appetitive stimuli: Considering the role of individual differences. *Psychophysiology, 45*(2), 275–278.

Goldman, R. I., Stern, J. M., Engel, J., & Cohen, M. S. (2002). Simultaneous EEG and fMRI of the alpha rhythm. *NeuroReport, 13*(18), 2487–2492.

Gonzalez Andino, S. L., Pascual-Marqui, R. D., Valdes Sosa, P. A., Biscay Lirio, R., Machado, C., Diaz, G., et al. (1990). Brain electrical field measurements unaffected by linked earlobes reference. *Electroencephalography and Clinical Neurophysiology, 75*, 155–160.

Gratton, G., Coles, M. G. H., & Donchin, E. (1983). A new method for off-line removal of ocular artifact. *Electroencephalography and Clinical Neurophysiology, 55*, 468–484.

Hagemann, D. (2004). Individual differences in anterior EEG asymmetry: Methodological problems and solutions. *Biological Psychology, 67*(1–2), 157–182.

Hagemann, D., & Naumann, E. (2001). The effects of ocular artifacts on (lateralized) broadband power in the EEG. *Clinical Neurophysiology, 112*(2), 215–231.

Hagemann, D., Naumann, E., Becker, G., Maier, S., & Bartussek, D. (1998). Frontal brain asymmetry and affective style: A conceptual replication. *Psychophysiology, 35*, 372–388.

Hagemann, D., Naumann, E., Thayer, J. F., & Bartussek, D. (2002). Does resting EEG asymmetry reflect a trait?: An application of latent state-trait theory. *Journal of Personality and Social Psychology, 82*, 619–641.

Harmon-Jones, E. (2003). Clarifying the emotive functions of asymmetrical frontal cortical activity. *Psychophysiology, 40*, 838–848.

Harmon-Jones, E. (2004). Contributions from research on anger and cognitive dissonance to understanding the motivational functions of asymmetrical frontal brain activity. *Biological Psychology, 67*, 51–76.

Harmon-Jones, E. (2006). Unilateral right-hand contractions cause contralateral alpha power suppression and approach motivational affective experience. *Psychophysiology*, *43*, 598–603.

Harmon-Jones, E., Abramson, L. Y., Nusslock, R., Sigelman, J. D., Urosevic, S., Turonie, L. D., et al. (2008). Effect of bipolar disorder on left frontal cortical responses to goals differing in valence and task difficulty. *Biological Psychiatry*, *63*(7), 693–698.

Harmon-Jones, E., Abramson, L. Y., Sigelman, J., Bohlig, A., Hogan, M. E., & Harmon-Jones, C. (2002). Proneness to hypomania/mania symptoms or depression symptoms and asymmetrical cortical responses to an anger-evoking event. *Journal of Personality and Social Psychology*, *82*, 610–618.

Harmon-Jones, E., & Allen, J. J. B. (1997). Behavioral activation sensitivity and resting frontal EEG asymmetry: Covariation of putative indicators related to risk for mood disorders. *Journal of Abnormal Psychology*, *106*, 159–163.

Harmon-Jones, E., & Allen, J. J. B. (1998). Anger and frontal brain activity: EEG asymmetry consistent with approach motivation despite negative affective valence. *Journal of Personality and Social Psychology*, *74*, 1310–1316.

Harmon-Jones, E., & Harmon-Jones, C. (2002). Testing the action-based model of cognitive dissonance: The effect of action-orientation on post-decisional attitudes. *Personality and Social Psychology Bulletin*, *28*, 711–723.

Harmon-Jones, E., Harmon-Jones, C., Fearn, M., Sigelman, J. D., & Johnson, P. (2008). Action orientation, relative left frontal cortical activation, and spreading of alternatives: A test of the action-based model of dissonance. *Journal of Personality and Social Psychology*, *94*, 1–15.

Harmon-Jones, E., Lueck, L., Fearn, M., & Harmon-Jones, C. (2006). The effect of personal relevance and approach-related action expectation on relative left frontal cortical activity. *Psychological Science*, *17*, 434–440.

Harmon-Jones, E., & Sigelman, J. (2001). State anger and prefrontal brain activity: Evidence that insult-related relative left prefrontal activation is associated with experienced anger and aggression. *Journal of Personality and Social Psychology*, *80*, 797–803.

Harmon-Jones, E., Sigelman, J. D., Bohlig, A., & Harmon-Jones, C. (2003). Anger, coping, and frontal cortical activity: The effect of coping potential on anger-induced left frontal activity. *Cognition and Emotion*, *17*, 1–24.

Harmon-Jones, E., Vaughn-Scott, K., Mohr, S., Sigelman, J., & Harmon-Jones, C. (2004). The effect of manipulated sympathy and anger on left and right frontal cortical activity. *Emotion*, *4*, 95–101.

Henderson, H. A., Fox, N. A., & Rubin, K. H. (2001). Temperamental contributions to social behavior: The moderating roles of frontal EEG asymmetry and gender. *Journal of the American Academy of Child and Adolescent Psychiatry*, *40*, 68–74.

Henriques, J. B., & Davidson, R. J. (1990). Regional brain electrical asymmetries discriminate between previously depressed and healthy control subjects. *Journal of Abnormal Psychology*, *99*, 22–31.

Henriques, J. B., & Davidson, R. J. (1991). Left frontal hypoactivation in depression. *Journal of Abnormal Psychology, 100*, 535–545.

Jasper, H. H. (1958). The ten–twenty electrode system of the International Federation. *Electroencephalography and Clinical Neurophysiology, 10*, 371–375.

Kano, K., Nakamura, M., Matsuoka, T., Iida, H., & Nakajima, T. (1992). The topographical features of EEGs in patients with affective disorders. *Electroencephalography and Clinical Neurophysiology, 83*, 124–129.

Kappenman, E. S., & Luck, S. J. (2007). Do high impedance ERP recording systems really save time? *Psychophysiology, 44*, S76.

Katznelson, R. D. (1981). Increased accuracy of EEG scalp localization by measurement of current source density using a Laplacian derivation. *Electroencephalography and Clinical Neurophysiology, 51*, 45.

Knyazev, G. G., & Slobodskaya, H. R. (2003). Personality trait of behavioral inhibition is associated with oscillatory systems reciprocal relationships. *International Journal of Psychophysiology, 48*, 247–261.

Mulert, C., Jager, L., Schmitt, R., Bussfeld, P., Pogarell, O., Moller, H. J., et al. (2004). Integration of fMRI and simultaneous EEG: Towards a comprehensive understanding of localization and time-course of brain activity in target detection. *NeuroImage, 22*, 83–94.

Nunez, P. L., & Silberstein, R. B. (2000). On the relationship of synaptic activity to macroscopic measurements: Does co-registration of EEG with fMRI make sense? *Brain Topography, 13*, 79–96.

Nunez, P. L., & Srinivasan, R. (2006). *Electrical fields of the brain: The neurophysics of EEG* (2nd ed.). Oxford, UK: Oxford University Press.

Nusslock, R., Abramson, L. Y., Harmon-Jones, E., Alloy, L. B., & Hogan, M. (2007). A goal-striving life event and the onset of hypomanic and depressive episodes and symptoms: Perspective from the behavioral approach system (BAS) dysregulation theory. *Journal of Abnormal Psychology, 116*, 105–115.

Olson, D. M., Chugani, H. T., Shewmon, D. A., Phelps, M. E., & Peacock, W. J. (1990). Electrocorticographic confirmation of focal positron emission tomography abnormalities in children with epilepsy. *Epilepsia, 31*, 731–739.

Pascual-Marqui, R. D., Lehmann, D., Koenig, T., Kochi, K., Merlo, M. C., Hell, D., et al. (1999). Low resolution brain electromagnetic tomography (LORETA) functional imaging in acute, neuroleptic-naive, first-episode, productive schizophrenia. *Psychiatry Research: Neuroimaging, 90*, 169–179.

Peterson, C. K., & Harmon-Jones, E. (2008a). *Circadian and seasonal variability of resting frontal EEG asymmetry.* Manuscript submitted for publication.

Peterson, C. K., & Harmon-Jones, E. (2008b). Proneness to hypomania predicts EEG coherence between left motor cortex and left prefrontal cortex. *Biological Psychology, 78*, 216–219.

Peterson, C. K., Shackman, A. J., & Harmon-Jones, E. (2008). The role of asymmetrical frontal cortical activity in aggression. *Psychophysiology,* *45,* 86–92.

Pfurtscheller, G., & Lopes da Silva, F. H. (1999). Event-related EEG/MEG synchronization and desynchronization: Basic principles. *Clinical Neurophysiology, 110,* 1842–1857.

Pizzagalli, D. A., Nitschke, J. B., Oakes, T. R., Hendrick, A. M., Horras, K. A., Larson, C. L., et al. (2002). Brain electrical tomography in depression: The importance of symptom severity, anxiety and melancholic features. *Biological Psychiatry, 52,* 73–85.

Pizzagalli, D. A., Oakes, T. R., Fox, A. S., Chung, M. K., Larson, C. L., Abercrombie, H. C., et al. (2004). Functional but not structural subgenual prefrontal cortex abnormalities in melancholia. *Molecular Psychiatry, 9,* 393–405.

Reid, S. A., Duke, L. M., & Allen, J. J. B. (1998). Resting frontal electroencephalographic asymmetry in depression: Inconsistencies suggest the need to identify mediating factors. *Psychophysiology, 35,* 389–404.

Reiman, E. M., Lane, R. D., van Petten, C., & Bandettini, P. A. (2000). Positron emission tomography and functional magnetic resonance imaging. In J. T. Cacioppo, L. G. Tassinary, & G. G. Berntson (Eds.), *Handbook of psychophysiology* (2nd ed., pp. 85–118). New York: Cambridge University Press.

Schaffer, C. E., Davidson, R. J., & Saron, C. (1983). Frontal and parietal electroencephalogram asymmetry in depressed and nondepressed subjects. *Biological Psychiatry, 18,* 753–762.

Schutter, D. J. L. G., & van Honk, J. (2005). Electrophysiological ratio markers for the balance between reward and punishment. *Cognitive Brain Research, 24,* 685–690.

Seecka, M., Lazeyrasb, F., Michela, C. M., Blankea, O., Gerickea, C. A., Ivesc, J., et al. (1998). Non-invasive epileptic focus localization using EEG-triggered functional MRI and electromagnetic tomography. *Electroencephalography and Clinical Neurophysiology, 106,* 508–512.

Semlitsch, H. V., Anderer, P., Schuster, P., & Presslich, O. (1986). A solution for reliable and valid reduction of ocular artifacts, applied to the P300 ERP. *Psychophysiology, 23,* 695–703.

Sutton, S. K., & Davidson, R. J. (1997). Prefrontal brain asymmetry: A biological substrate of the behavioral approach and inhibition systems. *Psychological Science, 8,* 204–210.

Taylor, S. E., & Gollwitzer, P. M. (1995). Effects of mindset on positive illusions. *Journal of Personality and Social Psychology, 69,* 213–226.

Thatcher, R. W., Krause, P. J., & Hrybyk, M. (1986). Corticocortical associations and EEG coherence: A 2-compartmental model. *Electroencephalography and Clinical Neurophysiology, 64,* 123–143.

Tomarken, A. J., Davidson, R. J., Wheeler, R. E., & Doss, R. C. (1992). Individual differences in anterior brain asymmetry and fundamental dimensions of emotion. *Journal of Personality and Social Psychology, 62,* 676–687.

Van Bogaert, P., Wikler, D., Damhaut, P., Szliwowski, H. B., & Goldman, S.

(1998). Cerebral glucose metabolism and centrotemporal spikes. *Epilepsy Research, 29*, 123–127.

Verleger, R. (1991). The instruction to refrain from blinking affects auditory P3 and N1 amplitudes. *Electroencephalography and Clinical Neurophysiology, 78*(3), 240–251.

Vitacco, D., Brandeis, D., Pascual-Marqui, R., & Martin, E. (2002). Correspondence of event-related potential tomography and functional magnetic resonance imaging during language processing. *Human Brain Mapping, 17*, 4–12.

Wallace, J. (1966). An abilities conception of personality: Some implications for personality measurement. *American Psychologist, 21*, 132–138.

Watson, D., Clark, L. A., & Tellegen, A. (1988). Development and validation of brief measures of positive and negative affect: The PANAS scales. *Journal of Personality and Social Psychology, 54*, 1063–1070.

Wheeler, R. E., Davidson, R. J., & Tomarken, A. J. (1993). Frontal brain asymmetry and emotional reactivity: A biological substrate of affective style. *Psychophysiology, 30*, 82–89.

Wilson, F. A., O'Scalaidhe, S. P., & Goldman-Rakic, P. S. (1994). Functional synergism between putative gamma-aminobutyrate containing neurons and pyramidal neurons in prefrontal cortex. *Proceedings of the National Academy of Sciences USA, 26*, 4009–4013.

Worrell, G. A., Lagerlund, T. D., Sharbrough, F. W., Brinkmann, B. H., Busacker, N.E., Cicora, K. M., et al. (2000). Localization of the epileptic focus by low-resolution electromagnetic tomography in patients with a lesion demonstrated by MRI. *Brain Topography, 12*, 273–282.

10

Using Event-Related Brain Potentials in Social Psychological Research
A Brief Review and Tutorial

Bruce D. Bartholow
David M. Amodio

The crowning achievement of the human mind is, arguably, its ability to negotiate the vast complexities of the social world. The current surge of interest in social neuroscience reflects the fascination of scientists from a wide range of disciplines with the neurocognitive mechanisms that give rise to social behavior (e.g., Cacioppo, Visser, & Pickett, 2005; Harmon-Jones & Winkielman, 2007). Of particular interest are questions such as these: How is information about social targets perceived? How does one manage conflicts between personal desires and social norms? What can functional neuroanatomy tell us about the social mind? What can an understanding of social cognition and motivation tell us about neural function? Social neuroscience research integrates theories and methods of the heretofore disparate approaches of social psychology, cognitive science, and cognitive–affective neuroscience, to address these and related core questions about the relationship between the brain and the social mind.

The present volume features methodological approaches used to measure activity of the brain in order to probe functions of the social mind. This chapter focuses on the event-related brain potential (ERP), a prominent method for observing patterns of brain activity associated with psychological events. ERPs are notable for their ability to assess rapid changes in neural processing, and they are the only noninvasive neuroimaging method that provides a direct measure of neural firing. Other prominent methods, such as functional magnetic resonance imaging (fMRI), provide indirect measures of neural activity by assessing, for example, the flow of oxygenated blood to neural tissue. Whereas traditional research on social cognition and motivation has had to infer the activity of underlying cognitive mechanisms only by the proxy of behavioral expressions (e.g., on reaction time tasks), ERPs and other neuroimaging methods allow researchers more direct access to the psychological mechanisms that drive social behavior, thereby providing a powerful tool for testing theories of psychological processes.

We begin this chapter with a brief overview of the theory and methods of the ERP (for a more thorough treatment, see Fabiani, Gratton, & Federmeier, 2007, or Luck, 2005). We then describe some of the ways in which ERPs have been used to address a range of questions concerning social perception, social cognition, and self-regulation. We conclude with some advice concerning experimental design and a discussion of the advantages and disadvantages of the ERP, relative to traditional behavioral measures and to other measures of brain function.

What Is the ERP?

The ERP is an index of brain activity derived from measures of electricity generated by the firing of cortical neurons. Although the existence of bioelectrical potentials in the brain had been established previously (e.g., R. Bartholow, 1882), Hans Berger (1929) first demonstrated that it is possible to measure electrical activity generated from within the living human brain, known as the electroencephalogram (EEG); he used two large, saline-soaked sponges held to the scalp and connected to a differential amplifier. The technology of EEG recording has advanced considerably since Berger's time, and modern methods permit high-quality measurement of scalp voltages from multiple scalp sites (Davidson, Jackson, & Larson, 2000). The continuous recording of EEG (e.g., during a psychological task) indexes changes in patterns of brain voltage over time, the amplitude of which normally ranges from approximately −100 to +100 μV (for more information on the EEG, see Harmon-Jones & Peterson, Chapter 9, this volume). When EEG is measured in the context of an experimental task involving specific events (e.g., stimuli or responses), it becomes possible to examine epochs of the EEG that reflect neural processes uniquely associated with those events. This event-related EEG response is called the ERP.

Physiologically, ERPs represent the summation of postsynaptic potentials from populations of synchronously active, primarily cortical neurons (see Allison, Wood, & McCarthy, 1986; Coles & Rugg, 1995). The columnar structure of cortical neurons aligns the electrical field orientation of their potentials, creating a summated signal that is strong enough to be detected at the scalp. The ERP reflects one end of the electrical dipole produced by firing neurons. The contrapolar dipole is oriented in the opposite direction (i.e., away from the scalp), and therefore typically is not measured. Not all neural signals are picked up by EEG; only those that produce dipoles oriented toward scalp electrodes are recorded. In addition, opposing dipoles from two or more generators (i.e., dipoles of opposite polarity that are oriented toward each other) can cancel each other out, so that neither is detected at the scalp.

A particular voltage deflection recorded at the scalp may comprise the activity of one or multiple sources located in different regions of the brain. Because the contours of the cerebral cortex are highly corrugated, there is substantial variability in the orientation of cortical neurons. As a result, the relative position of a neural source and the location at which it is detected at the scalp are also variable. For example, depending on the neuronal orientation, an ERP from activity in a similar region may be most pronounced at very different locations on the scalp. Finally, neural structures that are not organized in columns (e.g., subcortical structures like the amygdala) do not produce large summated dipoles that are evident at the scalp, and so activity from these neural regions cannot be assessed by using ERPs.

Psychologically, ERPs represent neural manifestations of specific information-processing activities associated with a stimulus or response event. The ERP waveform typically comprises a series of positive and negative voltage deflections, often referred to as "components" (see Figure 10.1). Specific ERP components are often associated with a particular information-processing operation or set of operations (see Fabiani et al., 2007), though it is quite likely that any given component represents numerous simultaneously occurring processes (see Coles & Rugg, 1995). In general, the amplitude of a given ERP component represents the extent to which those operations are engaged by a stimulus or response event, and the latency at which the component peaks is thought to index the time at which those operations have been completed (see Fabiani et al., 2007).

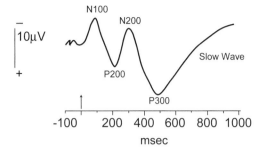

FIGURE 10.1. A schematic representation of an ERP waveform elicited by a novel visual stimulus. The vertical arrow on the time line (horizontal axis) represents stimulus onset time. The positive and negative deflections in the waveform represent typical ERP components, named here according to their polarity (P for positive deflections and N for negative deflections), and the approximate time (in milliseconds) following stimulus onset at which they peak. Note, however, that this temporal naming convention is based on broad generalities and often does not conform to observed peak latencies. Another method for component naming involves assigning numbers to the positive and negative deflections as a function of their serial order following stimulus onset (e.g., N1, P1, N2, etc.). Note also that negative voltage is plotted up here in accordance with convention, but that ERP waveforms sometimes are oriented with positive voltage up.

Measuring ERPs

ERPs can be measured noninvasively by using electrodes placed on the surface of the scalp, typically according to standard placement guidelines (see American Encephalographic Society, 1994); the electrodes are often embedded in a stretch-nylon cap that can be worn by the participant. Electrodes used to record ERPs are typically small disks of metal 4–8 mm in diameter, made either of tin (Sn) or of silver with a coating of silver chloride (Ag/AgCl), as these materials are highly conductive and resist polarization. These electrodes are connected to a set of preamplifiers, which in turn are connected to amplifiers that magnify the very weak electrical signals emitted by the neurons by a factor of 10,000–50,000, so they can be measured accurately. These analog signals are digitally sampled at a frequency ranging from 100 to about 10,000 Hz (samples per second) and stored to a computer hard drive. Sampling rates of 250–1000 Hz are common, and in principle should be at least twice as large as the largest waveform of interest (i.e., the Nyquist frequency) to avoid "aliasing," a type of sampling artifact (see Gratton, 2000). The amplified signal produces a waveform that appears as a continuous voltage waveform unfolding over time. The extent to which this "digitized" recording faithfully reproduces the original analog signal depends on the sampling rate, amplifier gain, and filtering parameters (see Luck, 2005, for more details).

Reducing Noise in ERP Measures

As with any measure used in psychological research, it is critical to limit measurement error as much as possible when one is recording EEG signals (from which ERPs are derived). Some important sources of error variance can be reduced by proper preparation of participants for electrophysiological recording (for details on preparation of participants for EEG recording, see Harmon-Jones & Peterson, Chapter 9, this volume), and by ensuring that the recording environment is free from sources of electrical interference, such as motors or unshielded power cables and computer monitors. EEG laboratories typically include two separate rooms, with computers and amplifiers located in a control room that is separate from the participant chamber. As an extra precaution, the participant chamber may be electrically shielded and soundproofed. Furthermore, the participant must be coached to remain still and focused on the experimental task during EEG recordings, in order to reduce movement artifacts (such as electromyographic activity) and distractions that can cause excessive eye movement artifacts.

Assuming that EEG data are recorded cleanly, steps must be taken to extract the relatively small ERP signal (a few microvolts) from the higher-amplitude background EEG (over 50 µV). The most common methods for extracting ERP "signal" from background EEG "noise" include filtering and averaging. Filtering involves passing the analog signal through a combination of capacitors and resistors designed to allow only signal within a particular range to pass through; a combination of high- and low-pass filters can be applied to narrow the range of frequencies recorded and to "filter out" signals that are not of interest (see Marshall-Goodell, Tassinary, & Cacioppo, 1990, for a review of bioelectrical measurement). For example, most components related to psychologically significant events tend to have a frequency range from about 0.5 to 30 Hz (see Fabiani et al., 2007; Luck, 2005). Thus, at the time of recording or later during data processing, digital or analog filter settings can be used to attenuate frequencies falling outside this range (however, for cautionary notes concerning excess use of filtering, see Luck, 2005). As a rule of thumb, most researchers record EEG from a relatively wide bandwidth (e.g., 0.01 to 100 Hz) with online analog filters, and then, in later offline processing, focus in on a narrower bandwidth capturing ERPs of interest with digital filters.

The averaging process capitalizes on the principle that EEG signals unrelated to a particular event will vary randomly across samples, and that after one centers the data in each epoch (typically by defining a preevent baseline period), these randomly varying aspects of the background EEG noise will average to zero. Meanwhile, aspects of the EEG that correspond to the event of interest will emerge as signal. In general, the inclusion of more samples will yield a better signal-to-noise ratio (but see Fabiani et al., 2007, and Luck, 2005, for qualifications). Figure 10.2 illustrates the concept of averaging. The ERP waveforms illustrated in Figure 10.2 were measured from four participants during an auditory discrimination task. For each of these four participants, four individual trial waveforms (first column), representing the response to four presentations of a particular stimulus, are averaged to form individual participant average waveforms (second column); in turn, these are averaged to form a grand average waveform (third column), representing the average response to this stimulus across these participants. Note, too, that adding more participants' responses (or more responses per participant) results in a cleaner ERP signal with less random EEG noise (fourth column).

Quantifying ERPs

Once an averaged waveform is computed for each participant, it can be scored for analysis with inferential statistics. The most common method of scoring is to determine the peak amplitude of the ERP component of interest, often defined as the minimum or maximum voltage within a predefined time window in which that component emerges. As an alternative, researchers will sometimes compute the average voltage within that time window. Whether peaks or means are used can depend on the specific questions being asked, the manner in which the EEG was measured and filtered, and (to some extent) on which components are being examined (see Fabiani, Gratton, Karis, & Donchin, 1987). Researchers may also be interested in the latency of an ERP component, in which case they would determine the time point at which the component reaches its peak value (for alternatives to peak and mean component amplitude measures, see Fabiani et al., 2007; Gratton, 2000). ERPs can be scored by using most commercially available ERP analysis software packages, which in turn will output the scores to a text (ASCII) file to be imported into a spreadsheet for statistical analysis. Alternatively, whole-waveform data may be exported as text into spreadsheets in statistical programs, and scoring and analysis can be accomplished by using user-created batch (i.e., macro) files.

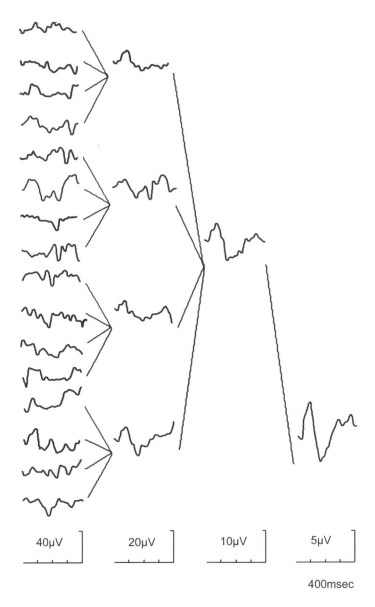

| 40µV] | 20µV] | 10µV] | 5µV] |

400msec

FIGURE 10.2. Effects of successive ERP averaging to an auditory stimulus. The far left column shows single-trial waveforms from each of four participants, recorded at the Cz (midline central) electrode location. The next column shows single-participant averages derived from each of the original four single trials. The third column shows the grand average of all participants and all single trials. The fourth column shows a grand average waveform derived from 64 trials of the same type. Comparison of this grand average with the grand average in the third column shows that inclusion of more trials results in less variance in the waveform (i.e., a cleaner, smoother signal). From Picton (1980). Copyright 1980 by John Wiley & Sons, Inc. Adapted by permission.

Interpreting ERP Data

The functional significance of different ERP components is inferred from a combination of factors, including the nature of the task used to elicit them; the timing, scalp location, and putative neural source(s) of components; and a researcher's particular theoretical perspective. In this section, we describe some commonly examined ERP components and discuss the types of questions that each class of ERP components is commonly used to address. These components include "stimulus-locked," "response-locked," and "anticipatory" ERP waves. This classification refers to the ways that epochs of EEG are combined during the averaging process. One method is to align all epochs of EEG to the time of stimulus onset, thereby rendering a stimulus-locked waveform. Alternatively, one may align EEG epochs to the moment when a task response is made (i.e., a response-locked waveform). Finally, EEG epochs may be aligned to a signal that indicates an upcoming stimulus, which we refer to as an anticipatory waveform. The method of averaging depends on the type of questions one wishes to ask and the nature of one's experimental task design. Note, too, that our list of components is incomplete, as the catalog of ERP components associated with specific processes continues to expand.

Stimulus-Locked Components

Stimulus-locked ERP components are generally associated with the engagement of attention toward a noteworthy stimulus. Larger stimulus-locked ERP amplitudes are typically interpreted as reflecting a stronger psychological response to the stimulus. Because ERPs can assess changes in such processes occurring on the order of milliseconds, and because they do not depend on verbal self-report, ERPs are very useful for measuring rapid and potentially implicit perceptual responses to a broad range of stimuli. Naming conventions for stimulus-locked ERPs typically refer to the polarity (positive or negative) and either the ordinal position following the event (e.g., the first positive-going deflection following stimulus onset is P1, then N1, then P2, etc.) or the approximate time at which the wave peaks (P100, N100, P200), as illustrated in Figure 10.1.

Early Components

Researchers interested in the extent to which attention is directed to a stimulus early in processing often focus on the amplitude of a set of early endogenous components. In particular, the N1 and the P1 have been linked to attentional processes (see Fabiani et al., 2007), in that increased amplitude of these components is thought to reflect increased direction of selective attention to stimulus processing (see Hillyard, Vogel, & Luck, 1998; Hopfinger & Mangun, 2001; Mangun, Hillyard, & Luck, 1993). The amplitude of the N2 component has also been associated with biased attention to social ingroup cues (see Dickter & Bartholow, 2007; Ito & Urland, 2003, 2005). Another relatively early negative component, the N170 (typically prominent at right-hemisphere occipital electrodes), is of particular interest to researchers interested in social perception, because it appears to be specific to face process-ing (e.g., Bentin, Allison, Puce, Perez, & McCarthy, 1996). The distinc-tion in psychological function between these early components is often unclear, beyond the notion that they reflect attentional engagement, and their neural sources are not well understood.

The "no-go" N2 is a special case of a stimulus-locked component that is elicited at about 300 msec following a no-go stimulus in a go/no-go task. Unlike most other stimulus-locked waves, the no-go N2 is associated with self-regulatory executive control processes such as inhi-bition (e.g., Kopp, Rist, & Mattler, 1996) and conflict detection (e.g., Nieuwenhuis, Yeung, van den Wildenberg, & Ridderinkhof, 2003), and has been shown to emerge from activity in the anterior cingulate cortex (ACC). However, there is reason to believe that the no-go N2 is associ-ated with the behavioral process of inhibition (i.e., muscle contractions that stop a response), which would explain why it has the characteristics of many response-locked components (see below).

Late Components

The widely studied P3 (also sometimes referred to as the P300 or, more generically, as the late positive potential or LPP; see Cacioppo, Crites, Gardner, & Berntson, 1994) is a relatively large positive deflection that typically peaks between 300 and 800 msec after a stimulus. The P3 has been associated with the processing of novelty (Friedman, Cycowicz, & Gaeta, 2001), in that its amplitude increases as the subjective probability of an event decreases (e.g., Donchin & Coles, 1988; Duncan-Johnson & Donchin, 1977; Squires, Wickens, Squires, & Donchin, 1976). The P3 also has been described as an index of working memory updating, based on numerous studies indicating better subsequent memory for stimuli that elicit larger P3 amplitudes (e.g., Donchin, 1981; Donchin & Coles, 1988; Friedman & Johnson, 2000). The latency at which the P3 peaks has been described as an indicator of stimulus evaluation or categoriza-tion time, with longer latencies indicating more effortful categorization (see Kutas, McCarthy, & Donchin, 1977; Magliero, Bashore, Coles, & Donchin, 1984). Although the neural source of the P3 has been elusive, recent research suggests that it may arise from multiple activations in the brain coordinated by norepinephrine signaling from the locus coeruleus in response to an arousing event (Nieuwenhuis, Ashton-Jones, & Cohen, 2005). Nieuwenhuis and colleagues' (2005) analysis provides a parsimonious explanation for the sometimes disparate functions ascribed to the P3.

A final stimulus-locked component that develops after the P3 has resolved is the negative slow wave (NSW). This component is typically most prominent over central or frontocentral electrode locations. It has been associated with the implementation of self-regulatory cognitive control processes, such as those required for inhibiting responses (Bartholow, Dickter, & Sestir, 2006) or overcoming cognitive conflict, such as that occurring on incongruent trials in a Stroop task (e.g., West & Alain, 1999; see also Curtin & Fairchild, 2003). Like the no-go N2, the NSW shares characteristics of response-locked waves, in that it is associated with self-regulation and may reflect a behavioral response rather than the processing of a stimulus.

Response-Locked Components

Whereas stimulus-locked components are typically associated with perception and attentional engagement, response-locked components are useful for examining mechanisms associated with the formation and regulation of a behavioral response. Response-locked waves tend to be named according to their polarity and the type of response that elicits them, such as the "error-related negativity" (ERN) and "error positivity" (P_e) components, and they tend to be pronounced at frontal or frontocentral scalp sites.

The ERN Component

The widely studied ERN component develops concurrently with the onset of a behavioral response, peaking at about 50–80 msec after the response, and is almost always larger for incorrect than for correct responses (Figure 10.3). Much research has localized the ERN's source to the dorsal ACC (Dehaene, Posner, & Tucker, 1994; van Veen & Carter, 2002). The fact that the ERN occurs specifically with response errors initially led researchers to interpret the ERN as a neural indicator of error detection (see Falkenstein, Hohnsbein, Hoormann, & Blanke, 1991; Gehring, Goss, Coles, Meyer, & Donchin, 1993). However, more recent reports of ERN-like negativity occurring on correct response trials under some conditions (i.e., correct-response negativity, or CRN) have led to the hypothesis that the ERN/CRN reflects a more general

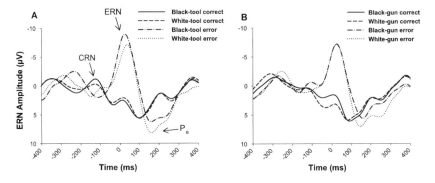

FIGURE 10.3. Response-locked ERP waveforms recorded from the FCz (midline frontocentral) channel during the weapons identification task (see Payne, 2001). ERPs are displayed for correct and incorrect tool (A) and gun (B) trials as a function of accuracy and the race (black vs. white) of the face prime. The ERN, CRN, and P_e components are labeled in panel A. On the x axis, 0 indicates the point at which responses were given. This figure shows that both the CRN and ERN waves were larger on black–tool trials, which required enhanced control over automatic stereotypes, compared with all other trial types. Data from Amodio et al. (2004).

process associated with conflict monitoring (e.g., Botvinick, Braver, Barch, Carter, & Cohen, 2001; Yeung, Botvinik, & Cohen, 2004), consistent with fMRI studies of the ACC (Carter et al., 1998). The ERN has also been interpreted as a neural "distress signal" sent by the ACC to other neural structures as an indication that enhanced cognitive control is required (see Bartholow et al., 2005; Bush, Luu, & Posner, 2000).

The P_e Component

The P_e component follows the ERN in the response-locked waveform, typically peaking between 250 and 400 msec after a response. Whereas the ERN has been shown to arise from activity in the dorsal ACC, the P_e has been localized to the rostral ACC and adjoining region of medial prefrontal cortex (PFC) (van Veen & Carter, 2002). Although considerably less research has been conducted on the P_e and its functional significance than on the ERN, research by Nieuwenhuis, Ridderinkhof, Blom, Band, and Kok (2001) suggests that the P_e is associated with the conscious awareness that one has made a response error, whereas the ERN occurs regardless of error awareness (but see Scheffers & Coles, 2000). More recent research (described in a later section) suggests that the P_e reflects the monitoring of conflict between one's behavior and external (e.g., normative) cues for response regulation (Amodio, Kubota, Harmon-Jones, & Devine, 2006).

Anticipatory ERP Components

A third class of ERP components consists of anticipatory waves, such as the "stimulus-preceding negativity" and "contingent negative variation" components. These components emerge as a participant prepares for an upcoming stimulus or response, and they are believed to reflect attentional engagement or preparatory control. These anticipatory ERP components are useful for examining participants' motivations for engaging in certain trials within a task. For example, a researcher may seek an unobtrusive measure of participants' motivation to respond to certain stimuli as a function of an experimental manipulation, such as the application of peer pressure, or of individual differences, such as motivations to respond without prejudice (e.g., Chiu, Ambady, & Deldin, 2004). As described above, the NSW also shares some characteristics of anticipatory waveforms, and thus one's interpretation of these waves relies on one's theoretical position and the design of the experimental task.

A related component is the "lateralized readiness potential" (LRP). Kornhuber and Deecke (1965) first noted that a negativity develops in the ERP during the warning interval preceding an imperative stimulus and is most pronounced over the motor cortex contralateral to the responding hand. Observing that this ERP appears to reflect preparation for a motor response, they labeled it a "readiness potential" (or *Bereitschaftspotential*). Approximately 20 years later, researchers began to use the LRP in choice reaction tasks to infer whether and when participants had preferentially prepared a particular motor response (e.g., Coles & Gratton, 1986; De Jong, Wierda, Mulder, & Mulder, 1988; Gratton, Coles, Sirevaag, Eriksen, & Donchin, 1988). Substantial evidence now indicates that the LRP indeed reflects activation in motor cortex associated with preparation to initiate a particular motor response (e.g., with the right or left hand; see Coles, 1989). In this regard, the LRP may be considered a special case of both anticipatory and stimulus-locked waveforms, as the LRP often develops as participants are anticipating a response to a target (e.g., following a warning cue or in a sequential priming task).

Interpretational Issues

An important caveat to the interpretation of ERP components is that a given component elicited in different modalities (e.g., visual vs. auditory), or in the context of different experimental tasks, probably reflects the activity of different neural structures and/or represents engagement of different psychological processes. For example, as noted by Luck (2005), the auditory P1 and N1 components appear to bear no relationship to the visual P1 and N1 components. Therefore, readers are cautioned against assuming that, for example, the N2 associated with an ingroup attention bias in social categorization tasks (e.g., Ito & Urland, 2003, 2005) reflects the same neural source or represents similar information-processing operations as does the prominent N2 often seen in tasks involving response conflict or inhibition. At present, no studies directly comparing the N2 in these different kinds of paradigms are available in the literature, and so this question has yet to be formally addressed.

Examples of ERP Research in Social Neuroscience

How can ERPs be used to elucidate social processes? As theories of social cognition have advanced, they have become increasingly sophisticated in their treatment of psychological processes underlying social judgments and behavior. However, it is often difficult to test hypotheses about underlying mechanisms by using only behavioral and self-report methods. First, these traditional research tools are unsuitable for assessing the rapidly changing processes believed to drive such phenomena as social perception, categorization, and stereotyping. Furthermore, implicit processes are by definition not amenable to explicit self-report, and the extent to which they can be clearly inferred from expressions of behavior is a matter of debate. Finally, it is difficult to measure subtle online changes in mental processes unobtrusively with these traditional tools, as these measures often interfere with the process of interest. However, we are happy to report that ERPs can provide a solution to these problems. In this section, we describe research that has used ERPs to address some enduring questions about social processes.

Attitudes and Evaluative Processes

Using ERPs to Assess Attitudes

In a seminal early report, Cacioppo, Crites, Berntson, and Coles (1993) applied the theory and methods of the P3 component of the ERP to examine attitudes. The authors noted that P3 amplitude often is increased when a given stimulus represents a category different from that of preceding stimuli (e.g., Donchin & Coles, 1988; Squires, Wickens, Squires, & Donchin, 1976). Their paradigm represented a modification of a classic "oddball" task often used to study the P3, in which relatively infrequent target stimuli (i.e., oddballs) are presented among more frequent context stimuli. This approach ensures an enhanced P3 to the targets, which represent an evaluatively different category from the context stimuli. They reasoned that because attitudes represent a type of evaluative categorization (e.g., good vs. bad), an evaluatively inconsistent attitude word (e.g., a negative word preceded by positive words) should elicit a larger P3 than should evaluatively consistent attitude words (e.g., a negative word preceded by other negative words). Cacioppo and colleagues' results confirmed this hypothesis, and opened the door to a method for studying attitudes that did not rely on participants' self-reports (see also Cacioppo et al., 1994; Cacioppo, Crites, & Gardner, 1996; Crites & Cacioppo, 1996; Ito, Larsen, Smith, & Cacioppo, 1998). Subsequent work suggested the promise of using ERPs as an implicit measure of attitudes (for a review, see Ito & Cacioppo, 2007). For example, Crites, Cacioppo, Gardner, and Berntson (1995) compared P3 amplitudes for conditions in which participants truthfully reported versus misreported their attitudes toward target objects. Across reporting conditions, the P3 was sensitive to the underlying evaluative nature of the stimuli and not to subjects' explicitly reported evaluations (see also Ito & Cacioppo, 2000). Similar work has shown that self-relevant stimuli elicit larger P3s than other stimuli do, even when participants' explicit task is to categorize stimuli along other dimensions (see Gray, Ambady, Lowenthal, & Deldin, 2004).

Mechanisms of Affective Priming

This issue (and similar issues) has recently been discussed within the context of affective or evaluative priming tasks. Fazio, Sanbonmatsu, Powell, and Kardes (1986) first demonstrated that the valence of affective target words is categorized more quickly when they are preceded by prime words of the same valence (i.e., congruent trials) than when they are preceded by prime words of the opposite valence (i.e., incongruent trials). Similar results have been reported by numerous other researchers (e.g., see Klauer & Musch, 2003). However, researchers continue to debate the underlying mechanism for this "affective congruency effect." Recently, some researchers have begun using ERPs to investigate the neural underpinnings of this effect. Zhang, Lawson, Guo, and Jiang (2006) were the first to use ERPs to study neural responses in an affective priming task. These authors reported more negativity to incongruent targets in two different ERP components, one corresponding to an N2 component (180–280 msec after the stimulus) and one referred to by the authors as an N400 component (480–680 msec). From these data, Zhang and colleagues concluded that the N400 component is sensitive not only to semantic mismatches (see Kutas & Hillyard, 1980), but also to affective mismatches, suggesting that affective priming and semantic priming have similar mechanisms.

More recently, Bartholow, Schepers, Saults, and Lust (2008) used ERPs to test competing theoretical models of affective congruency effects. One prominent model holds that the affective congruency effect stems from facilitation and inhibition within the evaluative categorization process (see Klauer, Musch, & Eder, 2005), while another model posits that the effect stems from conflict occurring during the response output stage of processing (e.g., Klinger, Burton, & Pitts, 2000). Bartholow and colleagues used ERPs to investigate the locus of the affective congruency effect within the information-processing system. Under conditions in which congruent trials were highly likely (80%) or were as likely as incongruent trials (50%), the amplitude of the LRP elicited by prime words showed that participants initially activated the incorrect response on incongruent trials (at prime onset) before ultimately activating the correct response (following target onset). These conflicting response activations influenced the amplitude of the N2 component, which was larger on incongruent than on congruent trials (again, when the probability of congruent trials was either 80% or 50%). Evidence in favor of the evaluative categorization hypothesis would be seen if the amplitude and/or latency of the P3 component mirrored the behavioral affective congruency effect (e.g., slower P3 latency on incongruent vs. congruent trials). However, this did not occur. Hence these findings were generally consistent with the idea that affective congruency effects were a result of conflict during the response output stage, rather than of simple evaluative match versus mismatch.

Person Perception

Numerous ERP components have been used to understand rapidly unfolding processes in person perception (see Bartholow & Dickter, 2007). Some early work in this area was carried out by Cacioppo and colleagues (1994), who extended the basic evaluative inconsistency paradigm (Cacioppo et al., 1993) to person perception by measuring variability in P3 amplitude as a function of positive and negative personality trait words. Inspired by this work, Bartholow, Fabiani, Gratton, and Bettencourt (2001) used ERPs to study the effects of expectancy violations associated with person perception. Bartholow and colleagues asked participants to form impressions of several fictitious characters by reading short paragraphs designed to induce a positive or negative trait inference. These paragraphs were followed by sentences depicting specific behaviors that either confirmed or violated the trait information presented previously. Consistent with their hypotheses, Bartholow and colleagues (2001; see also Bartholow, Pearson, Gratton, & Fabiani, 2003) found that expectancy-violating behaviors elicited larger

P3 amplitude than did expectancy-consistent behaviors. Expectancy-violating behaviors also were recalled better on a subsequent recall test than expectancy-consistent behaviors, supporting the hypothesized working memory updating function reflected in the P3 (see Donchin & Coles, 1988).

ERPs also have been used to track the time course and level of engagement of processes associated with social categorization (see Ito, Willadsen-Jensen, & Correll, 2007). Ito and Urland (2003) had white participants categorize faces of black and white men and women according to either race or gender. Different ERP responses as a function of target race were observed as early as 120 msec, in the N100 component, and effects for gender were observed at about 170 msec, in the P200 component. Similar to earlier work (see Mouchetant-Rostaing, Girard, Bentin, & Aguera, 2000), these effects occurred regardless of whether participants were explicitly categorizing race or gender (see also Ito & Urland, 2005). More recent research (Willadsen-Jensen & Ito, 2006) that has included an additional racial outgroup (Asians) observed a larger P200 to outgroup Asian faces than to white faces, but a larger N200 to white faces than to outgroup Asian faces.

Ito and colleagues also have used ERPs to clarify the relationship between spontaneous categorization processes and white participants' explicit, self-reported evaluations of blacks as a group. Ito, Thompson, and Cacioppo (2004) presented participants with equally infrequent pictures of white faces and black faces among more frequent negatively valenced context images (Experiment 1) or positive context images (Experiment 2) while ERPs were recorded. Across both experiments, the amplitude of the P3 indicated more negative evaluative categorization of black faces than of white faces. Moreover, the extent of this race bias in the P3 was positively correlated with more negative explicit evaluations of blacks.

The fact that all participants in these previous studies were white leaves some ambiguity with respect to whether the findings reflect biased processing of particular racial group cues or differential processing of ingroup and outgroup cues. For example, it could be that black and Asian faces attract more attention early in processing (N100 and P200) because they are relatively rare for white participants, or because the faces activate specific knowledge structures (e.g., stereotypes) that motivate attention. This issue was addressed in a study by Dickter and Bartholow (2007), which included both white and black male and female participants and white and black male and female target faces. Among white participants, black targets elicited larger P200 and smaller N200 than white targets did, replicating previous work (see Ito & Urland, 2003, 2005; Willadsen-Jensen & Ito, 2006). However, among black participants, these patterns were reversed (i.e., larger P200 to white targets and larger N200 to black targets), suggesting that these early ERP components are sensitive to general ingroup–outgroup distinctions rather than to specific features of any one racial group (for a similar demonstration with Asian participants, see also Willadsen-Jensen & Ito, 2008).

Stereotyping

In addition to revealing the neural correlates of social categorization, ERPs also have been used to investigate the consequences of category activation—namely, stereotyping. In an early example of this research, Osterhout, Bersick, and McLaughlin (1997) recorded ERPs while participants read sentences that violated definitional (e.g., "The mailman took a shower after *she* got home") or stereotypical (e.g., "Our aerobics instructor gave *himself* a break") noun–pronoun agreement (or violated neither). Their findings indicated that P3 amplitude was enhanced in response to both definitionally and stereotypically incongruent sentences (compared to control sentences), and that these effects were independent of participants' overt judgments of the grammatical and syntactical correctness of the sentences.

More recently, Bartholow and colleagues (2006, Experiment 1) used the P3 as a neurocognitive measure of stereotype violation effects within a stereotype-priming paradigm. Participants responded to trait words that were either stereotype-consistent or stereotype-inconsistent with (or irrelevant to) the race of black and white faces (primes) that preceded them (see Dovidio, Evans, & Tyler, 1986). Bartholow and colleagues replicated previous work showing faster responses to stereotype-consistent words (indicating that the face primes activated stereotypes), but they also showed that stereotype-inconsistent words (e.g., "athletic" following a white face) elicited larger and slower P3s than stereotype-consistent words did. These findings provide evidence that stereotype violations are more difficult for perceivers to categorize, and thus produce enhanced updating of working memory compared to stereotype confirmations (see also Macrae, Bodenhausen, Schloersheidt, & Milne, 1999).

Researchers also have used ERPs to study how stereotypes influence the processing of race cues. For example, Bartholow and Dickter (2008) had participants identify as quickly as possible the race of briefly presented black faces and white faces (targets). On each trial, the target faces were surrounded on four sides by "distracter" words that either were congruent with the stereotype for the target's race (e.g., the word "violent" presented with a black face) or were stereotype-incongruent with the target (e.g., the word "smart" presented with a black face).

The proportion of stereotype-congruent and stereotype-incongruent stimulus arrays was manipulated so that half of the trial blocks contained 80% congruent arrays and half contained 20% congruent arrays. Bartholow and Dickter reasoned that a high proportion of stereotype-congruent distracter trials would lead participants to use the distracter words as information to help categorize the race of the targets, and that doing so would create response conflict (i.e., the tendency to activate multiple responses on the same trial) when incongruent distracter trials were encountered (see Gratton, Coles, & Donchin, 1992). Their results confirmed this prediction, showing that incongruent trials encountered in the 80% congruent blocks were associated with initial activation of the incorrect categorization response, as seen in the amplitude of the LRP, and also elicited enhanced amplitude of the N2 conflict-monitoring component.

Self-Regulation

"Self-regulation" refers broadly to the process of coordinating goal-consistent responses. Most research on self-regulation focuses on the process of overriding a prepotent tendency with a competing intentional response. An initial ERP study examining mechanisms of self-regulation in social psychology addressed a long-standing question about the control of stereotyping: Do people sometimes fail to override automatic stereotypes because (1) they are unable to detect the unwanted influence of the stereotype, or (2) because they are unable to implement control, even though the unwanted influence of the stereotype was detected? Building on research in cognitive neuroscience (e.g., Botvinick et al., 2001), Amodio and colleagues (2004) suggested that the self-regulation of responses to stereotyped targets involves the coordination of two separate mechanisms: an initial conflict-monitoring mechanism subserved by activity in the dorsal ACC, and a subsequent regulative mechanism associated with activity in the lateral PFC (see Kerns et al., 2004), which strengthens the influence of intentional responses to override an unwanted tendency. Much research shows that the ERN and frontal N2 provide reliable indices of activity of the dorsal ACC, particularly in the context of cognitive control tasks such as the Stroop and Flankers tasks (Dehaene et al., 1994; Nieuwenhuis et al., 2001; van Veen & Carter, 2002), and that stronger activation of these components is associated with conflict processing (Yeung et al., 2004).

Amodio and colleagues (2004) sought to address the question of whether failures to override the influence of racial stereotypes were due to problems with conflict monitoring or with regulative function. Subjects in this study completed the weapons identification task (Payne,

2001), in which they quickly classified objects as either handguns or hand tools after briefly viewing the face of a black or white person. Consistent with stereotypes of black people as violent and dangerous (Devine & Elliot, 1995), black faces facilitated the correct classification of guns, and as a consequence interfered with the classification of tools, relative to white faces (Payne, 2001). As a result, subjects responded more accurately on black–gun trials, on which the black faces prime the correct "gun" response, but made more errors on black–tool trials, on which the black face prime conflicts with the correct "tool" response. This pattern suggests that responding accurately on black–tool trials requires greater control than on black–gun trials, due to the biasing effect of African American stereotypes.

To examine the role of conflict-related ACC activity, Amodio and colleagues (2004) compared ERN amplitudes on trials that required the inhibition of stereotypes (black–tool) or did not (black–gun). As expected, ERNs on black–tool trials were significantly larger than those on black–gun trials, indicating that stronger conflict was being registered on trials requiring the control of race bias. This finding indicated that stereotype-biased response errors were being made despite the detection of conflict, suggesting that failures to control were associated with a problem in engaging regulative processes. Analyses of the CRN component (sometimes referred to as the $N2_{correct}$) corroborated this finding, such that it was largest on the high-conflict black–tool trials and smallest on the low-conflict black–gun trials (cf. Bartholow et al., 2005).

A more recent, similar study by Bartholow and colleagues (2006, Experiment 2) used ERPs to more directly investigate the role of the regulative mechanism in the control of race bias. Bartholow et al. hypothesized that alcohol intoxication interferes with the regulative function of control, rather than with conflict monitoring. Participants in this study completed a version of the stop-signal task that was adapted to involve stereotype-consistent versus inconsistent responses. Specifically, participants were asked to indicate as quickly as possible whether trait words (some were stereotypic and some were counterstereotypic) could be used to describe black and white faces (primes), but on 25% of the trials (i.e., "stop" trials) a red "X" appeared shortly after the onset of the trait word, signaling participants to halt the response they had initiated. The primary ERP results from this study are shown in Figure 10.4. As predicted, the NSW was larger for sober than for intoxicated subjects, and this difference was largest for the more difficult stereotype-consistent stop trials, indicating that inhibiting responses on those trials required implementation of greater cognitive control than inhibiting responses on stereotype-inconsistent trials. Similarly, the amplitude of the no-go N2 component, associated with conflict monitoring, was

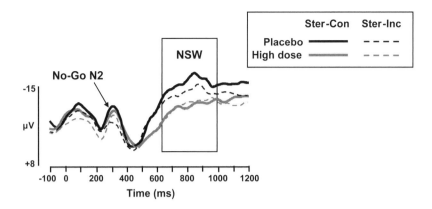

FIGURE 10.4. ERP waveforms recorded from the FCz (midline frontocentral) electrode on stop trials for participants who consumed either a placebo alcohol beverage (Placebo) or a 0.80-g/kg alcohol beverage (High dose) prior to completing the stereotype-related stop-signal task (see text for details). Time 0 represents the onset of the stop signal. NSW, negative slow wave; Ster-Con, stereotype-consistent trial; Ster-Inc., stereotype-inconsistent trial. This figure illustrates that withholding a stereotype-consistent response (solid line) elicited stronger engagement of cognitive control in prefrontal cortex (larger NSW amplitude) than did withholding a stereotype-incongruent response (dashed line). However, this did not occur in the high-dose group, indicating that alcohol impaired engagement of cognitive control. The no-go N2 was also larger on stereotype-consistent trials, indicating heightened conflict monitoring on those trials, but this effect was not significantly influenced by alcohol. Data from Bartholow, Dickter, and Sestir (2006).

larger on stereotype-consistent than on stereotype-inconsistent stop trials, but did not differ across beverage groups. The different patterns of results observed for the NSW and the no-go N2 components indicated that alcohol causes a selective impairment on the regulative function of control, while sparing conflict monitoring. These findings further supported the idea that the control of intergroup responses involves multiple dissociable mechanisms (see also Correll, Urland, & Ito, 2006).

Amodio and colleagues (2006) recently applied their ERN approach to examine different mechanisms involved in regulating responses in accordance with internal versus external cues. In this study, larger ERN amplitudes were associated with greater internally driven response control on the weapons identification task. However, when participants completed the task in public, the P_e component was more strongly associated with response control, but only among subjects who reported being highly sensitive to external pressures to respond without prejudice. These findings suggested that the P_e, and its associated rostral ACC/ medial PFC neural generator, was specifically involved in externally driven forms of response control, consistent with the theory that the rostral ACC/medial PFC region functions to regulate responses in accordance with social cues (Amodio & Frith, 2006).

A third set of studies in this program of research addressed the question of why egalitarians who hold positive attitudes toward black people nonetheless show substantial variability in their ability to respond without bias on reaction time measures of stereotyping (Amodio, Devine, & Harmon-Jones, 2008). The authors hypothesized that egalitarians vary in the extent to which the activation of stereotypes creates conflict with simultaneously activated motives to respond without bias. Consistent with this hypothesis, they found that among subjects with equally pro-black attitudes, failure to control stereotype-driven responses was associated with smaller ERNs when stereotype inhibition was needed. These findings suggest that some egalitarians are prone to unwanted race-biased expressions because activated stereotypes do not register cognitive conflict.

Other social neuroscience research has examined ERP responses on basic conflict tasks, such as the Stroop or go/no-go tasks, as a means to test hypotheses about self-regulation as being rooted in basic neurocognitive mechanisms (e.g., Amodio, Jost, Master, & Yee, 2007; Amodio, Master, Yee, & Taylor, 2008; Forbes, Schmader, & Allen, in press; Inzlicht & Gutsell, 2007). For example, Amodio and colleagues (2007) demonstrated that the individual differences in cognitive styles associated with more liberal versus more conservative political views (see Jost, Glaser, Kruglanski, & Sulloway, 2003) is related to the sensitivity of the conflict-monitoring system, as measured by the ERN. Other research has used ERPs to indicate the effects of a manipulation on self-regulatory capacity (Inzlicht & Gutsell, 2007), such that a regulatory load associated with stereotype threat led to diminished ERN amplitudes during incongruent Stroop trials.

It is notable that in the recent ERP research on the self-regulation of bias, ERPs have been used not simply as indicators of generic neural events, but as indices of specific underlying neural activations. For example, the ERN and P_e have been used to assess activation of the dorsal and rostral ACC, respectively, in much research (e.g., Amodio et al., 2004, 2006; Nieuwenhuis et al., 2001), and the NSW is believed to reflect activity of the PFC (e.g., Bartholow et al., 2006). Associations between ERP responses and neural substrates have been established through the combination of source localization studies and convergence with fMRI and patient data from studies using similar experimental tasks. By linking ERPs associated with psychological responses to specific neural substrates, researchers can draw from the vast literatures of behavioral and cognitive neuroscience to inform their theories abut psychological processes and to interpret their findings.

Another important feature of ERP research on self-regulation is the use of behavioral measures to validate interpretations of ERP effects. For example, Amodio and colleagues (2004) proposed that the ERN should be associated with controlled, but not automatic, patterns of behavior on the weapons identification task. Using a process dissociation method of computational modeling to create independent estimates of automatic and controlled responding (Jacoby, 1991; Payne, 2001), the authors demonstrated that ERN amplitudes were strongly associated with control, but were uncorrelated with automaticity. Thus, by combining ERPs with computational modeling of behavior, researchers can achieve a high level of theoretical and methodological precision (see also Gonsalkorale, Sherman, Allen, Amodio, & Bartholow, 2008).

Methodological Issues for ERP Research in Social Neuroscience

ERPs offer a powerful tool for probing mental processes associated with social cognition and social behavior, provided that they are used in the context of an appropriate theoretical question and experimental design. Because valid ERP measures require the averaging of responses to many (i.e., ~30–50) trials, ERPs are appropriate only for assessing psychological phenomena that can be measured repeatedly within a task. Psychological phenomena that are difficult to produce in the laboratory (e.g., an epiphany during problem solving), that can only be meaningfully experienced once or twice in a single sitting (i.e., before practice or habituation effects set in), or that involve sustained psychological processes are not good candidates for ERP experiments. ERPs are responses to independent, discrete events, and thus a good experimental task must contain several such events, each of which is psychologically meaningful. By contrast, manipulations that involve, say, freely reading a paragraph of text are inappropriate, because it is difficult to determine exactly when a significant psychological event (e.g., a sudden insight) might occur. Finally, ERP measurement relies on high-quality EEG recordings, and thus a participant must be able to complete a task while keeping his or her head and upper body still. Tasks should be designed to keep participants' attention, as mind wandering may diminish the effectiveness of the experimental manipulations on ERPs, and shifting eye gaze (e.g., looking around the room) will create electroocular artifacts that will interfere with ERP scoring. It is often a good idea to coach participants to keep their gaze fixed on the stimulus. Note that these same constraints also generally apply to other methods of neuroimaging, such as fMRI.

As described above, ERPs are an excellent means of assessing temporal changes in neural activity, but they provide poor spatial information concerning the source of neural activity. For this reason, ERP methods are not usually appropriate for addressing questions about the location of a neural process, for reasons outlined above (except in a few cases where the neural generator of a given component has been well characterized). However, recent advances in dipole modeling procedures have enhanced researchers' ability to estimate the neural generator of an ERP by modeling data obtained from a "dense array" of electrodes. That is, EEG signals recorded from an array of 64, 128, or 256 channels provide dipole modeling algorithms with relatively high spatial resolution that can be used to estimate the source of an ERP dipole. Such models are typically constrained by anatomical parameters (e.g., specifying that a signal may only emerge from cortex with columnar organizations of neurons), and also may be constrained by the number of possible generators.

In a previous section, we have described three broad classes of ERP components, each of which is associated with different types of theoretical questions. In what follows, we provide some methodological recommendations for research taking each approach, as well as research using the "special case" of LRPs.

Stimulus-Locked ERP Approaches

Stimulus-locked ERP methods are primarily useful for probing the timing of differential attentional responses to social stimuli. To use ERPs in this way, one must design an experimental task that permits perceptual processing of a stimulus without the interruption of other psychological processes, such as the preparation and implementation of a behavioral response. That is, an ideal task would involve presentation of single stimuli for a period of time that allows the full range of ERP components to unfold. For example, the P300/LPP wave often emerges 500–1000 msec after a stimulus, depending on various task parameters, and therefore it is important to allow participants to view the stimulus for that entire period of time without interruption or distraction. If some event, such as stimulus offset or a response, occurs before the later waveforms are able to emerge, these events will create their own ERP responses that will interfere with the scoring of the component of interest.

Alternatively, tasks can be designed so that ERP activity associated with extrastimulus events (e.g., responses) can be subtracted from the stimulus-locked ERP waveform, thus permitting the use of tasks in which, for example, speeded responses must be made. Many ERP studies of social psychological processes have used sequential priming tasks, in which a prime stimulus precedes the target. The use of sequential priming tasks in ERP research is somewhat novel and requires special care. The most common practice in such cases is to include a number (up to one-third of all trials; see Woldorff, 1993) of "prime-only" trials, in which a prime is presented without a subsequent target. This approach permits later subtraction of averaged prime-related ERP activity from the average target-locked waveforms, effectively removing the influence of prime-processing from target-processing ERP effects. This procedure also permits examination of prime processing that is not confounded by overlapping target-related ERP activity.

Response-Locked ERP Approaches

Response-locked ERPs are often used to address questions about the engagement of behavior and self-regulation. Research using response-locked ERP components depends on a good behavioral task. When preparing to conduct an ERP study, one should begin with a behavioral task that is effective in modeling the psychological variables of interest. It is often a good idea to conduct a behavioral experiment prior to the ERP study to ensure that the task is effective (i.e., that the task produces variability across conditions in behavioral outcomes of interest). The timing of components in the task is very important. In most cases, trials should begin with a fixation point to ensure that participants will be prepared to see the experimental stimulus. Participants should know ahead of time how to respond to each stimulus (e.g., through an initial set of practice trials), so that their responses are not interrupted by attempts to remember how to complete the task. After a response, time is needed for all response-locked components to unfold; this may take a second or more. Finally, it is often advisable to vary the timing of the intertrial intervals, so that ERPs associated with the response on one trial and stimulus onset on the subsequent trial are not confounded. The use of event-related designs in which different trial types are presented in random order, rather than in a single block, further aids in reducing ERP confounds associated with expectancy effects.

   In some cases, a researcher may be interested in examining ERPs associated with error responses (e.g., ERN components). In these cases, one must design a task that elicits a sufficient number of error responses to permit a valid average of error-related EEG epochs. This is often accomplished by imposing a time deadline on the participants' responses (e.g., 500 msec) that has proven effective for that particular task. When one is averaging epochs of EEG to create ERPs, epochs associated with correct and incorrect responses should be averaged separately within each trial condition. Response windows are also useful because they keep participants focused on the task and discourage mind wandering and inattentiveness.

Anticipatory ERP Approaches

Anticipatory ERPs are useful for examining participants' motivations for engaging in certain trials within a task. In order to examine anticipatory ERP waves, one must use a task that allows participants to anticipate the onset of an upcoming stimulus or signal to respond (e.g., a pretrial fixation point or warning cue). Because it takes nearly a second for these waves to emerge clearly, an appropriate task will present the anticipatory signal at least a second before the target stimulus. Note that many experimental tasks may inadvertently create response anticipation. That is, if a new trial always begins at a regular interval after the response to the previous trial, anticipatory ERPs may be observed, and the amplitudes of these ERPs may be related to features of the previous response. In order to separate activity associated with two consecutive trials, it is advisable to vary the intertrial intervals so that any systematic relationship between the anticipatory ERP and the participant's response to the previous trial will be removed in the averaging process.

LRP Approaches

As noted previously, LRPs are something of a special case, sharing features of both stimulus-locked waveforms and anticipatory waveforms. LRPs can be measured in numerous contexts, but often are used to characterize how an initial stimulus (e.g., a warning cue) influences preparation to response to a subsequent target stimulus (see Gehring, Gratton, Coles, & Donchin, 1992). However, stimulus-locked LRPs can also be derived in tasks involving only a single stimulus on every trial, as a way to shed light on how particular stimulus parameters or task features affect response activation (see Gratton et al., 1992). In either case, measurement and scoring of LRPs require, at a minimum, measurement of ERPs from electrodes positioned bilaterally over the motor cortex (i.e., just left and right of midline at central scalp locations); the researcher must also know which hand (i.e., left or right) each participant used to make correct overt responses in each experimental condition. This can be achieved most easily with two-alternative forced-choice tasks, in which participants use one hand to respond to targets in one condition and the other hand to respond to targets in the other condition, and in which response hand and stimulus type are counterbalanced across participants. (For a more detailed explanation of the LRP and its applications for understanding information processing, see Coles, 1989; Coles, Smid, Scheffers, & Otten, 1995.)

Practical Considerations for Conducting ERP Research

Like all methods used to study social behavior and its underlying mechanisms, the use of ERPs has both advantages and disadvantages. A major advantage of ERPs as a dependent measure is their unrivaled capacity for tracking the precise timing of neural processes. That is, ERPs provide a direct measure of neural firing with extremely high temporal resolution. In contrast, the temporal resolution of fMRI is limited by the much slower changes in blood flow that are believed to follow the firing of neurons. Another major advantage of ERPs over traditional behavioral measures, as mentioned previously, is the ability to measure psychological processes independently of, or in the absence of, any behavioral response. This property allows researchers to separate, for example, the latency of overt responses from the timing of underlying cognitive processes on which those responses are thought to depend (see McCarthy & Donchin, 1981), as well as processes associated with cognitive processing versus response implementation (see Coles et al., 1995).

Perhaps the most significant disadvantages of the ERP method for most social and/or personality psychologists are the time and resources required to implement it. Social and personality psychologists interested in incorporating ERPs into their research programs must typically augment their traditional training with additional training in a psychophysiology lab, often as postdoctoral fellows. Although this is still a common route, some graduate training programs now offer joint training in social–personality psychology and psychophysiology and/or cognitive neuroscience. Even in such programs, trainees must master additional theoretical background (e.g., foundations of cognitive or affective neuroscience; basics of electrical circuits and physiology) and acquire specific skill sets (e.g., knowledge of complex EEG recording hardware and software; troubleshooting electrophysiological measurement), beyond the basics of social psychological theory and experimental methodology that are required in all graduate training programs. For psychophysiologists or cognitive neuroscientists who wish to apply their skills to the study of social or personality processes, the challenge is reversed: They must seek additional training and experience in these fields.

An additional consideration is the cost required to set up and maintain an ERP laboratory. Although system costs can vary a great deal, it is not unusual for a modest ERP setup to cost $75,000 to $100,000, including amplifiers, data acquisition and analysis software, electrode caps, and other necessary equipment (e.g., computers), in addition to any necessary building renovations. Most major universities will provide sufficient startup funds for new faculty to outfit a lab, but some smaller universities and colleges will not. In such cases, researchers must obtain funds for setting up a lab from other sources (e.g., grants). Once a laboratory is equipped, costs for using the lab are continuous. For example, measuring ERPs requires a number of disposable laboratory supplies, including electrode gel, skin preparation materials (e.g., alcohol pads, skin cleansers), electrode collars (to hold facial electrodes in place), and so on, all of which represent ongoing laboratory costs (though the cost of maintaining an EEG lab is far less than that of an MRI center).

ERP research is also more time-consuming than behavioral research at virtually every step of the process. First, unlike many studies based on self-report or behavioral measures, participants in ERP experiments must be run individually. Moreover, each experimental session in an ERP study lasts considerably longer than a comparable session in a behavioral experiment. For example, a typical session in an ERP study will require additional time at each step—from the consent document (which generally requires extended explanation of the risks and discomforts associated with electrophysiological recording) to the instructions (which are often more elaborate), and especially the paradigm itself, which will need to include at least four times as many trials as in a behavioral study to ensure sufficiently stable ERP waveforms. Furthermore, additional time is required to apply the electrode cap (with even a simple electrode montage, this step itself takes 30–45 min) and to remove it and clean it after the session—not to mention allowing time for participants to clean up (e.g., rinsing conductive electrode gel from their hair). All in all, a typical experimental session of this kind will last approximately three to four times longer than a comparable behavioral experiment, and will garner only one participant's worth of data.

The good news is that ERP experiments typically require fewer participants overall than similar behavioral experiments; this is due in part to the larger number of trials used in ERP protocols, which results in less error variance. However, this advantage is greatly attenuated in between-subjects designs, which can limit the kinds of paradigms that reasonably can be used in an ERP lab. Other design considerations also must be carefully taken into account when one is contemplating the use of ERPs, as mentioned previously (see Luck, 2005, for an extended discussion).

Conclusions

We have provided an overview of how ERPs may be used to address a range of critical questions concerning social cognition and social behavior. Given the unique assessments afforded by ERPs, such as exquisite temporal measurement of neurocognitive processes and their versatile use with a range of experimental tasks, ERP methodology is a valuable tool in the social neuroscientist's toolbox. As the field of social neuroscience continues to grow, research will increasingly depend on scientists' ability to integrate a broad set of physiological and behavioral approaches and their associated theoretical models. Those who understand and incorporate cognitive and affective neuroscience with basic behavioral approaches will be well positioned to make significant contributions to the understanding of social behavior and, ultimately, to society.

References

Allison, T., Wood, C. C., & McCarthy, G. M. (1986). The central nervous system. In M. G. H. Coles, E. Donchin, & S. W. Porges (Eds.), *Psychophysiology: Systems, processes, and applications* (pp. 5–25). New York: Guilford Press.

American Encephalographic Society. (1994). Guideline thirteen: Guidelines for standard electrode position nomenclature. *Journal of Clinical Neurophysiology, 11*, 111–113.

Amodio, D. M., Devine, P. G., & Harmon-Jones, E. (2008). Individual differences in the regulation of intergroup bias: The role of conflict monitoring and neural signals for control. *Journal of Personality and Social Psychology, 94*, 60–74.

Amodio, D. M., & Frith, C. D. (2006). Meeting of minds: The medial frontal cortex and social cognition. *Nature Reviews Neuroscience, 7*, 268–277.

Amodio, D. M., Harmon-Jones, E., Devine, P. G., Curtin, J. J., Hartley, S. L., & Covert, A. E. (2004). Neural signals for the detection of unintentional race bias. *Psychological Science, 15*, 88–93.

Amodio, D. M., Jost, J. T., Master, S. L., & Yee, C. M. (2007). Neurocognitive correlates of liberalism and conservatism. *Nature Neuroscience, 10*, 1246–1247.

Amodio, D. M., Kubota, J. T., Harmon-Jones, E., & Devine, P. G. (2006). Alternative mechanisms for regulating racial responses according to internal vs. external cues. *Social Cognitive and Affective Neuroscience, 1*, 26–36.

Amodio, D. M., Master, S. L., Yee, C. M., & Taylor, S. E. (2008). Neurocognitive components of the behavioral inhibition and activation systems: Implications for theories of self-regulation. *Psychophysiology, 45*, 11–19.

Bartholow, B. D., & Dickter, C. L. (2007). Social cognitive neuroscience of person perception: A selective review focused on the event-related brain potential. In E. Harmon-Jones & P. Winkielman (Eds.), *Social neuroscience: Integrating biological and psychological explanations of social behavior* (pp. 376–400). New York: Guilford Press.

Bartholow, B. D., & Dickter, C. L. (2008). A response conflict account of the effects of stereotypes on racial categorization. *Social Cognition, 26* 314–332.

Bartholow, B. D., Dickter, C. L., & Sestir, M. A. (2006). Stereotype activation and control of race bias: Cognitive control of inhibition and its impairment by alcohol. *Journal of Personality and Social Psychology, 90,* 272–287.

Bartholow, B. D., Fabiani, M., Gratton, G., & Bettencourt, B. A. (2001). A psychophysiological analysis of cognitive processing of and affective responses to social expectancy violations. *Psychological Science, 12,* 197–204.

Bartholow, B. D., Pearson, M. A., Dickter, C. L., Sher, K. J., Fabiani, M., & Gratton, G. (2005). Strategic control and medial frontal negativity: Beyond errors and response conflict. *Psychophysiology, 42,* 33–42.

Bartholow, B. D., Pearson, M. A., Gratton, G., & Fabiani, M. (2003). Effects of alcohol on person perception: A social cognitive neuroscience approach. *Journal of Personality and Social Psychology, 85,* 627–638.

Bartholow, B. D., Schepers, M. A., Saults, J. S., & Lust, S. A. (2008). *Psychophysiological evidence of response conflict and strategic control of responses in affective priming.* Manuscript submitted for publication.

Bartholow, R. (1882). *Medical electricity: A practical treatise on the applications of electricity to medicine and surgery* (2nd ed.). Philadelphia: Lea.

Bentin, S., Allison, T., Puce, A., Perez, E., & McCarthy, G. (1996). Electrophysiological studies of face perception in humans. *Journal of Cognitive Neuroscience, 8,* 551–565.

Berger, H. (1929). Über das Elektrenkephalogramm das Menschen. *Archiv für Psychiatrie und Nervenkrankheiten, 87,* 527–570.

Botvinick, M. M., Braver, T. S., Barch, D. M., Carter, C. S., & Cohen, J. D. (2001). Conflict monitoring and cognitive control. *Psychological Review, 108,* 624–652.

Bush, G., Luu, P., & Posner, M. L. (2000). Cognitive and emotional influences in anterior cingulate cortex. *Trends in Cognitive Sciences, 4,* 215–222.

Cacioppo, J. T., Crites, S. L., Jr., Berntson, G. G., & Coles, M. G. H. (1993). If attitudes affect how stimuli are processed, should they not affect the event-related brain potential? *Psychological Science, 4,* 108–112.

Cacioppo, J. T., Crites, S. L., & Gardner, W. L. (1996). Attitudes to the right: Evaluative processing is associated with lateralized late positive event-related brain potentials. *Personality and Social Psychology Bulletin, 22,* 1205–1219.

Cacioppo, J. T., Crites, S. L., Gardner, W. L., & Berntson, G. G. (1994). Bioelectrical echoes from evaluative categorizations: I. A late positive brain potential that varies as a function of trait negativity and extremity. *Journal of Personality and Social Psychology, 67,* 115–125.

Cacioppo, J. T., Visser, P. S., & Pickett, C. L. (2005). *Social neuroscience: People thinking about thinking people.* Cambridge, MA: MIT Press.

Carter, C. S., Braver, T. S., Barch, D. M., Botvinick, M. M., Noll, D., & Cohen, J. D. (1998). Anterior cingulate cortex, error detection, and the online monitoring of performance. *Science, 280,* 747–749.

Chiu, P., Ambady, N., & Deldin, P. (2004). Contingent negative variation to emotional in- and out-group stimuli differentiates high- and low-prejudiced individuals. *Journal of Cognitive Neuroscience, 16,* 1830–1839.

Coles, M. G. H. (1989). Modern mind–brain reading: Psychophysiology, physiology, and cognition. *Psychophysiology, 26,* 251–269.

Coles, M. G. H., & Gratton, G. (1986). Cognitive psychophysiology and the study of states and processes. In G. R. J. Hockey, A. W. K. Gaillard, & M. G. H. Coles (Eds.), *Energetics and human information processing* (pp. 409–424). Dordrecht, The Netherlands: Nijhof.

Coles, M. G. H., & Rugg, M. D. (1995). Event-related brain potentials: An introduction. In M. D. Rugg & M. G. H. Coles (Eds.), *Electrophysiology of mind: Event-related brain potentials and cognition* (pp. 1–26). New York: Oxford University Press.

Coles, M. G. H., Smid, H. G. O. M., Scheffers, M. K., & Otten, L. J. (1995). Mental chronometry and the study of human information processing. In M. D. Rugg & M. G. H. Coles (Eds.), *Electrophysiology of mind: Event-related brain potentials and cognition* (pp. 86–131). New York: Oxford University Press.

Correll, J., Urland, G. R., & Ito, T. A. (2006). Event-related potentials and the decision to shoot: The role of threat perception and cognitive control. *Journal of Experimental Social Psychology, 42,* 120–128.

Crites, S. L., & Cacioppo, J. T. (1996). Electrocortical differentiation of evaluative and nonevaluative categorizations. *Psychological Science, 7,* 318–321.

Crites, S. L., Cacioppo, J. T., Gardner, W. L., & Berntson, G. G. (1995). Bioelectrical echoes from evaluative categorization: II. A late positive brain potential that varies as a function of attitude registration rather than attitude report. *Journal of Personality and Social Psychology, 68,* 997–1013.

Curtin, J. J., & Fairchild, B. A. (2003). Alcohol and cognitive control: Implications for regulation of behavior during response conflict. *Journal of Abnormal Psychology, 112,* 424–436.

Davidson, R. J., Jackson, D. C., & Larson, C. L. (2000). Human electroencephalography. In J. T. Cacioppo, L. G. Tassinary, & G. G. Berntson (Eds.), *Handbook of psychophysiology* (2nd ed., pp. 27–52). New York: Cambridge University Press.

Dehaene, S., Posner, M. I., & Tucker, D. M. (1994). Localization of a neural system for error detection and compensation. *Psychological Science, 5,* 303–305.

De Jong, R., Wierda, M., Mulder, G, & Mulder, L. J. M. (1988). Use of partial information in responding. *Journal of Experimental Psychology: Human Perception and Performance, 14,* 682–692.

Devine, P. G., & Elliot, A. J. (1995). Are racial stereotypes really fading?: The Princeton trilogy revisited. *Personality and Social Psychology Bulletin, 21,* 1139–1150.

Dickter, C. L., & Bartholow, B. D. (2007). Event-related brain potential evidence of ingroup and outgroup attention biases. *Social Cognitive and Affective Neuroscience, 2,* 189–198.

Donchin, E. (1981). Surprise! . . . Surprise? *Psychophysiology, 18,* 493–513.

Donchin, E., & Coles, M. G. (1988). Is the P300 component a manifestation of context updating? *Behavioral and Brain Sciences, 11,* 357–427.

Dovidio, J. F., Evans, N., & Tyler, R. B. (1986). Racial stereotypes: The contents of their cognitive representations. *Journal of Experimental Social Psychology, 22,* 22–37.

Duncan-Johnson, C. C., & Donchin, E. (1977). On quantifying surprise: The variation of event-related potentials with subjective probability. *Psychophysiology, 14,* 456–467.

Fabiani, M., Gratton, G., & Federmeier, K. (2007). Event related brain potentials. In J. T. Cacioppo, L. G. Tassinary, & G. G. Berntson (Eds.), *Handbook of psychophysiology* (3rd ed., pp. 85–119). New York: Cambridge University Press.

Fabiani, M., Gratton, G., Karis, D., & Donchin, E. (1987). The definition, identification, and reliability of measurement of the P300 component of the event-related brain potential. In P. K. Ackles, J. R. Jennings, & M. G. H. Coles (Eds.), *Advances in psychophysiology* (Vol. 1, pp. 1–78). Greenwich, CT: JAI Press.

Falkenstein, M., Hohnsbein, J., Hoormann, J., & Blanke, L. (1991). Effects of crossmodal divided attention on late ERP components: II. Error processing in choice reaction tasks. *Electroencephalography and Clinical Neurophysiology, 78,* 447–455.

Fazio, R. H., Sanbonmatsu, D. M., Powell, M. C., & Kardes, F. R. (1986). On the automatic activation of attitudes. *Journal of Personality and Social Psychology, 50,* 229–238.

Forbes, C. E., Schamder, T., & Allen, J. J. B. (in press). The role of devaluing and discounting in performance monitoring: A neurophysiological study of minorities under threat. *Social, Cognitive and Affective Neuroscience.*

Friedman, D., Cycowicz, Y. M., & Gaeta, H. (2001). The novelty P3: An event-related brain potential (ERP) sign of the brain's evaluation of novelty. *Neurosceince and Biobehavioral Reviews, 25,* 355–373.

Friedman, D., & Johnson, R., Jr. (2000). Event-related potential (ERP) studies of memory encoding and retrieval: A selective review. *Microscopy Research and Technique, 51,* 6–28.

Gehring, W. J., Goss, B., Coles, M. G. H., Meyer, D. E., & Donchin, E. (1993). A neural system for error detection and compensation. *Psychological Science, 4,* 385–390.

Gehring, W. J., Gratton, G., Coles, M. G. H., & Donchin, E. (1992). Probability effects on stimulus evaluation and response processes. *Journal of Experimental Psychology: Human Perception and Performance, 18,* 198–216.

Gonsalkorale, K., Sherman, J. W., Allen, T. J., Amodio, D. M., & Bartholow, B. D. (2008). *On the underlying bases of implicit attitude variability and malleability.* Manuscript submitted for publication.

Gratton, G. (2000). Biosignal processing. In J. T. Cacioppo, L. G. Tassinary, & G. G. Berntson (Eds.), *Handbook of psychophysiology* (2nd ed., pp. 900–923). New York: Cambridge University Press.

Gratton, G., Coles, M. G. H., & Donchin, E. (1992). Optimizing the use of information: Strategic control of activation of responses. *Journal of Experimental Psychology: General, 121*, 480–506.

Gratton, G., Coles, M. G., Sirevaag, E. J., Eriksen, C. W., & Donchin, E. (1988). Pre- and poststimulus activation of response channels: A psychophysiological analysis. *Journal of Experimental Psychology: Human Perception and Performance, 14*, 331–334.

Gray, H. M., Ambady, N., Lowenthal, W. T., & Deldin, P. (2004). P300 as an index of attention to self-relevant stimuli. *Journal of Experimental Social Psychology, 40*, 216–224.

Harmon-Jones, E., & Winkielman, P. (Eds.). (2007). *Social neuroscience: Integrating biological and psychological explanations of social behavior.* New York: Guilford Press.

Hillyard, S. A., Vogel, E. K., & Luck, S. J. (1998). Sensory gain control (amplification) as a mechanism of selective attention: Electrophysiological and neuroimaging evidence. *Philosophical Transactions of the Royal Society of London, Series B, 353*, 1257–1270.

Hopfinger, J. B., & Mangun, G. R. (2001). Electrophysiological studies of reflexive attention. In C. Folk & B. Gibson (Eds.), *Attraction, distraction, and action: Multiple perspectives on attentional capture* (pp. 3–26). Amsterdam: Elsevier.

Inzlicht, M., & Gutsell, J. N. (2007). Running on empty: Neural signals for self-control failure. *Psychological Science, 8*, 233–238.

Ito, T. A., & Cacioppo, J. T. (2000). Electrophysiological evidence of implicit and explicit categorization processes. *Journal of Experimental Social Psychology, 35*, 660–676.

Ito, T. A., & Cacioppo, J. T. (2007). Attitudes as mental and neural states of readiness: Using physiological measures to study implicit attitudes. In B. Wittenbrink & N. Schwarz (Eds.), *Implicit measures of attitudes* (pp. 125–158). New York: Guilford Press.

Ito, T. A., Larsen, J. T., Smith, N. K., & Cacioppo, J. T. (1998). Negative information weighs more heavily on the brain: The negativity bias in evaluative categorizations. *Journal of Personality and Social Psychology, 75*, 887–900.

Ito, T. A., Thompson, E., & Cacioppo, J. T. (2004). Tracking the timecourse of social perception: The effects of racial cues on event-related brain potentials. *Personality and Social Psychology Bulletin, 30*, 1267–1280.

Ito, T. A., & Urland, G. R. (2003). Race and gender on the brain: Electrocortical measures of attention to the race and gender of multiply categorizable individuals. *Journal of Personality and Social Psychology, 85(4)*, 616–626.

Ito, T. A., & Urland, G. R. (2005). The influence of processing objectives on the perception of faces: An ERP study of race and gender perception. *Cognitive, Affective, and Behavioral Neuroscience, 5*, 21–36.

Ito, T. A., Willadsen-Jensen, E. C., & Correll, J. (2007). Social neuroscience and social perception: New perspectives on categorization, prejudice, and stereotyping. In E. Harmon-Jones & P. Winkielman (Eds.), *Social neuroscience: Integrating biological and psychological explanations of social behavior* (pp. 401–421). New York: Guilford Press.

Jacoby, L. L. (1991). A process dissociation framework: Separating automatic from intentional uses of memory. *Journal of Memory and Language, 30*, 513–541.

Jost, J. T., Glaser, J., Kruglanski, A. W., & Sulloway, F. (2003). Political conservatism as motivated social cognition. *Psychological Bulletin, 129*, 339–375.

Kerns, J. G., Cohen, J. D., MacDonald, A. W., III, Cho, R. Y., Stenger, V. A., & Carter, C. S. (2004). Anterior cingulate conflict monitoring predicts adjustments in control. *Science, 303*, 1023–1026.

Klauer, K. C., & Musch, J. (2003). Affective priming: Findings and theories. In J. Musch & K. C. Klauer (Eds.), *The psychology of evaluation: Affective processes in cognition and emotion* (pp. 7–49). Mahwah, NJ: Erlbaum.

Klauer, K. C., Musch, J., & Eder, A. B. (2005). Priming of semantic classifications: Late and response related, or earlier and more central? *Psychonomic Bulletin and Review, 12*, 897–903.

Klinger, M. R., Burton, P. C., & Pitts, G. S. (2000). Mechanisms of unconscious priming: I. Response competition not spreading activation. *Journal of Experimental Psychology: Learning, Memory, and Cognition, 26*, 441–455.

Kopp, B., Rist, F., & Mattler, U. (1996). N200 in the flanker task as a neurobehavioral tool for investigating executive control. *Psychophysiology, 33*, 282–294.

Kornhuber, H. H., & Deecke, L. (1965). Hirnpotentialanderungen bei willkarbewegungen und passiven bewegungen des Menschen: Bereitschaftspotential und reafferente Potentiale. *Pflügers Archiv, 284*, 1–17.

Kutas, M., & Hillyard, S. A. (1980). Reading senseless sentences: Brain potentials reflect semantic incongruity. *Science, 207*, 203–205.

Kutas, M., McCarthy, G., & Donchin, E. (1977). Augmenting mental chronometry: The P300 as a measure of stimulus evaluation time. *Science, 197*, 792–795.

Luck, S. J. (2005). *An introduction to the event-related potential technique.* Cambridge, MA: MIT Press.

Macrae, C. N., Bodenhausen, G. V., Schloersheidt, A. M., & Milne, A. B. (1999). Tales of the unexpected: Executive function and person perception. *Journal of Personality and Social Psychology, 76*, 200–213.

Magliero, A., Bashore, T. R., Coles, M. G. H., & Donchin, E. (1984). On the dependence of P300 latency on stimulus evaluation processes. *Psychophysiology, 21*, 171–186.

Mangun, G. R., Hillyard, S. A., & Luck, S. J. (1993). Electrocortical substrates of visual selective attention. In D. Meyer & S. Kornblum (Eds.), *Attention and performance XIV* (pp. 219–243). Cambridge, MA: MIT Press.

Marshall-Goodell, B. S., Tassinary, L. G., & Cacioppo, J. T. (1990). Principles of bioelectrical measurement. In J. T. Cacioppo & L. G. Tassinary (Eds.), *Principles of psychophysiology: Physical, social, and inferential elements* (pp. 113–148). New York: Cambridge University Press.

McCarthy, G., & Donchin, E. (1981). A metric of thought: A comparison of P300 latency and reaction time. *Science, 21,* 171–186.

Mouchetant-Rostaing, Y., Girard, M. H., Bentin, S., & Aguera, P. E. (2000). Neurophysiological correlates of face gender processing in humans. *European Journal of Neuroscience, 12,* 303–310.

Nieuwenhuis, S., Aston-Jones, G., & Cohen, J. D. (2005). Decision making, the P3, and the locus coeruleus–norepinephrine system. *Psychological Bulletin, 131,* 510–532.

Nieuwenhuis, S., Ridderinkhof, K. R., Blom, J., Band, G. P. H., & Kok, A. (2001). Error-related brain potentials are differently related to awareness of response errors: Evidence from an antisaccade task. *Psychophysiology, 38,* 752–760.

Nieuwenhuis, S., Yeung, N., van den Wildenberg, W., & Ridderinkhof, K. R. (2003). Electrophysiological correlates of anterior cingulate function in a go/nogo task: Effects of response conflict and trial type frequency. *Cognitive, Affective, and Behavioral Neuroscience, 3,* 17–26.

Osterhout, L., Bersick, M., & McLaughlin, J. (1997). Brain potentials reflect violations of gender stereotypes. *Memory and Cognition, 25,* 273–285.

Payne, B. K. (2001). Prejudice and perception: The role of automatic and controlled processes in misperceiving a weapon. *Journal of Personality and Social Psychology, 81,* 181–192.

Picton, T. W. (1980). The use of human event-related potentials in psychology. In I. Martin & P. H. Venables (Eds.), *Techniques in psychophysiology* (pp. 357–395). New York: Wiley.

Scheffers, M. K., & Coles, M. G. H. (2000). Performance monitoring in a confusing world: Event-related brain activity, judgments of response accuracy, and types of errors. *Journal of Experimental Psychology: Human Perception and Performance, 26,* 141–151.

Squires, K. C., Wickens, C., Squires, N. K., & Donchin, E. (1976). The effect of stimulus sequence on the waveform of the cortical event-related potential. *Science, 193,* 1142–1146.

van Veen, V., & Carter, C. S. (2002). The timing of action-monitoring processes in the anterior cingulate cortex. *Journal of Cognitive Neuroscience, 14,* 593–602.

West, R., & Alain, C. (1999). Event-related neural activity associated with the Stroop task. *Cognitive Brain Research, 8,* 157–164.

Willadesn-Jensen, E., & Ito, T. A. (2006). Ambiguity and the timecourse of racial perception. *Social Cognition, 24,* 580–606.

Willadesn-Jensen, E., & Ito, T. A. (2008). A foot in both worlds: Asian Americans' perceptions of Asian, white and racially ambiguous faces. *Group Processes and Intergroup Relations, 11,* 182–200.

Woldorff, M. G. (1993). Distortion of ERP averages due to overlap from temporally adjacent ERPs: Analysis and correction. *Psychophysiology, 30,* 98–119.

Yeung, N., Botvinick, M. M., & Cohen, J. D. (2004). The neural basis of error detection: Conflict monitoring and the error-related negativity. *Psychological Review, 111,* 931–959.

Zhang, Q., Lawson, A., Guo, C., & Jiang, Y. (2006). Electrophysiological correlates of visual affective priming. *Brain Research Bulletin, 71,* 316–323.

11

Transcranial Magnetic Stimulation

Dennis J. L. G. Schutter

Historical Background

The attractive force of lodestone was already known to the Chinese and the ancient Greeks by about 1000 B.C. The story goes that the shepherd Magnes discovered the mineral magnetite in the mountains of Mysia, a region in the northwest part of modern Turkey, as the nails in his shoes and his metal cap of his staff literally pinned him to the ground. It is, however, more likely that the term "magnetism" was derived from the name of the Greek city Magnesia in Thessalia, where local inhabitants found these strange stones that could attract iron. These stones were rich in the mineral magnetite (Fe_3O_4). (Interestingly, an electric current of at least 1,000,000 A is needed to magnetize ordinary stones. The only phenomenon existing in nature that is capable of developing such electric currents is lightning.) The first scientific report of electrical and magnetic phenomena, however, did not appear until 1600 A.D. English physician William Gilbert (1544–1603) was the first to use the term "electric force" in studying the attractive properties of substances, such as rubbed amber. Furthermore, he inferred that electricity and magnetism were unrelated, and he distinguished between electric and magnetic action. His argument was based on the false assumption that, contrary to magnetic attraction, electric attraction depended on heat production during rubbing.

The groundbreaking discoveries of one of the most distinguished scientists of the 19th century, Danish physicist and chemist Hans Christian Ørsted (1755–1851), were what laid the foundation of our modern understanding of electromagnetism. In 1820, he observed that the needle of an ordinary compass diverges from the magnetic north when an electrical current is passed through a wire and held near the compass. Ørsted's observation demonstrated that electricity and magnetism are closely related phenomena. Soon afterward, he discovered that an electric current flowing through a wire produces a magnetic field surrounding the electric current. Eleven years later, Michael Faraday (1791–1867) showed that an electric current will be generated in a conductor whenever this conductor is placed inside a rapidly changing magnetic field. This principle is known as "Faraday's law of electromagnetic induction," and lies at the heart of noninvasive magnetic stimulation of the human brain. Figure 11.1 shows the founding father of modern transcranial magnetic stimulation (TMS).

Scottish physicist James Clerk Maxwell (1831–1879) finally provided the mathematical unifying proof for the reciprocal relation between electricity and magnetism, known nowadays as the "Maxwell equations of electromagnetism." Near the turn of the century (1896), French physicist and physician Jacques Arsène d'Arsonval (1851–1940) was among the first to describe the effects of electromagnetic induction

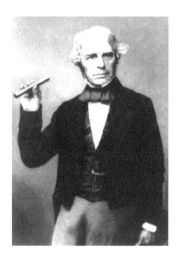

FIGURE 11.1. Michael Faraday (1791–1867).

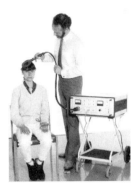

FIGURE 11.2. Anthony Barker performing TMS over the primary motor cortex. From Barker (1991). Copyright 1991 by Lippincott Williams & Wilkins. Reprinted by permission.

on the human brain. Volunteers whose heads were placed inside a large induction coil experienced phosphenes (light flashes/auras), vertigo, and even syncope. These effects were replicated by others multiple times at the beginning of the 20th century.

The first documented demonstration of noninvasive stimulation of the human brain in conscious subjects was by Merton and Morton (1980), who applied short high-voltage electric pulse via small scalp electrodes. Unfortunately, the use of electrical stimulation has remained limited, because high voltages are needed to overcome the poor conducting properties of scalp and skull; the high voltages in turn cause considerable discomfort and pain, due to the stimulation of nerve endings in the skin and superficial muscles. In 1985, Faraday's law of electromagnetic induction provided the solution to the impedance problem, and for the first time the human primary motor cortex was stimulated by applying magnetic pulses to the scalp in a noninvasive and painless manner (Barker, Jalinous, & Freeston, 1985). Figure 11.2 shows Anthony Barker applying TMS to the primary motor cortex of a healthy volunteer.

Basic Characteristics of TMS

The fundamental principle underlying TMS is Faraday's law, which states (as noted above) that situated near conductors, a magnetic pulse oriented in the right direction is transformed into an electric current. When the magnitude of this magnetic pulse varies in the order of a few hundred microseconds, a secondary current is generated (Pascual-Leone, Walsh, & Rothwell, 2000). "Transcranial" literally means "through the skull." When TMS is applied over the scalp, the secondary electric current creates so-called "transmembrane potentials," which, if strong enough, will result in the depolarization of underlying cortical nerve cells that are tangentially oriented to the magnetic field (Bohning, 2000). The axons excited are oriented in the plane of the induced electric field parallel to the curvature of the head at the stimulated area. Figure 11.3 illustrates the current flows involved in magnetic stimulation of neurons (Hallett, 2007).

The magnetic field strength directly under the coil can be as large as 2.5 T (Stewart, Ellison, Walsh, & Cowey, 2001), which is approximately 40,000 times the intensity of the earth's magnetic field (Bohning, 2000). Although the size of the effective stimulating field and the amount of current spread in the tissue of the head depends on level of cortical excitability and the intensity of TMS, the technique allows researchers to map cortical functions on the scalp with a spatial resolution of about 1 cm^2. It should, however, be noted that according to the Biot–Savart law of physics, the strength of the magnetic field deteriorates exponentially with distance. As a result, the *direct* local effects of TMS are confined to the areas that face the cranium, but because the brain consists of highly functionally interconnected structures, TMS can also have *indirect* distal effects (Ilmoniemi et al., 1997).

Whereas functional magnetic resonance imaging (fMRI) has excellent spatial resolution, and electroencephalography (EEG) is excep-

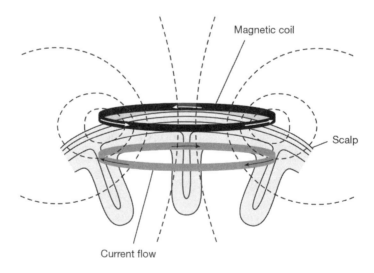

FIGURE 11.3. Magnetic and electric current flows in the brain. From Hallett (2007). Copyright 2007 by Elsevier, Inc. Adapted by permission.

tionally well suited for studying the temporal characteristics of brain signals (for reviews, see Whalen & Johnstone, Chapter 14; Bartholow & Amodio, Chapter 10; and Harmon-Jones & Peterson, Chapter 9, all this volume), TMS has so-called "functional resolution," in which the spatial and temporal aspects of activation in the outer brain structures can be combined and causally related to its function. The macroscopic responses to TMS can be measured with the brain imaging tools reviewed in this book, as well as with surface electromyography (for details, see Hess, Chapter 5, this volume) and changes in behavior. Since its introduction in 1985, TMS has been used to examine the functional integrity of the motor system in neurological patients (e.g., Werhahn, Conforto, Kadom, Hallett, & Cohen, 2003); to evaluate the effects of pharmacological agents on cortical physiology (Ziemann, 2004); and to study the cortical dynamics of speech, vision, and movement (for a comprehensive review, see Stewart, Ellison, et al., 2001). In addition, with the publication of two case reports in which it was suggested that TMS could improve mood (Hoflich, Kaper, Hufnagel, Ruhrmann, & Moller, 1993), psychiatrists commenced to investigate the applicability of TMS in the treatment of depression (George et al., 1997). The ability of TMS to tap directly into the brain's circuitry and examine its functional correlates makes it a unique method to study the neurobiological underpinnings of emotions, mood, and personality. The remainder of this chapter presents an overview of how TMS technology has contributed to our current understanding of how the social brain operates.

Repetitive TMS

Although the duration of effects induced by a single magnetic pulse or a train of such pulses is usually very short, when TMS is applied in a repetitive, continuous fashion for an extended period of time (e.g., 20 min), its effects can easily outlast the stimulation itself, providing a time window for studying the effects of TMS on emotive processes. Depending on the intensity and frequency of stimulation, repetitive TMS (rTMS) can either reduce or increase neural excitability in the area being stimulated. Repetitive stimulation at about 1 Hz, termed "slow-frequency rTMS," attenuates neural excitability, whereas repetitive stimulation of 5 Hz and higher, termed "fast-frequency rTMS," augments neural excitability (Wassermann & Lisanby, 2001). Even though the physiological working mechanisms are still unclear, it has been suggested that, analogous to models of long-term depression and long-term potentiation in animals, slow-frequency rTMS induces states of relative hyperpolarization, whereas fast-frequency rTMS causes relative depolarization of neurons.

Alternatively, it has been speculated that the opposite effects of slow- and fast-frequency rTMS at least partially depend on changes in the activity of inhibitory gamma-aminobutyric acid (GABA) interneurons (Daskalakis et al., 2006; Khedr, Rothwell, Ahmed, Shawky, & Farouk, 2007). At the psychological level of analysis, slow- and fast-frequency rTMS have been found useful for studying brain–behavior relationships by way of disturbing and enhancing neuronal functioning, respectively. Importantly, however, the behavioral effects also depend on which type of mental process is under investigation (Walsh & Pascual-Leone, 2005). For example, some researchers have proposed that disrupting the inhibitory function of the prefrontal cortex with slow-frequency rTMS will augment participants' creativity (Snyder, Bossomaier, & Mitchell, 2004).

The power intensity of rTMS is an another important feature that contributes to its effects on the brain. Intensity of stimulation is usually established by finding the lowest threshold for eliciting small finger movements by applying single-pulse TMS to the hand area of the motor cortex—the so-called "motor threshold" (Wassermann, 1998). It has been demonstrated that low-intensity (subthreshold) rTMS mainly targets the underlying tissue, whereas higher-intensity (suprathreshold) rTMS produces additional remote effects (Speer et al., 2000). Ilmoniemi and colleagues (1997), for instance, recorded increases in brain activity over the right motor cortex starting approximately 20 msec following a focal high-intensity TMS pulse to the left motor cortex. These so-called "transsynaptic effects" are established via white matter fibers in functionally interconnected regions resulting from local activation of neurons, and enable researchers to study networks in the brain.

rTMS Studies of the Prefrontal Cortex

In the first published rTMS experiment addressing the lateralized role of the frontal lobes in human emotion, slow-frequency suprathreshold rTMS was applied continuously for 20 min over the left and the right dorsolateral prefrontal cortex (PFC) on separate occasions in a random and counterbalanced fashion (d'Alfonso, van Honk, Hermans, Postma, & de Haans, 2000). Afterward, emotional responses to angry facial expressions were investigated (for a review, see van Honk & Schutter, 2007). The results showed emotionally vigilant responses to angry facial expressions after right-PFC rTMS, and emotionally avoidant responses to angry facial expressions after left-PFC rTMS. This was the first study to provide direct evidence to support Harmon-Jones's (2003) frontal lateralization model of motivational direction. Citing an extensive line of studies showing links between the left PFC and anger/aggression, Harmon-Jones proposed that approach-related emotions are processed by the left PFC and avoidance-related emotions by the right PFC. Moreover, additional analyses of sympathetic and parasympathetic activity of the heart showed that vigilant responses to angry facial expressions after right- compared to left-PFC rTMS were paralleled by higher levels of sympathetic activity (van Honk et al., 2002).

In a follow-up study, the involvement of the right PFC in the avoidance-related emotion of fear was investigated in a sham-controlled slow-frequency suprathreshold rTMS design (van Honk et al., 2002). In earlier studies, sham control was achieved by tilting the coil 45° to prevent the TMS pulse from reaching the target tissue, but keeping other variables (including the sound of the pulse and coil pressure on the scalp) similar to real rTMS. Nowadays, specially designed sham coils that are physically indistinguishable from real coils are used; these effectively shield the brain from magnetic pulses, but they mimic the clicking sounds and the sensations of real TMS. In two separate sessions, healthy volunteers received either 20 min of real or sham rTMS over the right PFC in a counterbalanced order, and emotional responses to fearful facial expressions were investigated. In line with the motivational direction model, inhibition of the right PFC yielded a significant decrease in vigilant responses to fearful facial expressions.

Ignoring a threat signal is a risky behavioral strategy and is most likely to be observed in low-anxiety, anger-prone, and possibly left-PFC-dominant individuals (d'Alfonso et al., 2000; Fox, 1991). Empirical evidence supporting these assumptions was provided by a study that studied frontal electric brain activity and mood states after real and sham slow-frequency suprathreshold rTMS to the right PFC in healthy volunteers (Schutter, van Honk, d'Alfonso, Postma, & de Haan, 2001). Right-PFC rTMS induced significant left-sided increases in theta (4–7 Hz) EEG activity, accompanied by decreases in self-reported anxiety (see also Plate 11.1). Notably, frontal theta EEG activity has been found to be inversely related to state anxiety (Mizuki, Suetsugi, Ushijima, & Yamada, 1997).

Finally, in a recent sham-controlled TMS study, significant reductions in the processing of anger were observed after rTMS deactivated the left PFC, compared to both placebo and right-PFC rTMS (van Honk & Schutter, 2006). Neither left- nor right-PFC deactivation influenced the processing of happiness. The latter finding further supports Harmon-Jones's model of the frontal asymmetry of emotion, and has led to the hypothesis that happiness may be the result of frontal homeostasis rather than asymmetry.

This series of studies shows that rTMS can induce predictable changes in motivational states and, in combination with neuroimaging methods, can be used to characterize the cortical dynamics associated with these changes. Furthermore, combining rTMS with other modern neuroimaging techniques makes it feasible to visualize the effects of rTMS in distal subcortical brain structures as well. For example, as shown in Plate 11.2, robust changes in metabolism have been observed in the parahippocampus, medial temporal lobe, and cerebellum following slow-frequency rTMS to the left PFC with positron emission tomography (PET) (Speer et al., 2003). More recently, a combined TMS–PET experiment showed that fast-frequency rTMS over the left PFC can influence serotonin-related activity in limbic brain structures (Sibon et al., 2007). Even though these studies did not examine emotion directly, the data provide a functional neuroanatomical basis for studying corticolimbic interactions in, for instance, the regulation of emotions and mood. Issues concerning depth of stimulation and interconnectivity are discussed later in this chapter.

rTMS Studies of the Parietal Cortex

Although social neuroscientists have traditionally focused on studying the frontal lobes and amygdala, there is increasing evidence that the parietal cortex (Pctx) also contributes to various aspects of emotive processes. Earlier studies established relationships between right-Pctx hyperactivity and anxious depression (e.g., Heller, Nitschke, Etienne, & Miller, 1997). In more recent studies, evidence was found for parietal involvement in the processing of angry facial expressions, and it was shown that relative right-to-left Pctx EEG asymmetries predicted avoidant responses to angry faces (Schutter, de Haan, & van Honk, 2004; Schutter, Putman, Hermans, & van Honk, 2001). Even though the right parietal hyperactivity could be explained in terms of elevated psychological arousal, which contributes to negative thoughts, ruminations, worrying, vigilant attention, and a weak approach system, the evidence for right-Pctx involvement remained correlational in nature. To address this issue, slow-frequency subthreshold rTMS was applied over the right Pctx of healthy volunteers for 20 min in a sham-controlled design (van Honk, Schutter, Putman, de Haan, & d'Alfonso, 2003). Results showed that right-Pctx rTMS caused reductions in phenomenological, physiological, and attentional indices of depression. Participants showed not only reductions in self-reported depressive mood, but also more vigilant responses to the angry facial expression. Furthermore, these vigilant responses were accompanied by significant heart rate elevations. Together, these findings suggest that the right Pctx is an important node in the cortical circuit of the approach system. As shown in Plate 11.3, increases in functional "cross-talk" (i.e., EEG coherence) between the left PFC and right Pctx following fast-frequency suprathreshold rTMS to the left PFC provide additional support for this notion (Jing & Takigawa, 2001).

rTMS Studies of the Cerebellum

The cerebellum is a structure located in the back of the brain and is well known for its involvement in posture, balance, and movement. The first evidence for cerebellar involvement in emotion was provided by Robert G. Heath during the early 1950s. Although Heath's initial work consisted predominantly of electrical stimulation of the septum, he later commenced stimulating the cortical surface of the cerebellum, which, according to him, provided a better entry to the emotional circuitry of the brain. He found positive effects on mood and personality (Heath, 1977; Heath, Dempsey, Fontana, & Myers, 1978). In particular, the medial part of the cerebellum, called the vermis, has multiple connections with midbrain and limbic structures. For comprehensive reviews of the cerebellum's involvement in emotion and emotional disorders, see Schutter and van Honk (2005) and Schmahmann (2004).

Inspired by the studies of Heath and the notion that TMS is basically the noninvasive variant of electrical stimulation, we applied fast-frequency rTMS to the medial cerebellum in a sham-controlled within-subject design. Additional active control sites included the lateral cerebellum and the occipital cortex. It was found that fast-frequency rTMS over the medial cerebellum showed increases in alertness and positive affect, and changes in resting state EEG activity, compared to the three control conditions. These results were interpreted as evidence in favor of cerebellar involvement in the brain's emotion circuit (Schutter, van Honk, d'Alfonso, Peper, & Panksepp, 2003). More recently, in a slow-frequency rTMS experiment involving healthy volunteers, it was demonstrated that inhibiting cerebellar activity caused impaired emotion regulation. Whereas subjects were able to successfully "neutralize" their negative feelings in response to highly aversive scenes in the sham and occipital rTMS condition, they were less able to do so in the cerebellar rTMS condition (Schutter, Enter, & van Honk, 2007). These findings and those of another study, in which it was found that single-pulse TMS over the medial cerebellum evokes theta EEG responses over the frontal cortex (Schutter & van Honk, 2006), suggest that cerebellar dysregulation of corticolimbic interactions underlies impaired emotion regulation. Furthermore, in our most recent placebo-controlled double-blind study, fast-frequency rTMS to the cerebellum resulted in increased emotional responses to happy facial expressions (Schutter, Enter, & Hoppenbrouwers, in press). For targeting the medial and lateral parts of the cerebellum, the inion is often used as an anatomical landmark. As can be seen

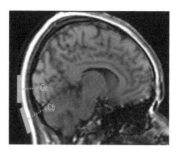

FIGURE 11.4. Inion-referenced target sites for TMS to the cerebellum, overlying a T1-weighted structural brain scan of a healthy volunteer. Occ, occipital region; Cb, medial cerebellum. From Schutter, Kammers, Enter, & van Honk (2006). Copyright 2006 by Taylor & Francis. Reprinted by permission.

from Figure 11.4, structural MRI shows that this approach produces reliable estimations.

This series of rTMS studies demonstrates that the cerebellum is directly implicated in emotion and the regulation of emotion. However, the exact underlying physiological mechanisms remain unclear, and studies using a combination of rTMS and functional neuroimaging are warranted in the near future.

Summary of rTMS Research

rTMS is a basic research method that is mostly used to inhibit or facilitate cortical activity, allowing researchers to study brain–function relationships and changes in cognitive and emotional behavior. When combined with modern neuroimaging techniques, rTMS can be used to investigate complex brain networks and obtain unique insights into the neural basis of emotions, mood, and personality.

Single- and Paired-Pulse TMS

TMS can also be applied to the scalp in single- and paired-pulse fashion. This allows researchers to obtain direct insights into certain aspects of cortical physiology. In a typical single-pulse TMS paradigm, a suprathreshold pulse is given to the primary motor cortex, which produces a motor evoked potential (MEP) that can be readily recorded from the contralateral thumb muscle (abductor pollicis brevis) or index finger muscle (first dorsal interosseus). The latency and amplitude of the MEP can be used to index processing speed and excitability of the frontal cortex and the corticospinal motor tract. In paired-pulse TMS paradigms, a subthreshold conditioning pulse is preceded by a suprathreshold test pulse to the motor cortex. The test pulse MEP will be inhibited if the interval between pulses is between 1 and 6 msec; this is referred to as "intracortical inhibition" (ICI). In contrast, the MEP will be larger if the test pulse precedes the conditioning pulse 8–30 msec; this is referred to as "intracortical facilitation" (ICF) (Chen et al., 1998). Pharmacological studies have shown that ICI is related to activation of GABAergic interneurons, whereas ICF is linked to glutamatergic action in the cortex (for a comprehensive review, see Ziemann, 2004). These paradigms can provide valuable information on cortical brain physiology in relation to emotions and mood states. For example, reduced GABAergic tone as evidenced by reduced ICI has been found in medication-free patients with major depression in a study using a paired-pulse TMS design (Bajbouj et al., 2006). Significant deficits in ICI have also been found in unmedicated patients with schizophrenia (Daskalakis et al., 2002); interestingly, the reductions in GABAergic inhibition were correlated with the severity of psychotic symptoms. These studies are exemplary for demonstrating direct correlates between aberrant cortical function and altered mood states. In Figure 11.5, the MEPs to single- and paired-pulse TMS are shown.

Although commonly used in psychiatry, the single- and paired-pulse TMS paradigms are relatively new research tools in the social neurosciences. In spite of this, they permit examination of certain aspects of the brain's communication pathways.

Single- and Paired-Pulse Studies of Cortical Excitability

Previous EEG and more recent rTMS studies have provided ample evidence for involvement of the left frontal cortex in approach-related emotions, and of the right frontal cortex in withdrawal-related emotions. However, among the remaining unknowns concerning the frontal asymmetry model of emotion is the role of cortical excitability in motivational tendencies. Frontal asymmetrical EEG resting states and motivational tendencies indexed by the Carver and White (1994) questionnaire were compared to cortical excitability of the left and right primary motor cortex (MT) as assessed by TMS in young, healthy right-handed volunteers. Results showed that predominant left frontal cortical excitability was correlated with enhanced emotional approach relative to avoidance. These findings concur with those of an earlier study, in which higher right- than left-sided levels of cortical excitability as determined by MT measurement were observed in patients with depression—a disorder characterized by increased avoidance and reduced approach-

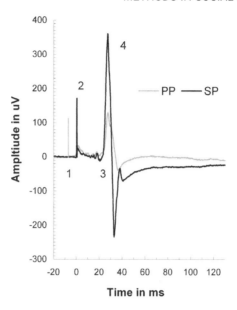

FIGURE 11.5. Motor evoked potentials (MEPs) recorded from abductor pollicis brevis to contralateral single-pulse (SP) and paired-pulse (PP) TMS over the primary motor cortex. 1, subthreshold conditioning pulse in PP condition; 2, suprathreshold test pulse; 3, onset of MEPs at ~24 msec; 4, MEPs.

related motivation. Furthermore, asymmetries of brain excitability and approach–avoidance motivational predispositions were both reflected by frontal beta EEG (13–30 Hz) asymmetries (Schutter, Weijer, Meuwese, Morgan, & van Honk, 2008). The findings not only provide strong support for the frontal asymmetry model of emotion, but also offer a new entry point into the neural substrates of motivation, personality, and action.

The close connections among perception, emotion, and action (Frijda, 1986; Hajcak et al., 2007) were further investigated by measuring changes in corticospinal motor tract excitability to fearful facial expressions (Schutter, Hofman, & van Honk, 2008). In this study, a single suprathreshold TMS pulse was given to the primary motor cortex 300 msec after presentation of a fearful, happy, or neutral facial expression. MEPs were measured from the abductor pollicis brevis to record changes in cortical excitability to face presentation. In agreement with evolutionary views on the relation between threat signals and action readiness (Öhman, 1986), significant MEP increases were observed after fearful as compared to happy and neutral facial expressions (Figure 11.6). The

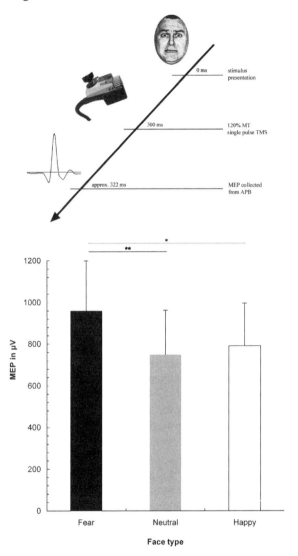

FIGURE 11.6. Single-pulse TMS delivered to the primary motor cortex 300 msec after presentation of emotional facial expressions (upper panel). There were significant increases in MEPs to fearful as compared to neutral and happy facial expressions (lower panel). From Schutter, Hofman, & van Honk (2008). Copyright 2008 by Blackwell Publishing. Reprinted by permission.

data demonstrate direct activation of the defensive brain circuits devoted to attention and action preparation (Davis & Whalen, 2001).

Future paired-pulse TMS studies may be able to delineate whether the threat-related increase of the MEP results from reduced GABAergic input, elevated glutamatergic input, or a combination of both.

Single- and Paired-Pulse Studies of Interhemispheric Connectivity

A physiological basis for investigating frontal brain communication, balance, and asymmetries requires the study of white matter fiber connections between the cerebral hemispheres. This bundle of fiber connections is called the corpus callosum and constitutes the main trajectory for information transfer between the cerebral hemispheres. Communication between the hemispheres is based on a cortical mechanism of excitatory transcallosal fibers targeting inhibitory interneurons, which is known as "transcallosal inhibition" (TCI). The vast majority of techniques used in functional studies of the human brain provide only indirect information about TCI, but it can be directly studied with two TMS paradigms. In the first (paired-pulse) variant, the MEP to a single unilateral pulse is compared to the MEP to a unilateral magnetic (test) pulse that is preceded by a contralateral magnetic (conditioning) pulse. When the test pulse is given ~10 msec after the conditioned stimulus, a significant reduction in size of the MEP test response is observed (Figure 11.7).

In the second (single-pulse) TMS variant, as depicted in Figure 11.8, TCI can be demonstrated by suppressing ongoing voluntary muscle activity in the ipsilateral hand to a unilateral magnetic pulse; this suppression is known as the "ipsilateral silent period" (iSP). This inhibitory process starts ~30–40 msec following a contralateral magnetic pulse. TCI has been demonstrated to be absent in acallosal patients, but is preserved in patients with lesions in the descending corticospinal motor tract, suggesting that TCI is a phenomenon of the corpus callosum (Meyer, Roricht, & Woiciechowsky, 1998).

Interestingly, abnormalities in TCI as evidenced by a longer iSP have been observed attention-deficit/hyperactivity disorder (ADHD) in children and attributed to delayed brain maturation (Garvey et al., 2005). Deceased interhemispheric functional connectivity may explain some of the behavioral disturbances observed in ADHD, including impulsivity, motor disinhibition, and impaired emotion regulation. Reduced bidirectional TCI has also been demonstrated in females and males with alexthymia (Richter et al., 2006). "Alexithymia" literally means "without words for emotions" and refers to persons who have difficulties in identifying, understanding, and describing their emotions. According

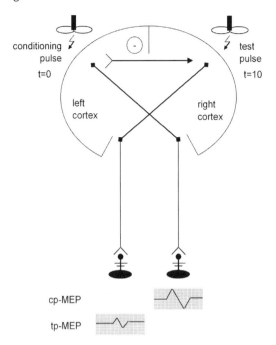

FIGURE 11.7. Paired-pulse TMS paradigm for quantifying transcallosal inhibition (TCI) between the cerebral hemispheres. –, inhibitory projections; cp, conditioning pulse (t = 0 msec); tp, test pulse (t = ~10 msec); MEP, motor evoked potential.

to Richter and colleagues (2006), reduced communication between the "verbal" left hemisphere and the "emotional" right hemisphere may result in a failure to integrate verbalization with emotion-related processing streams. Although the lateralized effect of emotions in the right hemisphere is not consistent with the frontal asymmetry model, the TCI abnormalities associated with alexithymia are notable and warrant further research.

Paired-Pulse Studies of Cerebellocortical Interactions

Similar to the interhemispheric connections via the corpus callosum, projections between the cerebellum and frontal cortex are inhibitory; hence the term "cerebellocortical inhibition" (CCI). CCI can be demonstrated by applying magnetic pulses in brief succession to the cerebellum and motor cortex. The MEP to a unilateral pulse is compared with the MEP to a unilateral magnetic (test) pulse that is preceded by a contral-

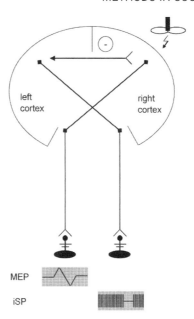

FIGURE 11.8. Single-pulse TMS paradigm for quantifying TCI between the cerebral hemispheres. –, inhibitory projections; tp, test pulse (t = ~10 msec); MEP, motor evoked potential; iSP, ipsilateral silent period.

ateral magnetic (conditioning) pulse applied to cerebellum. When the test pulse is given ~5–7 msec after the conditioned stimulus, a significant reduction in size of the MEP test response is observed (Figure 11.9). CCI is the unilateral test pulse MEP minus the unilateral test pulse MEP preceded by the contralateral conditioning pulse.

Reduced CCI has recently been demonstrated in patients with schizophrenia (Daskalakis, Christensen, Fitzgerald, Fountain, & Chen, 2005). Impaired cerebellocortical connectivity may play an important role in disturbed thinking patterns, psychoses, and emotion dysregulation. In particular, since reduced ICI has also been observed in patients with schizophrenia, the findings support abnormalities in either cerebellar output or cerebellocortical connectivity. Interestingly, a growing body of evidence suggests that rTMS over the cerebellum can modulate CCI (Chen, 2004). This would, for instance, provide the opportunity to examine the relation between cerebellar involvement in emotion regulation (Schutter et al., 2007) and changes in cerebellocortical connectivity. In particular, since emotions, mood, and personality are unlikely to be localizable in discrete regions, studying the brain's connectivity patterns with TMS may be a more powerful approach.

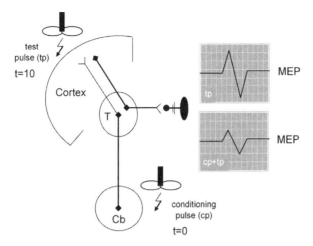

FIGURE 11.9. Paired-pulse TMS paradigm for quantifying cerebellar inhibition of the cortex (CCI). Cb, cerebellum; T, thalamus; t, time in milliseconds; cp, conditioning pulse (t = 0 msec); tp, test pulse (t = 5–7 msec); MEP, motor evoked potential.

Summary of Single- and Paired-Pulse Research

TMS can be used to study cortical physiology and functional connectivity. Single-pulse TMS can index changes in cortical excitability to emotional information entering the system, or can measure cortical excitability related to internal motivational or emotional states. Paired-pulse TMS ICI and ICF can give insights into GABAergic and glutamatergic activity in relation to emotive processes and motivational tendencies. Furthermore, ICI and CCI can be used as measures of functional connectivity. Abnormalities in functional connectivity have been associated with several psychopathological disorders, including schizophrenia and depression. These measures can offer exclusive insights into the neurophysiological underpinnings of human affect.

Discussion

Since its introduction in 1985, TMS has become an established research tool in studying brain–function relationships. By decomposing complex cognitive functions into separate units and localizations, TMS can help researchers determine which brain areas are actively involved in specific functions, as well as when they are participating. Although the potential contribution of such approaches to the understanding of the relation between structure and function is generally acknowledged, critics argue that, similar to neuroimaging techniques, TMS has certain conceptual difficulties. The term "new phrenology" has been coined to highlight a fundamental problem with the modern neuroscientific approaches (Uttal, 2002): It may not be possible to dissect the workings of complex emotive and cognitive behaviors on the basis of these approaches, for the assumption of a one-to-one relation between a function and the localization of its underlying neural representations may be false. Although TMS methods cannot account for the explanatory gap between neurophysiological dynamics and the ways in which subjective experiences arise from such functions of the brain, these new and innovative techniques can identify and locate certain psychoneural entities, or at least key nodes within the greater whole, by means of true causal analyses (Schutter, van Honk, & Panksepp, 2004). Furthermore, TMS technology enables researchers to directly investigate functional brain connectivity, which goes beyond the localization and mapping of brain function. In spite of its strengths, magnetic brain stimulation does have a number of limitations; these and other points of interest are discussed in more detail below.

Safety

An important practical issue in TMS research is safety. TMS is a noninvasive way of conveying electric charges into the brain, and therefore is capable of eliciting adverse events (Wassermann, 1998). Accidental seizures are considered the most serious adverse events, and cases of TMS-related seizures were reported before the mid-1990s. Even though these cases could be explained in terms of family histories of epilepsy, medication, and high stimulation intensities, general safety guidelines for TMS were introduced in 1996 by the International Federation of Clinical Neurophysiology (IFCN) (see Wassermann, 1998). The guidelines include contraindications (including a family history of epilepsy and a personal history of brain trauma), as well as safe stimulation parameters. It is estimated that tens of thousands of subjects around the world have participated in TMS research since the introduction of the IFCN guidelines, and reports of accidental seizures since then have been extremely rare. Furthermore, results from a recent review on the incidence of adverse events show that the chance of an adverse event in patients with epilepsy is approximately 1.4% (Bae et al., 2007). In fact, slow-frequency rTMS is now actually used in treating epilepsy (Tassinari, Cincotta, Zaccara, & Michelucci, 2003). Finally, there is even some evidence suggesting that rTMS has neuroprotective properties (Post, Müller, Engelmann, & Keck, 1999). In sum, TMS is a safe technique as long as the IFCN guidelines are followed.

Localization

Another important aspect of TMS research is the issue of localization. One way to determine the target region on the scalp is by using the scalp site that overlies the thumb representation ("hot spot") of the motor cortex as a marker for estimating the cortical region of interest. For example, the dorsolateral PFC is then approximated by moving 4.5 cm anterior to the thumb hot spot. The international 10–20 EEG system is another strategy that is often used in TMS research. The 10–20 EEG system is based on the relationship between electrode location and underlying area of cerebral cortex. The distances between neighboring electrodes are either 10% or 20% of the total front-to-back or right-to-left distance on the scalp. Anatomical brain scans and the 10–20 EEG system show a good fit for regions located in the frontal cortex, but variability increases toward the back of the head (Herwig, Satrapi, & Schonfeldt-Lecuona, 2003). Although both localization methods are sufficient for addressing research questions on lateralization and anterior–posterior distinctions, these methods are not suitable for finer-grained positioning. To overcome this limitation, structural brain scans can be used to navigate the TMS coil over the scalp, to target the underlying cortical region of interest to the nearest centimeter. In addition, data from functional neuroimaging experiments can be used to target clusters or "blobs" of activation with TMS, as well as to examine the functional nature of these activations.

Depth of Stimulation

The vast majority of commercially available TMS machines deliver magnetic pulses that penetrate the brain approximately 2–3 cm. As a result, the direct physiological effects of TMS are confined to the superficial layers of the cerebral cortex and cerebellum.

Although these brain areas evidently play important roles in the experience and regulation of emotion and motivation, subcortical brain structures such as the amygdala and the nucleus accumbens cannot be reached with TMS directly. However, distal effects in response to focal TMS have been well described in the literature. Strafella, Paus, Barrett, and Dagher (2001), for instance, found changes in dopaminergic activity of the striatum in response to PFC rTMS, suggesting that rTMS is a suitable approach for studying the cortical and subcortical components of the brain's reward circuitry. It should be pointed out that these type of studies show that the effects of rTMS are not limited to the area being targeted. The changes in emotional and motivational behavior are therefore more likely to be the results of changes in functionally connected networks.

An exciting new development in the field of magnetic brain stimulation is the construction of a new type of coil, named the Hesed coil (H-coil) (Roth, Amir, Levkovitz, & Zangen, 2007). The unique configuration of the H-coil allows researchers to stimulate deep brain regions directly. The efficacy of this coil was demonstrated by activating the primary motor cortex at a distance of 5–6 cm (Zangen, Roth, Voller, & Hallett, 2005). Although the magnetic field is less focal than that of the traditional coils, the development of this coil type holds great promise for noninvasive stimulation of deep brain structures.

Generalizability

The primary motor cortex is commonly used as the reference region for estimating an excitability index for the cerebral cortex and is used to calibrate TMS intensities. Electric responses recorded over the primary motor cortex have been shown to correlate with the electric responses over the PFC evoked by single pulses of TMS (Kähkönen, Komssi, Wilenius, & Ilmoniemi, 2005). Even though the similarities between the brain responses suggest common underlying neurophysiological properties, this assumption is by no means indisputable (for a review, see Komssi & Kähkönen, 2006). In an earlier study, no evidence was found that primary motor cortex excitability and visual cortex excitability were correlated (Stewart, Walsh, & Rothwell, 2001). Visual cortex excitability can be assessed by quantifying the presence or absence of auras to single-pulse TMS over the occipital area—the so-called "phosphene threshold." However, more recently, a positive relationship between phosphene and motor thresholds was observed; these results support the view of a shared responsiveness to TMS across the cortical surface (Deblieck, Thompson, Iacoboni, & Wu, 2008). It is suggested that differences in scalp-to-cortex distance and brain anatomy may at least partially explain the variations found across the cerebral cortex. Although the generalization of primary motor cortex excitability to other cortical brain regions should be made with caution, several studies suggest that the physiological properties measured from the primary motor cortex may provide a useful index for other cortical areas as well.

Conclusion

Despite the fact that TMS is a relatively new research tool, it has already made significant contributions to the field of social neuroscience. With TMS, researchers no longer have to rely on mere causal suppositions that can arise in abundance from correlations between structure and function derived from modern brain imaging. Furthermore, the integration of rTMS technology with modern neuroimaging methods is an ongoing development that will allow researchers to combine the strengths of the different brain techniques, and to develop stronger neurobiological models of motivation, emotion, mood, and personality. Finally, TMS can also be employed to study aspects of cortical physiology and functional connectivity, which provide a strong framework and direct approach for tapping into the central nervous system.

In conclusion, TMS is a technique that "can serve as a heuristic method for resolving causal issues in an arena where only correlative tools have traditionally been available" (Schutter, van Honk, & Panksepp, 2004, p. 151). As such, it is a unique tool for studying the neurobiological basis of human social behavior.

Acknowledgment

The writing of this chapter was supported by an Innovational Research Grant (No. VIDI 452-07-012) from the Netherlands Organization for Scientific Research.

References

Bae, E. H., Schrader, L. M., Machii, K., Alonso-Alonso, M., Riviello, J. J., Pascual-Leone, A., et al. (2007). Safety and tolerability of repetitive transcranial magnetic stimulation in patients with epilepsy: A review of the literature. *Epilepsy and Behavior, 10*, 521–528.

Bajbouj, M., Lisanby, S. H., Lang, U. E., Danker-Hopfe, H., Heuser, I., & Neu, P. (2006). Evidence for impaired cortical inhibition in patients with unipolar major depression. *Biological Psychiatry, 59*, 395–400.

Barker, A. T. (1991). An introduction to the basic principles of magnetic nerve stimulation. *Journal of Clinical Neurophysiology, 8*, 26–37.

Barker, A. T., Jalinous, R., & Freeston, I. L. (1985). Non-invasive magnetic stimulation of human motor cortex. *Lancet, 325*, 1106–1107.

Bohning, D. E. (2000). Introduction and overview of TMS physics. In M. S. George & R. H. Belmaker (Eds.), *Transcranial magnetic stimulation in neuropsychiatry* (pp. 3–44). Washington, DC: American Psychiatric Press.

Carver, C. S., & White, T. L. (1994). Behavioral inhibition, behavioral activation, and affective responses to impending reward and punishment: The BIS/BAS scales. *Journal of Personality and Social Psychology, 67*, 319–333.

Chen, R. (2004). Interactions between inhibitory and excitatory circuits in the human motor cortex. *Experimental Brain Research, 154*, 1–10.

Chen, R., Tam, A., Butefisch, C., Corwell, B., Ziemann, U., Rothwell, J. C., et al. (1998). Intracortical inhibition and facilitation in different representations of the human motor cortex. *Journal of Neurophysiology, 80,* 2870–2881.

d'Alfonso, A. A. L., van Honk, J., Hermans, E. J., Postma, A., & de Haan, E. H. F. (2000). Laterality effects in selective attention to threat after repetitive transcranial magnetic stimulation at the prefrontal cortex in female subjects. *Neuroscience Letters, 280,* 195–198.

Daskalakis, Z. J., Christensen, B. K., Chen, R., Fitzgerald, P. B., Zipursky, R. B., & Kapur, S. (2002). Evidence for impaired cortical inhibition in schizophrenia using transcranial magnetic stimulation. *Archives of General Psychiatry, 59,* 347–354.

Daskalakis, Z. J., Christensen, B. K., Fitzgerald, P. B., Fountain, S. I., & Chen, R. (2005). Reduced cerebellar inhibition in schizophrenia: A preliminary study. *American Journal of Psychiatry, 162,* 1203–1205.

Daskalakis, Z. J., Möller, B., Christensen, B. K., Fitzgerald, P. B., Gunraj, C., & Chen, R. (2006). The effects of repetitive transcranial magnetic stimulation on cortical inhibition in healthy human subjects. *Experimental Brain Research, 174,* 403–412.

Davis, M., & Whalen, P. J. (2001). The amygdala: Vigilance and emotion. *Molecular Psychiatry, 6,* 13–34.

Deblieck, C., Thompson, B., Iacoboni, M., & Wu, A. D. (2008). Correlation between motor and phosphene thresholds: A transcranial magnetic stimulation study. *Human Brain Mapping, 29*(6), 662–670.

Fox, N. A. (1991). If it's not left, it's right: Electroencephalograph asymmetry and the development of emotion. *American Psychologist, 46,* 863–872.

Frijda, N. (1986). *The emotions.* Cambridge, UK: Cambridge University Press.

Garvey, M. A., Ziemann, U., Bartko, J. J., Denckla, M. B., Barker, C. A., & Wassermann, E. M. (2005). The ipsilateral silent period in boys with attention-deficit/hyperactivity disorder. *Clinical Neurophysiology, 116,* 1889–1896.

George, M. S., Wassermann, E. M., Kimbrell, T. A., Little, J. T., Williams, W. E., Danielson, A. L., et al. (1997). Mood improvement following daily left prefrontal repetitive transcranial magnetic stimulation in patients with depression: A placebo-controlled crossover trial. *American Journal of Psychiatry, 154,* 1752–1756.

Hajcak, G., Molnar, C., George, M. S., Bolger, K., Koola, J., & Nahas, Z. (2007). Emotion facilitates action: A transcranial magnetic stimulation study of motor cortex excitability during picture viewing. *Psychophysiology, 44,* 91–97.

Hallett, M. (2007). Transcranial magnetic stimulation: A primer. *Neuron, 55,* 187–199.

Harmon-Jones, E. (2003). Clarifying the emotive functions of asymmetrical frontal cortical activity. *Psychophysiology, 40,* 838–848.

Heath, R. G. (1977). Modulation of emotion with a brain pacemaker: Treatment for intractable psychiatric illness. *Journal of Nervous and Mental Disease, 165,* 300–317.

Heath, R. G., Dempsey, C. W., Fontana, C. J., & Myers, W. A. (1978). Cerebellar stimulation: Effects on septal region, hippocampus and amygdala of cats and rats. *Biological Psychiatry, 13*, 501–529.

Heller, W., Nitschke, J. B., Etienne, M. A., & Miller, G. A. (1997). Patterns of regional brain activity differentiate types of anxiety. *Journal of Abnormal Psychology, 106*, 376–385.

Herwig, U., Satrapi, P., & Schonfeldt-Lecuona, C. (2003). Using the international 10–20 EEG system for positioning of transcranial magnetic stimulation. *Brain Topography, 16*, 95–99.

Hoflich, G., Kaper, S., Hufnagel, A., Ruhrmann, S., & Moller, H. J. (1993). Application of transcranial magnetic stimulation in treatment of drug-resistant major depression: A report of two cases. *Human Psychopharmacology, 8*, 361–365.

Ilmoniemi, R. J., Virtanen, J., Ruohonen, J., Karhu, J., Aronen, H. J., Naätanen, R., et al. (1997). Neuronal responses to magnetic stimulation reveal cortical reactivity and connectivity. *NeuroReport, 8*, 3537–3540.

Jing, H., & Takigawa, M. (2001). Observation of EEG coherence after repetitive transcranial magnetic stimulation. *Clinical Neurophysiology, 111*, 1620–1631.

Kähkönen, S., Komssi, S., Wilenius, J., & Ilmoniemi, R. J. (2005). Prefrontal TMS produces smaller EEG responses than motor-cortex TMS: Implications for rTMS treatment in depression. *Psychopharmacology, 181*, 16–20.

Khedr, E. M., Rothwell, J. C., Ahmed, M. A., Shawky, O. A., & Farouk, M. (2007). Modulation of motor cortical excitability following rapid-rate transcranial magnetic stimulation. *Clinical Neurophysiology, 118*, 140–145.

Komssi, S., & Kähkönen, S. (2006). The novelty value of the combined use of electroencephalography and transcranial magnetic stimulation for neuroscience research. *Brain Research Reviews, 52*, 183–192.

Merton, P. A., & Morton, H. B. (1980). Stimulation of the cerebral cortex in the intact human subject. *Nature, 285*, 227.

Meyer, B. U., Roricht, S., & Woiciechowsky, C. (1998). Topography of fibers in the human corpus callosum mediating interhemispheric inhibition between the motor cortices. *Annals of Neurology, 43*, 360–369.

Mizuki, Y., Suetsugi, M., Ushijima, I., & Yamada, M. (1997). Differential effects of dopaminergic drugs on anxiety and arousal in healthy volunteers with high and low anxiety. *Progress in Neuropsychopharmacology and Biological Psychiatry, 21*, 573–590.

Öhman, A. (1986). Face the beast and fear the face: Animal and social fears as prototypes for evolutionary analyses of emotion. *Psychophysiology, 23*, 123–145.

Pascual-Leone, A., Walsh, V., & Rothwell, J. (2000). Transcranial magnetic stimulation in cognitive neuroscience: Virtual lesion, chronometry, and functional connectivity. *Current Opinion in Neurobiology, 10*, 232–237.

Post, A., Müller, M. B., Engelmann, M., & Keck, M. E. (1999). Repetitive transcranial magnetic stimulation in rats: Evidence for a neuroprotective effect *in vitro* and *in vivo*. *European Journal of Neuroscience, 11*, 3247–3254.

Richter, J., Möller, B., Spitzer, C., Letzel, S., Bartols, S., Barnow, S., et al. (2006). Transcallosal inhibition in patients with and without alexithymia. *Neuropsychobiology, 53,* 101–107.

Roth, Y., Amir, A., Levkovitz, Y., & Zangen, A. (2007). Three-dimensional distribution of the electric field induced in the brain by transcranial magnetic stimulation using figure-8 and deep H-coils. *Journal of Clinical Neurophysiology, 24,* 31–38.

Schmahmann, J. D. (2004). Disorders of the cerebellum: Ataxia, dysmetria of thought, and the cerebellar cognitive affective syndrome. *Journal of Neuropsychiatry and Clinical Neurosciences, 16,* 367–378.

Schutter, D. J. L. G., de Haan, E. H. F., & van Honk, J. (2004). Functionally dissociated aspects in anterior and posterior electrocortical processing of facial threat. *International Journal of Psychophysiology, 53,* 29–36.

Schutter, D. J. L. G., Enter, D., & Hoppenbrouwers, S. S. (in press). High frequency transcranial magnetic stimulation to the cerebellum and implicit information processing of happy facial expressions. *Journal of Psychiatry and Neuroscience.*

Schutter, D. J. L. G., Enter, D., & van Honk, J. (2007). Cerebellar involvement in emotion regulation: A transcranial magnetic stimulation study *NeuroImage, 36,* S62 .

Schutter, D. J. L. G., Hofman, D., & van Honk, J. (2008). Fearful faces selectively increase corticospinal motor tract excitability: A transcranial magnetic stimulation study. *Psychophysiology, 45*(3), 345–348.

Schutter, D. J. L. G., Kammers, M. P. M., Enter, D., & van Honk, J. (2006). A case of illusory own-body perceptions after transcranial magnetic stimulation of the cerebellum. *Cerebellum, 5,* 238–240.

Schutter, D. J. L. G., Putman, P., Hermans, E. J., & van Honk, J. (2001). Parietal electroencephalogram beta asymmetry and selective attention for angry facial expressions. *Neuroscience Letters, 314,* 13–16.

Schutter, D. J. L. G., & van Honk, J. (2005). The cerebellum on the rise in human emotion. *Cerebellum, 4,* 290–294.

Schutter, D. J. L. G., & van Honk, J. (2006). An electrophysiological link between the cerebellum, cognition and emotion: Frontal theta EEG activity to single-pulse cerebellar TMS. *NeuroImage, 33,* 1227–1231

Schutter, D. J. L. G., van Honk, J., d'Alfonso, A. A. L., Peper, J. S., & Panksepp, J. (2003). High frequency repetitive transcranial magnetic over the medial cerebellum induces a shift in the prefrontal electroencephalography gamma spectrum: A pilot study in humans. *Neuroscience Letters, 336,* 73–76.

Schutter, D. J. L. G., van Honk, J., d'Alfonso, A. A. L., Postma, A., & de Haan, E. H. F. (2001). Effects of slow rTMS at the right dorsolateral prefrontal cortex on EEG asymmetry and mood. *NeuroReport, 12,* 445–447.

Schutter, D. J. L. G., van Honk, J., & Panksepp, J. (2004). Introducing transcranial magnetic stimulation (TMS) and its property of causal inference in investigating brain–function relationships. *Synthese, 141,* 151–173.

Schutter, D. J. L. G., Weijer, A. D., Meuwese, J. D. I., Morgan, B., & van Honk,

J. (2008). Interrelations between motivational stance, cortical excitability, and the frontal electroencephalogram asymmetry of emotion: A transcranial magnetic stimulation study. *Human Brain Mapping, 29*(5), 574–580.

Sibon, I., Strafella, A. P., Gravel, P., Ko, J. H., Booij, L., Soucy, J. P., et al. (2007). Acute prefrontal cortex TMS in healthy volunteers: Effects on brain 11C-aMtrp trapping. *NeuroImage, 34,* 1658–1664.

Snyder, A., Bossomaier, T., & Mitchell, D. J. (2004). Concept formation: "Object" attributes dynamically inhibited from conscious awareness. *Journal of Integrative Neuroscience, 3,* 31–46.

Speer, A. M., Kimbrell, T. A., Wassermann, E. M., Repella, J. D., Willis, M. W., Herscovitch, P., et al. (2000). Opposite effects of high and low frequency rTMS on regional brain activity in depressed patients. *Biological Psychiatry, 48,* 1133–1141.

Speer, A. M., Willis, M. W., Herscovitch, P., Daube-Witherspoon, M., Shelton, J. R., Benson, B. E., et al. (2003). Intensity-dependent regional cerebral blood flow during 1–Hz repetitive transcranial magnetic stimulation (rTMS) in healthy volunteers studied with H215O positron emission tomography: II. Effects of prefrontal cortex rTMS. *Biological Psychiatry, 54,* 826–832.

Stewart, L. M., Ellison, A., Walsh, V., & Cowey, A. (2001). The role of transcranial magnetic stimulation (TMS) in studies of vision, attention and cognition. *Acta Psychologica, 107,* 275–291.

Stewart, L. M., Walsh, V., & Rothwell, J. C. (2001). Motor and phosphene thresholds: A transcranial magnetic stimulation correlation study. *Neuropsychologia, 39,* 415–419.

Strafella, A., Paus, T., Barrett, J., & Dagher, A. (2001). Repetitive transcranial magnetic stimulation of the human prefrontal cortex induces dopamine release in the caudate nucleus. *Journal of Neuroscience, 21,* 1–4.

Tassinari, C. A., Cincotta, M., Zaccara, G., & Michelucci, R. (2003). Transcranial magnetic stimulation and epilepsy. *Clinical Neurophysiology, 114,* 777–798.

Uttal, W. R. (2002). Précis of *The new phrenology: The limits of localizing cognitive processes in the brain. Brain and Mind, 3,* 221–228.

van Honk, J., Hermans, E. J., d'Alfonso, A. A. L., Schutter, D. J. L. G., van Doornen, L., & de Haan, E. H. F. (2002). A left-prefrontal lateralized, sympathetic mechanism directs attention towards social threat in humans: Evidence from repetitive transcranial magnetic stimulation. *Neuroscience Letters, 319,* 99–102.

van Honk, J., & Schutter, D. J. L. G. (2006). From affective valence to motivational direction: The frontal asymmetry of emotion revised. *Psychological Science, 17,* 963–965.

van Honk, J., & Schutter, D. J. L. G. (2007). Vigilant and avoidant responses to angry facial expressions: Dominance and submissive motives. In E. Harmon-Jones & P. Winkielman (Eds.), *Social neuroscience: Integrating biological and psychological explanations of social behavior* (pp. 197–226). New York: Guilford Press.

van Honk, J., Schutter, D. J. L. G., Putman, P., de Haan, E. H. F., & d'Alfonso,

A. A. L. (2003). Reductions in phenomenological, physiological and attentional indices of depression after 2 Hz rTMS over the right parietal cortex in healthy human subjects. *Psychiatry Research, 120,* 95–101.

Walsh, V., & Pascual-Leone, A. (2003). *Transcranial magnetic stimulation: A neurochronometrics of mind.* Cambridge, MA: MIT Press.

Wassermann, E. M. (1998). Risk and safety of repetitive transcranial magnetic stimulation: Report and suggested guidelines from the International Workshop on the Safety of Repetitive Transcranial Magnetic Stimulation, June 5–7, 1996. *Electroencephalography and Clinical Neurophysiology, 108,* 1–16.

Wassermann, E. M., & Lisanby, S. H. (2001). Therapeutic application of repetitive transcranial magnetic stimulation: A review. *Clinical Neurophysiology, 112,* 1367–1377.

Werhahn, K. J., Conforto, A. B., Kadom, N., Hallett, M., & Cohen, L. G. (2003). Contribution of the ipsilateral motor cortex to recovery after chronic stroke. *Annals of Neurology, 54,* 464–472.

Zangen, A., Roth, Y., Voller, B., & Hallett, M. (2005). Transcranial magnetic stimulation of deep brain regions: Evidence for efficacy of the H-coil. *Clinical Neurophysiology, 116,* 775–779.

Ziemann, U. (2004). TMS and drugs. *Clinical Neurophysiology, 115,* 1717–1729.

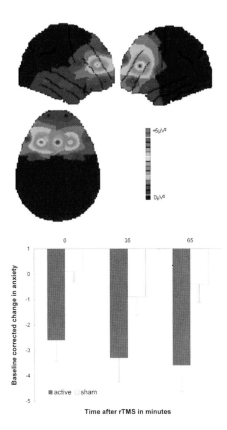

PLATE 11.1. Contralateral increases in frontal theta EEG activity (upper panel), and reductions in anxiety after 1-Hz rTMS over the right dorsolateral PFC (lower panel). Lower panel from Schutter, van Honk, et al. (2001). Copyright 2001 by Lippincott Williams & Wilkins. Reprinted by permission.

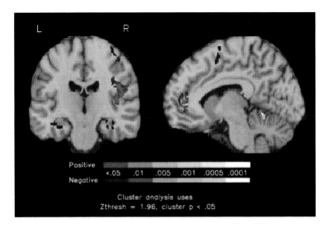

PLATE 11.2. Pattern of neural activity following slow-frequency rTMS over the left PFC. From Speer et al. (2003). Copyright 2003 by Elsevier, Inc. Adapted by permission.

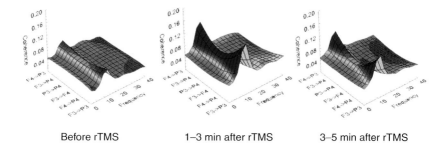

Before rTMS   1–3 min after rTMS   3–5 min after rTMS

PLATE 11.3. Significant increases in brain connectivity after fast-frequency rTMS to the left PFC. From Jing and Takigawa (2001). Copyright 2001 by Elsevier, Inc. Adapted by permission.

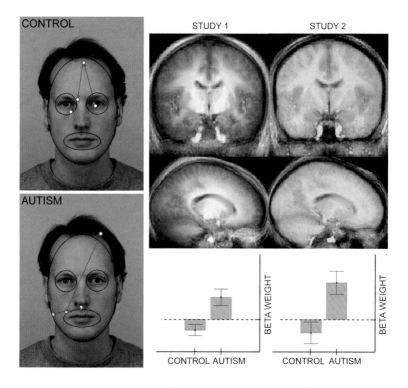

PLATE 14.1. An example of combining fMRI data with behavioral measures. In this study, fMRI was used to measure brain activation while a group of individuals with autism and a matched control group looked at pictures of faces. Eye gaze was tracked concurrently with fMRI. Left: Examples of eye gaze trajectories while individuals with autism (bottom) and controls (top) looked at the faces. Top right: Blue regions depict areas of the amygdala in which increased visual fixation on the eye region of faces predicted increased brain activation in the autism group, but not in the control group. Bottom right: Beta weights from the regression of eye fixation on brain activation in the amygdala show positive betas for the autism group only, implying that amygdala activation in the autism group, but not the control group, was related to the amount of time participants spent fixating on the eye region. Data from Dalton et al. (2005).

12

Using Connectionist Networks to Understand Neurobiological Processes in Social and Personality Psychology

Stephen J. Read
Brian M. Monroe

The other chapters in this book describe a wide range of different techniques for gathering data on how the brain supports and enables personality, social perception, social reasoning, and social behavior. This chapter is quite different: Here we focus on a particular class of techniques for building models of how various brain regions function and how they interact with one another. These techniques go by the name of "neural network modeling" or "connectionist modeling." Although some modeling approaches in neuroscience seek to model the behavior of individual neurons in detail, that is not the approach we take here. We are considering approaches in which we try to model the behavior of brain systems and their interactions—approaches that we believe to be critical for social and personality neuroscientists.

Much recent social–personality neuroscience has provided evidence that particular brain regions, particular systems, or particular responses play an important role in many different aspects of social perception and social reasoning. For example, researchers have demonstrated that the amygdala seems to play a role in stereotyping and negative evaluation of members of negatively stereotyped groups (Phelps et al., 2000). More generally, the amygdala seems to play a broad role in both positive and negative evaluations (e.g., Adolphs & Damasio, 2001; Cunningham, Raye, & Johnson, 2004.) For example, work by Bechara, Tranel, Damasio, and Damasio (1996) has provided evidence that a circuit involving the amygdala and the prefrontal cortex plays an important role in the ability to represent and experience anticipatory negative emotions in anticipation of taking a particular action, and that damage to elements in this circuit has a negative impact on appropriate and successful social functioning. Other work has provided evidence that various parts of the prefrontal cortex and other related brain regions play a critical role in various aspects of social perception, such as the activation of the superior temporal sulcus during judgments of intentionality (Pelphrey, Morris, & McCarthy, 2004) and the relation of the anterior paracingulate cortex to representation of others' beliefs (Walter et al., 2004). Still other work has identified some of the regions in the prefrontal cortex involved in self-regulation (Banfield, Wyland, Macrae, Münte, & Heatherton, 2004). Work by Eisenberger, Lieberman, and Williams (2003) has provided evidence that brain regions (e.g., anterior cingulate cortex, right ventral prefrontal cortex) that have been implicated in the perception of physical pain are also activated when people experience the "pain" of social rejection and ostracism. Other work has shown that the anterior cingulate cortex is active during episodes of cognitive dissonance (Harmon-Jones, 2004) and unintended race bias (Amodio et al. 2004).

Social reasoning, social perception, and social behavior clearly involve the interaction of many different brain centers, each doing a different kind of processing. Each region takes its inputs and processes them in certain ways, transforming that information in various ways and then sending it along to other centers. However, these relationships are by no means one-way. The brain, especially the human brain, is massively bidirectionally connected, enabling a wide array of feedback relationships among different brain centers. Not only do numerous "lower-level" brain regions send signals to various parts of the frontal cortex; the frontal cortex also has massive sets of connections back to the lower-level brain centers (e.g., Cunningham & Zelazo, 2007; O'Reilly & Munakata, 2000). For example, there is evidence that activation of the right lateral and orbital prefrontal cortex can inhibit the activation of lower-level systems (e.g., the amygdala) involved in emotional responding (Ochsner et al., 2004). And this is only one example of the massive bidirectionality of connections in the brain.

These extensive feedback relationships result in a highly dynamic system, with many different regions continually interacting with one another. But how such massive feedback relationships affect the brain and how numerous brain centers interact with each other cannot be adequately captured in verbal models or graphic representations, such as flowcharts or brain circuits. Verbal and graphic representations and intuition are weak tools for trying to understand such interacting, dynamic systems. To adequately understand such dynamic systems requires the development of adequate computational and mathematical models. One widely used technique for modeling such dynamically interacting brain systems is the construction of neural network models of the systems hypothesized to underlie particular psychological phenomena.

Neural network models have been extensively used in cognitive psychology and cognitive neuroscience to model a wide range of different tasks—from vision to reading to categorization, to attention, to short- and long-term memory (e.g., Botvinick & Plaut, 2006; for a review, see O'Reilly & Munakata, 2003). However, they are rarely used to model personality and aspects of social perception and social behavior. In this chapter, we describe the applications of such modeling approaches to personality and to attitudes and social evaluation. These models can represent how specific systems perform specific computations and transform their inputs, as well as how these systems interact with one another. In these models, a particular task can be broken down into a set of individual subtasks whose processing takes place in specific regions and the interactions among those regions.

Until recently, work in cognitive neuroscience that used imaging techniques (functional magnetic resonance imaging [fMRI], positron emission tomography [PET], etc.) has tended to focus on presenting evidence for specific systems that are uniquely identified with a particular kind of processing task, and have not provided accounts of the entire circuit in which those specific systems are involved. These techniques rely on a subtractive methodology; that is, they compare activation given the target task to activation given a control task that is hypothesized to be similar in all but the critical processes. However, there has recently been an increasing focus on building computational models, often in the form of neural network models, of such tasks.

The advantages of building computational models of how the brain achieves its various tasks are severalfold. First, one can model the computations performed by a specific system or brain region. Second, and perhaps more importantly, one can model circuits of brain systems, rather than simply focusing on isolated regions. In other words, one can model how various systems interact with one another in performing different tasks. For example, such modeling enables one to address questions about the extent to which various systems may compete with one another, or what kinds of information provided by one system are used in the computations performed by another and how this informational input is transformed by the computations performed in the subsequent systems. Third, one can build a computational, dynamic model of the circuit that can be computationally tested, rather than having to rely on a verbal or graphic model that cannot adequately capture either the transformations computed by specific regions or the dynamic interactions among regions that characterize real brains. Fourth, one can model the impact of the massive bidirectional connectivity of the human brain. As noted earlier, this massive bidirectionality leads to highly interactive and dynamic systems, whose behavior cannot be adequately captured with verbal models.

In this chapter, we outline the basic concepts of a neural network model and provide two examples of neural network models of phenomena in personality and social psychology. In doing so, we rely on a specific neural network architecture that is much more biologically inspired than most such architectures, although it does not get to the level of building detailed models of individual neurons—a level of analysis that is largely unnecessary for social neuroscientists. This architecture is called Leabra (O'Reilly & Munakata, 2000), an acronym for "local, error-driven and associative, biologically realistic algorithm."

After discussing Leabra, we present a detailed account of our recent neural network model of personality. This model integrates a wide range of evidence, both neurobiological and behavioral, to create a model in which personality is based on the behavior of underlying, interacting motivational systems. In other words, this model integrates a variety of approaches to personality into a common approach. We then present an initial sketch of a model of implicit and explicit evaluation that draws on both Cunningham and Zelazo's (2007) iterative reprocessing model and our recent neural network model of attitudes and attitude change (Monroe & Read, 2008).

Other work that is not discussed here, but which is relevant to the current enterprise, is the work of Eiser, Fazio, Stafford, and Prescott (2003) on modeling the development of attitudes in terms of learning from reward and punishment. Also relevant is Zebrowitz's work (e.g., Zebrowitz, Fellous, Mignault, & Andreoletti, 2003) showing that simple neural network models can learn to extract the features relevant to her ecological approach (e.g., features defining baby-facedness or different emotions) and will then overgeneralize from those features.

Description of a Neural Network Model

A neural network model is ultimately just a group of interconnected nodes that influence each other by passing activation back and forth through the connections between these nodes. The power of such a network comes from the ways in which a large number of simple units can interact to form powerful processing systems that can perform a wide variety of very complex computations. These nodes (interchangeably called "units") can range along a continuum of anatomical and biophysical fidelity, from being extremely biologically realistic to capturing only the most abstract features of a neuron's behavior. In most models, the nodes are designed simply to capture the central, abstract features of neurons—the ability to integrate a wide range of inputs and output a signal that is the result of those inputs—rather than to capture biological realism. The widely shared assumption is that when networks of "neurons" perform relatively high-level psychological tasks, what is important is how they behave as a system and the computations they can perform as an ensemble, and that at that level of analysis biological realism is unnecessary and computationally extremely expensive.

One important distinction to be made is whether a model is a "distributed" model of cognition or a "localist" model. Distributed models preserve the idea that information is learned and distributed over a group of nodes, rather than representing the entirety of information about a single "item" in one node. Localist models embody more of an approximation in this sense, in that they do tend to represent distinct items or concepts with a single node.

The type of network one should use depends on the level at which it is most useful to examine a particular phenomenon. For applications like discriminating shapes, for example, where the particular portion of the visual field on which a stimulus lands is important, representing individual neurons (or at least small groups of neurons) in the model will be more important.

However, when one is trying to examine a problem in higher-order cognition, like causal reasoning, the patterns of neural activity are far richer and complex; it is typically advantageous to consolidate a block of neurons, operating together to represent a rich concept, into one node, and to sacrifice a small amount of fidelity in order to keep the model manageable and understandable. For example, if one's central focus is on representing associative learning between a possible cause and an effect, as in trying to model causal learning and attribution or certain aspects of person perception, one should probably just use one node for the cause and one for the effect. Creating a detailed distributed representation of the two concepts will not, in most circumstances, provide any further insight into associative learning in this context, but it will make the modeling task immeasurably harder and more difficult to understand.

But to the degree that varying stimulus patterns (such as contextual cues) may alter the interpretation of features or concepts represented in the model, such as when one wants to model how pieces of information about a target in a stereotyping study may be processed, these features should be separately represented so that one can examine how they are processed and interact with one another. Unless one makes the claim that each node in the model represents an individual neuron, approximations are being made. For most problems of interest to social psychologists, individual neurons are not of primary interest; social concepts are likely to be encoded over large groups of associated neurons, and they are likely to behave with some degree of coherence, so some degree of consolidation is appropriate.

Neural network models also must represent how nodes are connected to each other. Individual connections between two nodes can be either unidirectional or bidirectional. Bidirectional connections result in feedback relationships, and networks with such connections are referred to as "recurrent" networks. The strength of individual connections can change over time, as a result of learning. Groups of units can be organized into "layers" that can represent a particular subsystem with some pattern of connectivity (e.g., the amygdala, or part of a hypothesized emotional circuit); or they can also represent units organized together by the modeler for practical reasons (perhaps comprehensibility of the model).

Furthermore, a model must specify the "activation function"—rules that govern the activation flow in individual nodes and throughout the whole network. Typically, the activation function determines how the input to a unit (that it receives from the other units) is transformed into the output (which it then sends to other connected units). The rules must also specify how the output from other sending units is combined to produce the input at a receiving unit.

Processing in a neural network proceeds by presenting an input pattern to the network and then allowing activation to flow among the nodes until the activations of the nodes stop changing. The strengths of the connections between nodes often change as a result of the pattern of activation flow. The "learning rule" dictates how these connections are changed during learning. This ability of the connections to change allows the network to learn the patterns of associations among the activation of nodes in the network.

Description of Leabra Implementation

The particular neural network architecture we focus on here is Leabra (O'Reilly & Munakata, 2000), which is designed to be faithful to general aspects of the actual biophysical processes that govern the behavior of real neurons, although it does makes certain abstractions and simplifications. For example, instead of putting out a set of firing spikes, the nodes output a continually varying activation, which abstractly represents the frequency of firing of the node. The essential features of Leabra are its activation function, its implementation of inhibitory processes, and the nature of learning. We consider each of these in more detail below.

Activation Function

Leabra's activation function results in an S- or sigmoid-shaped pattern of output activation. Sigmoidal functions are commonly used because they have a constrained range of activations, and because they are more powerful computationally than linear functions (see Read, Vanman, & Miller, 1997). The shape of a sigmoidal function is steeper near low inputs and flatter near high inputs. This represents a form of soft bounding: When a unit's activation gets higher, there are diminishing returns on adding more input to the unit.

Activation ranges from a minimum of 0 to a maximum of 1. The degree of activation represents the summed firing frequency of a neuron; thus it cannot have a negative activation. Leabra's activation equation is

$$y_j = \frac{\gamma[V_m - \Theta]_+}{\gamma[V_m - \Theta]_+ + 1} \tag{1}$$

where V_m stands for the "membrane potential" of the neuron and is the sum of the baseline (or resting) input of the unit, the input from the other nodes to which it is connected, and input from the bias node for the unit. (The bias node can represent the baseline activation of the node in the absence of any inputs.) Θ is the threshold for the firing of the unit, which V_m must exceed for the node to fire. γ is the gain of the node and represents its sensitivity to its inputs. Higher γ results in more steeply accelerated output activation. The + subscript indicates that the difference between the membrane potential and the firing threshold is set to 0 if the difference is negative.

The membrane potential itself (V_m) is governed by another equation describing the relationship between excitatory and inhibitory electrical forces within a neuron. For brevity, the equation is not presented here, but those interested should see O'Reilly and Munakata (2000, p. 39). The equation indicates that the total membrane potential is a weighted average of three "conductances" from the excitatory, inhibitory, and leak channels (in the actual neuron, these channels are governed by separate chemical ions—sodium, chlorine, and potassium, respectively). These inputs can be thought of as electrical currents (they are in fact directly related). The excitatory conductance drives the membrane potential up (makes it more active); the inhibitory conductance drives the membrane potential down (makes it less active); and the leak current acts like a drag coefficient. We refer to the excitatory conductance as g_e, which can be thought of as the net input sent from the outputs of the other connected units. Inhibitory processes are discussed in detail below.

The net input to a unit, which is considered to be the same as the excitatory conductance just described, is

$$g_e = (1 - dt_{net})g_e(t - 1) + dt_{net}\left(\frac{1}{\eta_p}\sum_k\frac{1}{\alpha_k}\left\langle x_i w_{ij}\right\rangle_k + \frac{\beta}{N}\right) \tag{2}$$

so it is the product of the activations of sending units (x_j) and the strength of connections to those units (the weights, w_{ij}), summed over all connected units. Note that activation at time t is a weighted average of the activation on the previous time step and the input at the current time, with the weighting indicated by dt_{net}. β refers to the input from the bias unit and is scaled by the number of projections, so that the bias activation has roughly the same influence as one synaptic input. From this equation, one can see how outputs (activations) are integrated into inputs, and ultimately turned back into outputs in other units. This is how activation flows through the network.

Several parameters in these equations are particularly important if one wants to vary the properties of a model. First, the gain parameter (γ) can be used to vary a node's sensitivity to inputs and resulting differences in its activation or firing strength. Higher gains produce more steeply accelerated activation functions, since higher gains result in greater output per unit input. Note that the gain parameter only applies to the amount by which the membrane potential exceeds the threshold; thus it has no impact on the likelihood that the membrane potential will exceed the firing threshold. The conductance ($\bar{g}_e$) can also be used to capture differences in sensitivity of the unit to inputs, but because the conductance directly affects the membrane potential, it can affect the likelihood that the membrane potential will exceed the threshold and "fire." The threshold (Θ) determines how high the incoming excitation (V_m) must be before the node will "fire." The threshold controls for the effect of random noise in the system and allows one to control the sensitivity of the node. The likelihood of firing is determined by the relative values of the threshold of the node (Θ) and by the baseline input of the node (which contributes to V_m).

Inhibition

Inhibitory connections in a network play an important role in the behavior of the network as a whole. Inhibition represents competition between nodes, and allows the network to "select" a preferred state given a particular input, based on the more strongly activated nodes in the network inhibiting the ones with weaker associations. In addition, more global inhibition in the network can improve the signal-to-noise ratio in the firing of the nodes. High levels of global inhibition result in only the most strongly activated nodes' remaining active, whereas weakly activated nodes move toward 0. This reduces the likelihood that a node can be influential simply as a result of random noisy inputs.

A frequent finding is that when one concept is highly activated, it tends to compete with and inhibit other concepts with which it is inconsistent. For example, in reading, when there are multiple senses of a word, there is good evidence that as the most likely sense becomes strongly activated, it inhibits the activation of alternative senses. Or when multiple possible interpretations can be applied to a social behavior, the most likely one inhibits alternative interpretations. Inhibition in such situations can be captured by using a large number of inhibitory neurons among the nodes to explicitly represent all the possible inhibitory relationships. However, because this incurs a large computational cost in reasonably large models, O'Reilly and Munakata (2000) have developed an implementation of the k-winners-take-all (kWTA) algorithm, which achieves the same outcome at much less cost. Essentially, this algorithm only allows a user-specified number of nodes to become activated, and it sets the values of all other nodes to 0. This captures the impact of a large network of inhibitory interneurons, without having to actually represent them or compute their effects.

Leabra models inhibition by a version of the kWTA algorithm (Majani, Erlarson, & Abu-Mostafa, 1989), and provides both a strict version and a more lenient variation of this algorithm. The strict version of the kWTA algorithm allows no more than k nodes out of the total n (in a layer) to become active. The more lenient version, average kWTA, allows k nodes to be active on *average*, but if the input activations are sufficiently strong it will allow more than k nodes to be active. Different layers can have different maximum numbers of nodes active, because inhibition is set for each individual layer.

One way to think about this way of implementing inhibition within a layer is that a lower value of k represents stronger competition between units, with only the k most active nodes remaining activated and influencing other nodes. This increases the selectivity of the network. In contrast, a network that allows many more units to remain active will not be very selective (but may be more flexible). Because inhibition can be set differently on different layers, it allows one to implement different subsystems with different degrees of selectivity.

Learning

In Leabra, the learning rule combines error-correcting learning with an associative, Hebbian form of learning. Hebbian learning enables the learning of the correlational or statistical structure of the environment (i.e., the more stable and consistent aspects of the environment). For example, it is relevant to learning what characteristics co-occur in different types of individuals, such as when learning what features go together in defining different person categories or stereotypes.

Error-correcting learning enables the network to learn task structure (i.e., whether the output in response to a given input is right or wrong). For example, it is relevant to such things as learning whether an action will be punished or rewarded, or learning a relatively arbitrary association between a situation and a behavior—something that happens quite frequently as one is socialized into a particular culture. Error-correcting learning is also important in learning to update predictions or expectations about one's own or other people's behavior. Error-correcting learning in Leabra is similar, although not identical, to delta rule learning (Widrow & Hoff, 1960). It uses a contrastive Hebbian learning (CHL) algorithm developed for the Boltzmann machine and then generalized by O'Reilly (1996). CHL compares the activation of the network in a plus phase (when both inputs and desired outputs are presented to the network) to its activation in a minus phase (when only the inputs are presented). CHL then adjusts weights to reduce the difference in activation between the two phases. One way to think about CHL is that in the minus phase, the network uses its inputs to *predict* its outputs, and the plus phase represents what the inputs actually lead to. CHL applies to situations in which individuals can make predictions (either implicitly or explicitly) about what will happen next, and can then update their predictions based on the difference between what they predicted and what actually happened.

As O'Reilly and Munakata (2000) demonstrate, sometimes task structure and correlational structure provide different kinds of information; thus combining the two kinds of information provides a more powerful learning mechanism. There are some problems that Hebbian learning fails to solve, and others that error-correcting learning has trouble solving by itself, but together they can overcome their individual limitations. In Leabra, weight change is calculated as a weighted average of the amount calculated by each of these two learning rules. Typically, the weight for the Hebbian component is much smaller (about .05 or less) than the weight for the error-correcting component (.95 or higher).

Importantly, CHL enables learning in multilayer networks with hidden units. O'Reilly and Munakata (2000) note that this provides the same kind of learning ability as does the better-known back-propagation rule, but does it in a more biologically plausible way. One major problem with back-propagation is that it requires the use of a nonlocal error term, such that the error must be propagated backward from the outputs to the preceding layers. But there is no known biological mechanism for this propagation of error to occur. In contrast, CHL only requires a local error term; there is no need to propagate error across multiple layers. (Hidden units are found in layers between input and output layers. Their function is to re-represent inputs in ways that help networks recognize critical combinations of features and find solutions to tasks— for example, to recognize that the letter combination "oo" makes a different sound in English than two individual "o"s placed together do.) The interested reader can find a detailed description of these learning mechanisms in O'Reilly and Munakata.

Two Examples of Neural Network Simulations of Personality and Social Behavior

In this section, we present two different neural network simulations. The first simulation is our virtual personalities II model (Read et al., 2008). Following this, we present an outline of a neural network account of Cunningham and Zelazo's (2007) iterative reprocessing model.

The Virtual Personality Model

The goal of our virtual personality model is to model both the structure and dynamics of personality in terms of an organized set of underlying motivational systems. We assume that personality and social behavior arise from such structured and organized motivational systems. Our goal, insofar as it is possible, is to rely on what is known about the neurobiology of motivational systems in building this model. In what follows, we describe the theoretical basis of our model.

In the personality literature, the study of personality structure (e.g., the dominant paradigm of the "Big Five" personality dimensions: extraversion, agreeableness, conscientiousness, neuroticism, and openness to experience/intellect; see Saucier & Simonds, 2006, for a recent review) and the study of personality dynamics have remained relatively separate. Researchers who focus on personality structure do not typically seek to provide an account of the underlying psychological and neurobiological mechanisms that may be responsible for that structure. And researchers who have focused on the dynamics of personality have spent relatively little effort trying to explain how the structure of personality may arise from underlying dynamics (for discussions of these issues, see Funder, 2001; Mischel & Shoda, 1998). Our model of personality aims to account for the mapping between dynamics and structure by using a neural network. Not only are we aiming to provide an account of personality dynamics in terms of the behavior of a structured and organized motivational system; we are also aiming to show how the structure of personality (as revealed in the lexicon and in personality measures) can arise from the behavior of such organized motivational systems.

In developing our model, we drew on central literatures in personality and neuroscience. These literatures enabled us to develop a model with a core set of processing systems that simulates the patterning of personality and social behavior, and so captures a number of individual differences in social behavior. The model we propose is heavily goal- and motive-based. According to this approach, individual differences in personality and behavior can be understood largely in terms of the behavior of underlying motivational systems.

The lexical analysis of trait terms (e.g., Digman, 1997; Goldberg, 1981; John & Srivastava, 1999; Peabody & De Raad, 2002; Saucier & Ostendorf, 1999) and the development of general personality measures (e.g., Eysenck, 1983, 1994; Lee & Ashton, 2004; McCrae & Costa, 1999; Tellegen & Waller, in press; Wiggins & Trapnell, 1996; Zuckerman, 2002) provide a wealth of information about personality structure. This work points to a structure of personality that contains five major factors: extraversion, neuroticism, conscientiousness, agreeableness, and openness to experience (but see Ashton et al., 2004). Work on personality structure also provides a great deal of information about the correlations between traits, but it does not focus as much on the underlying mechanisms that drive them.

Some of our previous work has argued that a trait is a mental structure tied to the goals, plans, resources, beliefs, and behavioral styles of the type of individual who can be characterized by the trait (Miller & Read, 1987, 1991; see also Read & Miller, 1989). For example, the trait "helpful" can be represented in terms of a goal of helping others, plans for achieving that goal, resources needed to achieve the goal, and beliefs related to the goal (e.g., whether one's actions would actually assist the other and whether the other desired assistance). Operating at a somewhat more general level of analysis, Mischel and Shoda's (1995) cognitive–affective processing system model also suggests that personality can be understood in terms of similar, although less differentiated, basic components.

In addition to the lexical and conceptual analyses described above, we have drawn heavily on work on the neurobiological bases of personality. These potential neurobiological bases of motivation include models of temperament (biologically based individual differences), evolutionary systems, and evidence from cognitive and affective neuroscience.

In the temperament literature, researchers such as Gray (1987, 1991; Gray & McNaughton, 2000) and Depue and Collins (1999) have argued that underlying extraversion is a behavioral approach system (BAS) (Gray, 1987, 1991) or a behavioral facilitation system (Depue & Collins, 1999), and that underlying neuroticism is a behavioral inhibition system (BIS) (Gray, 1987; Gray & McNaughton, 2000). Other authors have argued for similar approach and avoidance systems (e.g., Cacioppo, Gardner, & Berntson, 1999; Clark & Watson, 1999). The BAS system is sensitive to cues signaling rewards, and when activated it results in active approach, accompanied by feelings of energization and positive affect. It has been argued (e.g., Depue & Collins, 1999; Panksepp, 1998) that increasing levels of dopamine lead to greater activation of this system, resulting in increased exploration and vigor of approach. In contrast, the BIS is sensitive to cues of punishment or threat, and manages avoidance in threatening situations. Activation of this system is characterized by anxiety and fear.

Still other evidence is based on direct or indirect observations of neural activity. Davidson, Jackson, and Kalin (2000) reviewed considerable evidence demonstrating that the left prefrontal cortex processes approach-related emotions, whereas the right prefrontal cortex processes withdrawal-related emotions such as sadness, disgust, and fear (see also Davidson, 2003; Harmon-Jones & Sigelman, 2001).

An additional proposed broad system is the disinhibition–constraint system (e.g., Clark & Watson, 1999; Rothbart & Bates, 1998; Tellegen & Waller, in press), which is particularly related to self-control and emotion regulation. Individual differences in this system manifest themselves in terms of impulsivity and recklessness for low levels of inhibition, versus careful planning and avoiding risk and danger for high levels of inhibition. Serotonin levels are thought to influence this system, and roughly correspond to levels of inhibition (Clark & Watson, 1999; Depue & Collins, 1999; Spoont, 1992).

In addition to these broad systems, there is considerable evidence for more specific motivational systems that may be influenced by these broader systems. For example, on the basis of evolutionary arguments, some researchers (Bugental, 2000; Fiske, 1992; Kenrick & Trost, 1997) have proposed that humans have evolved specific brain systems specialized for handling our most important social tasks. They argue, based on both evolutionary and empirical considerations, that a variety of tasks need to be solved by human beings to survive and reproduce. these include (1) status and dominance; (2) coalition formation, communal sharing, and affectional relationships; (3) reciprocity; (4) self-protection; (5) mate choice; (6) parenting; (7) attachment; and (8) play or exploration. Some of these motives are approach related, whereas others are avoidance-related. These are among the more specific motives that underlie the two broader motivational systems in our model.

Altogether, there is a wealth of evidence that individual differences are related to specific neural systems. Simulations provide a microscope on the underlying complex personality dynamics in response to changing situations; they allow us to see how these elements may interact with each other, in ways that are not possible with more traditional methods. From this, we designed a model that we hoped would allow us to see how the dynamics of these systems would give rise to the observable properties of personalities.

Basic Network Architecture

The basic network architecture can be seen in Figure 12.1, and a description of the meaning of the different nodes in the network can be found in Table 12.1. There are two initial input layers: a situational feature layer and a personal resource layer. The situational feature layer defines the different situations to which the model responds. It uses a localist representation consisting of the different features (see Table 12.1 for lists of these and the other labeled nodes in the model) that are used to specify a wide variety of specific situations that can arise in two general contexts: work and parties.

The resource layer represents personal resources (e.g., wit, money, etc.) that are directly possessed by or part of an individual. Things that may be present in the environment, but that are not part of an individual, are represented in the situational feature layer rather than the resource layer. We view personal resources as a component of personality that should influence the kinds of behaviors most likely to be enacted (Read & Miller, 1989).

The situational feature layer connects, through a hidden layer, to two goal layers: an approach layer and an avoidance layer. Organiz-

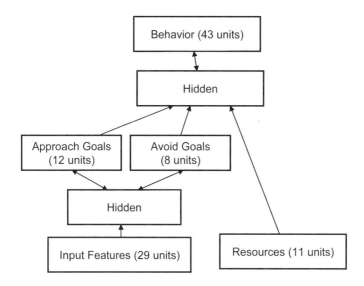

FIGURE 12.1. Structure of the virtual personalities neural network model.

ing the goals into two separate goal layers represents the idea that the approach and avoidance systems (BAS and BIS) are functionally separate systems with different characteristics. This organization into two separate layers also makes it easier to set certain parameters (e.g., gains) differently for the two systems, and to model processes of inhibition separately within the two goal systems.

The situational features, the goal layers, and the personal resource layer are all directly connected to a hidden layer, which then connects to the behavior layer. The behavior layer has a wide variety of different behaviors that can be enacted in work and party settings (e.g., give orders, work extra hard, dance, drink alcohol, tell jokes, etc.).

The situational features, resources, and behaviors in the model are not intended to be representative of the entire range of possibilities for social situations and social behavior. Rather, they are intended to enable us to provide a demonstration of the plausibility of the current approach, using relatively realistic representations.

The hidden layers mediate the transformation from the input to the output layers. As mentioned earlier, the various hidden layers should allow the network to learn to respond to conjunctions of inputs. For example, some goals should only be activated when a conjunction of certain situational features is present, or some behaviors should be activated only when a conjunction of certain situational features, goals, and personal resources is present.

**TABLE 12.1. Lists of Features at Different Layers
of the Virtual Personality II Model**

Situational feature list

At home	At party
In conference room	At work
Urgent work	Work to do
With friends	With strangers
With subordinates	With disliked acquaintance
With boss	In break room
In office/at desk	In a conflict situation
Watching TV	With potential date
With relatives	With date
With kids	At restaurant
Without others	At bar
With one other	Drinking alcohol
With two or more others	Dancing
With romantic partner	At wedding/formal party
With a person > 7 years older/younger	

Resource list

Social skills
Job skills
Face-saving skills
Quick thinking
Wit
Intelligence
Things to talk about
Money
Attention span
Status
Time

Goal list

Approach goals		Avoidance goals	
Friendship	Mastery	Avoiding rejection/ embarrassment	Avoiding loss of control
Sex/romance	Exploring	Avoiding guilt	Avoiding interpersonal conflict
Being liked	Fun	Avoiding failure	Avoiding effort
Helping others	Fairness/ equality/justice	Avoiding physical harm	Avoiding risk/ uncertainty
Dominance	Uniqueness		
Achievement	Material gain		

*(continued)*t

TABLE 12.1. *(continued)*

Behavior list

Eat/drink	Stay at periphery	Help others with work	Ensure that work is distributed fairly
Drink alcohol	Self-disclose	Order others what to do	Wear something distinctive
Relax	Ask others about self	Dance	Steal
Play practical joke	Talk politics	Ask other to dance	Kiss up
Tease/make fun of another	Gossip/talk about others	Ask for date	Be cheap
Try new dance steps	Talk about work (job-related)	Kiss	Mediate
Introduce self to others	Tell jokes	Do job	Give in
Surf Web	Compliment others	Work extra hard	Procrastinate
Explore environment	Ignore others	Find new way to do job	Pretend to work
Leave	Insult others	Improve skills	Stay with comfortable others
Be silent	Clean up	Confront another about slacking	

In Figure 12.1, double-headed arrows represent bidirectional connections among layers, whereas single-headed arrows represent unidirectional connections in the directions of these arrows. Bidirectional connections represent feedback relations among nodes and enable the network to function as a recurrent or parallel constraint satisfaction network.

Training Procedure

In the case that we were trying to model (social behavior), the model itself was not learning something de novo, but represented an individual with a life history. So before simulations could be run, the model had to be trained to learn the basic associations that represented its general knowledge about the world. Individual features were combined into a set of 15 situations (in this case, work or social situations) that the individual would be exposed to over the course of training. The model was trained on input–output patterns for each of the following pairings of input and output layers: situations–goals, situations–behaviors, goals–behaviors, and resources–behaviors. In addition, the model was trained on a set of events that involved pairing the simultaneous activation of three input layers (situations + goals + resources) with the behavior layer. An example of a training event was pairing the goal "avoiding interpersonal conflict" with the behavior "be silent," which seems a reasonable strategy that the average person would have learned. Further details of the training are beyond the scope of this chapter; it is only important to know that the model was trained so that given a set of inputs, a reasonable set of outputs was obtained. We tested the model against the training set to make sure it learned all the associations well and gave reasonable goals and behaviors for a particular situation.

Assessing Multiple Behaviors in One Situation

A final aspect of a node's behavior that is important in Leabra (although it is not represented in the activation function) is accommodation. Accommodation can be thought of as the tendency for a node to "fatigue" after constant firing. Biological neurons are unable to continue firing at a high level, and after some time they fire less strongly, even with the same input. In our personality model, we used accommodation to capture the idea that after the same behavior is enacted for a while, the behavior and associated goals will start to "fatigue," and their activation will decrease relative to other behaviors and goals. Although this is probably not the precise mechanism that determines when one switches behaviors, this property of the network was useful for seeing which behaviors were the second and third choices of the model in a given situation, allowing us to assess a wider variety of behaviors than if the model had just settled into one behavior and the network settled (and thus stopped processing).

We now present two sample simulations of different aspects of our personality model.

Sample Simulation 1: Impact of Differences in Gains of the Approach and Avoidance Layers on Approach and Avoidance Behaviors

METHOD

The aim of this simulation was to demonstrate that differences in the gains or sensitivity for the activation function of the goals in the two goal layers could allow us to capture individual differences in the strength of approach and avoidance motivations, and correspondingly capture individual differences in the degree of extraversion and neuroticism. For this test, we manipulated the gain parameter on the goals in the approach and avoidance layers. We had one condition in which the approach and avoidance layers had equal gains, one in which the approach layer had substantially higher gains than the avoidance layer, and one in which the avoidance layer had substantially higher gains than the approach layer.

The control or comparison condition had gains of 100 (a moderate level) on both the approach and avoidance layers. In a second condition, we set the gain for the approach layer to 200 (a high level) and the gain for the avoidance layer to 20 (a low level); in the third condition, we reversed the gains and set the gain for the approach layer to 20 and the gain for the avoidance layer to 200. The precise values chosen here were not critical. Our major interest was in demonstrating the ordinal relationships between gains and behaviors of the layers.

This test assessed the effect of differences in gain of the activation function of approach and avoidance goals on the behavioral outputs. We hypothesized that higher gain of the goals in the approach or avoidance layer should lead to increased impact of those goals on the model's outputs, and lower gain should lead to decreased impact. These differences in goal outputs should affect the likelihood of generating different behaviors. Specifically, the model should be more likely to generate approach-oriented behaviors when the approach layer had a higher gain and more likely to generate avoidance-oriented behaviors when the avoidance layer had a higher gain. In coding the results of these tests, we coded whether a behavior was an approach or an avoidance behavior by determining what proportion of approach or avoidance goals were paired with the behavior during training. If a behavior was paired only with approach goals during training, or with more approach goals than avoidance goals, it was coded as an approach behavior. Conversely, if a behavior was paired only with avoidance goals during training, or with more avoidance goals than approach goals, it was coded as an avoidance behavior. Of the 43 behaviors in the model, 33 were related to more approach goals than avoidance goals, and 8 were related only to avoidance goals during training (the other 2 behaviors were equally associated with both types of goals).

We tested the model with the set of 15 training situations and recorded the number of approach and avoidance behaviors activated under the different conditions. We tested the models with accommodation and recorded the first three behaviors generated by the models in response to each situation. We predicted that changes in gain should lead to corresponding differences in the frequency of activation of the corresponding types of behaviors.

RESULTS

As predicted, the relative gains of the approach and avoidance layers had a strong impact on the likelihood of generating approach-related and avoidance-related behaviors, even though all conditions were put through an identical series of situations. In the simulation where the approach gain was high and the avoidance gain was low, 16% of the behaviors were avoidance-related (behaviors related to avoidance goals during training); when the gain was moderate for both approach and avoidance layers, 24% of the behaviors were avoidance-related; and when the approach gain was low and the avoidance gain was high, 42% of the behaviors were avoidance-related. Furthermore, if we just looked at the first behavior generated, then when approach was high and avoidance low, none of the behaviors were avoidance-related; when approach and avoidance were both moderate, then 13% of the behaviors were avoidance-related; and when approach was low and avoidance high, then 20% of the behaviors were avoidance-related. This pattern is even more impressive than it appears on the surface, as there were approximately four times as many approach behaviors as avoidance behaviors.

Sample Simulation 2: Positivity Offset, Negativity Bias in the Approach and Avoidance Layers

Cacioppo, Gardner, and Berntson (1997) have reviewed evidence that positive and negative evaluation do not form a bipolar single dimension, but instead can be more accurately conceptualized in terms of a bivariate space with separate dimensions for positive and negative activation. This is consistent with neuroimaging evidence showing possible differences in representation of reward and punishment (O'Doherty, Kringelbach, Rolls, Hornak, & Andrews, 2001). Although we have not yet discussed this explicitly, this is a clear implication of the current model. In the current model, we have separate approach and avoidance layers, each with its own activation dynamics. Thus our model currently represents two separate motivational mechanisms, which is consistent with the idea of two separate evaluation systems or dimensions for positive and negative evaluation.

One conclusion of Cacioppo and colleagues' (1997) analysis is that not only are positive and negative evaluation the result of somewhat separate systems, but they also have somewhat different functional forms: a positivity offset and a negativity bias. "Positivity offset" means that the positive evaluation system has somewhat higher baseline activation than the negative evaluation system. Thus, in the presence of weak input activations, the positive evaluation system will be more highly activated than the negative evaluation system. And "negativity bias" means that the negative evaluation system has much higher gain, or is much more sensitive to input, than the positive evaluation system is. That is, each unit of input to the negative evaluation system results in a higher level of output than does the same unit of input to the positive evaluation system. Taken together, these two things mean that in the absence of any strong situational cues, there will tend to be a mild positive evaluation and a tendency to approach or explore interesting things in the environment. However, as the strength of situational cues increases, the greater negativity bias or gain means that the negative evaluation system will respond more strongly to negative cues than the positive evaluation system will to equally strong positive cues. Furthermore, the stronger sensitivity or "ramp-up" of the negative evaluation system makes it possible for strong negative cues to override the effect of strong positive cues.

One thing this means behaviorally is that in the absence of strong inputs, an organism will tend to explore. However, as both types of cues become stronger, the organism will be more sensitive to negative cues than positive cues. For example, given equally strong cues to reward and punishment, the organism should be much more likely to respond to the punishment cues. In fact, under some circumstances, even though the negative cues may be weaker than the positive cues, the negative evaluation system will override the positive system because of the stronger gain of the negative evaluation system. Obviously, by no means will negative cues always outweigh positive cues. Rather, to the extent that cues to negative outcomes are available, each unit increase in the strength of a negative cue will have a stronger effect than each unit increase in the strength of a positive cue.

METHOD

Our second sample simulation examined the relative impact of positivity offset and negativity bias or gain. The basic idea was to show that with relatively weak inputs to both the approach and avoidance layers, the positivity offset would tend to lead to approach-related behaviors, but as BAS- and BIS-related inputs start to increase equally, there would be a shift to avoidance-related behaviors.

To simulate the impact of positivity offset, we manipulated the baseline activation of the BAS layer so that it was higher than that for the BIS layer. If the baseline activation of one layer was higher, it would take less input for the nodes in that layer to be activated. We manipulated baseline activation by changing the resting "membrane potential" of nodes in a layer, using the $V_{m\_}$init parameter. In Leabra, all nodes have such a baseline or resting membrane potential, which is the default activation of the node, in the absence of any specific inputs. Nodes send activation or "fire" only when the membrane potential (V_m) exceeds the threshold value (θ) (see Equation 1 in the section on Leabra). Thus, if the threshold value is held constant, higher baseline activations reduce the distance to the threshold, and nodes with higher $V_m\_$init or resting membrane potentials require less input to "fire." In the current simulations, the $V_m\_$init for the BAS was 0.27 and for the BIS $V_m\_$init was 0.20, with the threshold (θ) for the goal layers set at 0.3.

To capture negativity bias or greater sensitivity of the BIS, we manipulated the *maximum* excitatory conductance ($\bar{g}_e$) for the nodes. This parameter controls the sensitivity of the unit to its incoming excitation. This is a way of manipulating the sensitivity of the system that is an alternative to the gain parameter. In this simulation, ($\bar{g}_e$) for the approach layer was 0.9 and for the avoidance layer was 1.2.

Once we had set the baseline activation to be higher for the BAS and the sensitivity to be higher for the BIS, we then manipulated the strength of the input cues to the two goal layers. We did this by taking the hidden layer between the situational inputs and the goal layers, and then by varying the weight scaling from this hidden layer to the goal layer across three levels: 0.5, 1, and 1.5. The scaling factor is multiplied by the existing weights to give the acting weights. That is, a weight scaling of 0.5 halves the existing weights, and a weight scaling of 1.5 increases the weights by 50%. This scaling then varies the strength of the impact of the input cues on the activation of the goal layer. In other words, it allowed us to create strong and weak stimuli in this simulation.

RESULTS

We then presented the network with each of the 15 test situations and recorded the number of avoidance behaviors that were activated in response. In this simulation, as in previous simulations, an avoidance behavior was defined as any behavior that was paired with more avoidance goals than approach goals during initial learning. With weak stimuli, 1 out of 15 behaviors was an avoidance behavior; with moderate stimuli, 7 out of 15 behaviors were avoidance behaviors; and with strong stimuli, 7 out of 15 behaviors were avoidance behaviors. Thus, as predicted, as the strength of the inputs increased, the relative impact of the BIS layer also increased. This is consistent with Cacioppo and colleagues' (1997) characterization of the relative behavior of the positive and negative evaluation systems.

Summary of Simulations

These two sample simulations showed how the model responded differently in terms of approach- versus avoidance-related behaviors, depending on the manipulation of parameters that influenced the response sensitivity of the approach and avoidance systems. However, we do not make strong claims that the parameters in our model that we manipulated correspond directly to the actual reasons why one system is more sensitive than another. These are merely reasonable ways to change the response and influence of these systems in an attempt to model the observations faithfully. More importantly, we hope it is clear that although we mainly manipulated the sensitivity of the goal systems, it was not only the goal systems that were important. The behavior of the model was also constrained to act in a certain way in a given situation because of its previously learned situation–behavior knowledge. In other words, the model was unlikely to perform a behavior solely because it was related to an active goal; it also took the situational constraints into account. Systems often work in parallel with each other, and it is important to look at their interaction to ultimately explain the behavior. For example, even though a goal strongly associated with social bonding might have been active, this might not have been the most important determinant of behavior, because the situation demanded work-focused activities.

This kind of interaction between situation–behavior associations and goal processes has been noted recently with respect to behavioral data (Wood & Neal, 2007). Another point we hope has been illustrated is that knowing (or assuming) two different systems exist may not be enough for one to accurately model and replicate the behavioral data; one must also know the degree to which each of the systems influences the resulting behavior. It is thus important to be able to change parameters so as to fit real data as closely as possible.

A Neural Network Account of the Iterative Reprocessing Model

Attitudes are a good fit for modeling by means of a neural network. They can be strongly influenced by what information is active in memory (Schwarz, 2007), but at the same time they are thought to be (somewhat) stable structures in memory (Pratkanis, Breckler, & Greenwald, 1989). This behavior corresponds closely to the features of neural networks, where different nodes can be active to varying degrees at different times, yet the pathway through which activation flows is guided by relatively stable patterns of weights between the nodes. Essentially, neural networks represent things in terms of both dynamically changing activation patterns and relatively stable weights among nodes. Interestingly, this dichotomy maps onto the ongoing question in attitude research as to whether (or to what degree) attitudes are constructed "on the fly" or retrieved from memory. Recent attempts have been made to account for limited sets of attitude phenomena in terms of computations of simple neural-like processing nodes (Van Overwalle & Siebler, 2005).

The aim of creating a neural network model of attitudes is to account for the attitudinal processes in terms of computational processes. But at the same time, it would be ideal to incorporate both neuroscientific evidence (such as fMRI findings) and behavioral data to inform and constrain the model. We show that these three existing approaches to examining attitudes already converge significantly, and that this convergence can be used to design a hypothetical neuroanatomically inspired model of attitudes. In our discussion, we examine how a neural network can be used to model the processes outlined in Cunningham and Zelazo's (2007) iterative reprocessing (IR) neurobiological model of attitudes. In general terms, the IR model suggests that evaluative responses to a stimulus develop over time as the result of iterative reprocessing in a set of brain systems that are bidirectionally connected. Activation is first sent to lower-level sensory and evaluative systems, and from there to higher-level systems that produce more complex representations; then activation is sent back to the lower-level systems, which in turn send updated activation back to the higher-level systems. This bidirectional flow of activation occurs over multiple cycles, with the number of cycles being influenced by frequently competing needs to accurately represent the environment and to conserve computational resources.

More specifically, the IR model (see Figure 12.2) suggests that upon initial interpretation of the stimulus, activation is immediately sent to the brain centers (e.g., the amygdala and then the orbitofrontal cortex) that are involved in affective and evaluative processes. As activity continues, more brain circuits are recruited (e.g., portions of the prefrontal cortex), and more complex representations are activated in these higher-order systems. These higher-order systems have bidirectional connections back to the orbitofrontal cortex and the amygdala, which can then further influence the evaluative responses in the orbitofrontal cortex and the amygdala. These affective areas of the brain, in addition to receiving information from higher-order areas, may also transmit activation to them, influencing activation patterns in those areas in the process, and so on. Thus there is a recurrent flow of activation, with each brain area able to reciprocally influence the others to which it is connected. This process can continue until the brain is "satisfied" with its evaluation; that is, it settles into a stable state. The early evaluation—which is predominantly the result of early activation in the primary evaluative systems, such as the amygdala and the orbitofrontal cortex—is proposed to be responsible for implicit attitude responses (which are typically time-limited responses), whereas later consideration of more complex information maps onto explicit attitude responses (which are not constrained by time limits).

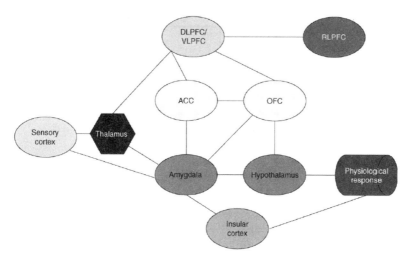

FIGURE 12.2. The iterative reprocessing (IR) model. From Cunningham and Zelazo (2007). Copyright 2007 by Elsevier Ltd. Reprinted by permission.

This proposed model is conceptually strikingly similar to our recent computational model of attitudes, the attitudes as constraint satisfaction (ACS) model (Monroe & Read, 2008), which relies on a minimal set of assumptions about the evaluation process. Figure 12.3 provides a graphic representation of the basic components of the ACS model. In this computational model of attitudes, there are three important classes of nodes: (1) the attitude object itself; (2) the evaluation/affect node(s); and (3) other cognitions associated with the attitude object, which are collectively organized in what we call the "cognitorium." In this model, operationalization of the evaluation process relevant to an attitude goes as follows: The attitude object itself is externally activated, corresponding to stimulus information in the environment (possibly either seeing a visual representation of the object, or reading about it, or hearing about it). Since the attitude object is associated with the evaluation directly, and with other cognitions that are also relevant to an evaluation, activation spreads in both these directions—into the evaluation node and into the cognitorium. As these connected units become more active themselves, they will pass on their activation to other connected units throughout all the layers. In this way, activation continues to spread throughout the model until some stopping criterion is reached (e.g., until activation stops changing because it has reached a stable configuration).

When activation first spreads in a model like this, the first thing that will become most active is the evaluation itself, since the attitude object is

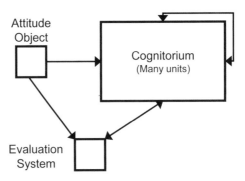

FIGURE 12.3. The attitude as constant satisfaction (ACS) model. From Monroe and Read (2008). Copyright by the American Psychological Association. Reprinted by permission.

directly connected to the evaluation. The strength of this association has probably developed through repeated physical and mental experiences. The next opportunity to influence the evaluation is for those things (represented in the cognitorium) that are directly associated with the attitude object, and that also have direct associations to affect, to send their activation to the evaluation unit. In other words, activation flows from the attitude object to a unit in the cognitorium, and then from there to the evaluation node. This corresponds to fairly concrete attributes of the attitude object. But complex patterns of connections between units representing structures in memory can also influence evaluation. As the activation flows through the model, it tends to settle into stable coherent configurations. These complex patterns of connections can represent propositional configurations and more abstract concepts. But it takes time for these activation patterns to form, because activation has to flow through many units and generate the complex representation, and only then can the influence of the complex concept reach its full extent on the evaluation. It should also be noted that during this complex processing, activation can flow from the evaluation node back into the cognitorium, allowing the initial evaluation to influence further processing.

This simple model captures many of the insights of the IR model. Simulations with this model (Monroe & Read, 2008) show that it is able to reproduce such phenomena as the difference between implicit and explicit attitudes, and to show how one type of evaluation may be influenced more than the other by different types of information. This ability is mainly a result of activation spreading first into the evaluation node, resulting in an early evaluation, and then through the cognitorium route, resulting in later influence on the evaluation. It also can account for dual-process models of persuasion, whereby a low amount of processing actually confers greater effectiveness on persuasive attempts based on simple heuristic relations, while in contrast, a greater amount of processing increases the effectiveness of more complex arguments and at the same time decreases the effectiveness of weak arguments.

This model of spreading activation leading to more complex cognitions is based on a simple idea—that cognitions exist in a network that allows activation to flow between units. This conceptualization is widely shared in cognitive psychology and cognitive science. It is consistent with other recent process models of attitude change, such as the cognition in persuasion model (Albarracin, 2002). This model is concerned with the order in which particular types of attitude-relevant processes and judgments occur. Consistent with a spreading-activation-based account of attitudes, the first process to occur (beyond interpretation of the stimulus) is retrieval of prior knowledge from memory. This information is subsequently used for a variety of judgments. Behavioral evidence suggests that conflict detection during these cognitive processes spurs more scrutiny of persuasive information (e.g., Baker & Petty, 1994) and can prolong the duration of processing, leading to even more complex and integrative judgments. We surmise that this temporal ordering of complexity may have significant consequences for the type of attitude object being considered. Greenwald (1989) and others have proposed an important conceptual distinction in the complexity of attitude objects, in order from simple to complex: feature, object, category, proposition, and schema. It seems likely that the more complex the attitude object is, the more processing has to occur to arrive at a coherent evaluative response, and thus the more opportunity intervening cognitive systems may have to alter the course of processing and the evaluative result.

This remarkably simple process of spreading activation has many implications. We see it as responsible for many of the important constructs and dynamic processes in which attitude researchers are interested. The types of constructs that can have evaluative implications include evaluations directly associated with (conditioned with) the attitude object; concrete attributes or features of an attitude object (e.g., the pleasing aroma of coffee); propositional relations (e.g., a politician's claims of what he or she will do after taking office, and what results these actions might have on one's welfare); and then other abstract concepts (e.g., world peace) and higher-order relations that may govern the interactions between elements such as the ones just mentioned.

Although a simple network model such as the ACS model can seemingly capture many of the same phenomena as the IR model, it lacks much of the structure that Cunningham and Zelazo's (2007) model suggests is important in capturing the details and the time course of evaluative processing. A more detailed neural network model, which is an extension of the ACS model, might be able to inform a neurological model of attitudes and evaluation. We present one hypothetical version of what this model might look like (Figure 12.4). Although the basic version of the ACS model uses a single layer to contain all the attitude-relevant information, a multilayer approach could be more powerful and allow for more complex representations. In this model, a hidden layer and another "higher-order" layer would be used for re-representing concepts, resulting in more complex, higher-order representations that have evaluative implications. Thus there would be one layer for more concrete constructs that have evaluations more directly associated with them, such as features that result from more detailed processing in sensory cortices, and another layer for more abstract, less affect-laden mental constructs. When the lower-order constructs became active, they would send their activation to the evaluative system, providing a relatively earlier evaluation. But at the same time they would activate the higher-order concepts through the intervening hidden layer, resulting in more complex higher-order representations, which would then send activation by bidirectional connections to the lower-order concepts and evaluative system, and change the activation subsequently. This bidirectional flow of activation would continue until the model settled or until processing was interrupted to handle another task or situation. A computational scheme to detect conflict and further control processing, like the one implemented by Botvinick, Braver, Barch, Carter, and Cohen (2001),

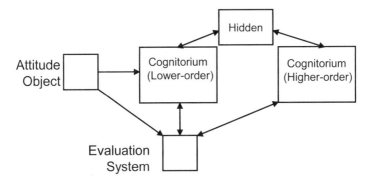

FIGURE 12.4. A hypothetical computational attitude model architecture based on the IR and ACS models. Although the connectivity patterns would be the same as in the ACS model, lateral connections between units in the same cognitorium layers are not shown, for the sake of simplicity.

could be added to correspond to the anterior cingulate cortex's function in directing processing in the IR model.

We believe that in this case the computational and neurological perspectives would have things to offer each other. The IR model might have an advantage in terms of specifying the patterns of connectivity between subsystems, but the computational model would be able to specify much more precise attitudinal and cognitive content. Modeling the way the specific contents interact could allow us to constrain the possible effects of a certain pattern of connectivity. And if computational modeling explorations would allow us to infer how long certain judgments take to unfold, we might then draw conclusions about whether activity in a certain cortical brain region (measured with functional neuroimaging) is antecedent to or a consequence of the evaluative system response—in essence, helping map the flow of activation through the evaluative brain circuit. This might be important, if, for example, a simple attitude object like a morning cup of coffee takes less time to influence the evaluation than a complex object like world peace, where presumably the evaluation system has had several iterations to influence the type of information that is active. Finally, when combining the recurrent nature of this processing with specific content and a learning mechanism, like the one used in the ACS model, we might attempt to account for the patterns of activation and the resulting weight change that influence long-term attitude change—something the IR model is currently silent on.

Concerns for Potential Modelers

Experimental Design Considerations

Many different software packages now exist for building neural network models. Several quite comprehensive packages are currently available for free and run on the major operating systems. For the simulations presented here and other simulations we have recently done, we have used PDP++ (*psych.colorado.edu/~oreilly/PDP++*) and its descendant Emergent (*grey.colorado.edu/emergent*). These packages are available for Windows, MacOSX, and various versions of Linux, and provide many of the most widely used algorithms. PDP++ is still available, but it is no longer being developed. Development and support have switched to its descendant Emergent, which is being actively developed and has an active user community. Other freely available packages are the Stuttgart Neural Network Simulator (SNNS) and JavaNNS, which has a Java-based front end to the SNNS computational kernel. However, it does not seem that this package is being further developed. Another package is the FIT package provided by Frank Van Overwalle (*www.vub. ac.be/FIT*), in conjunction with his recent book *Social Connectionism: A Reader and Handbook for Simulations* (Van Overwalle, 2007).

In addition to these freely available packages, there are several commercial packages, including a very extensive Neural Network Toolbox for MATLAB and a neural network toolbox for Mathematica. Both MATLAB and Mathematica have academic pricing, which makes them affordable for researchers. A number of other packages and add-ons for Microsoft Excel can be found searching the Web. If researchers' needs are met by one of these packages or others, then we strongly suggest working with a program such as Emergent, which has an active user community and provides extensive documentation and tutorials. However, given that the basic computations for most neural network models are relatively straightforward, it is also possible for researchers with reasonable programming knowledge to build their own neural network models. Nevertheless, if researchers are tempted to build their own models, we would suggest investing in either MATLAB or Mathematica and using the chosen package's toolboxes, which can be modified as desired.

Advantages and Disadvantages of the Method for Studying Social and Personality Questions

We hope that the advantages of this method have been made clear in the previous discussions. First, it allows researchers to build models of the computations performed by particular brain regions. Second, it enables them to build models of circuits of systems—of how the systems interact with one another in performing a particular task. Third, as a result of this, it allows them to begin examining the dynamics of the interactions of these regions.

Probably the main disadvantages of this method are threefold. First, social and personality psychologists are not typically used to thinking about psychological phenomena in computational terms. Their models are almost always stated in verbal or graphic (e.g., flowchart) form. Thus, before building a computational model of a task or phenomena, a researcher must start to frame a model in terms of the necessary representations and computations, and to identify the relevant systems and their potential interactions. In this light, one potential advantage of using neural network models, as opposed to other computational modeling techniques, is that there is a rough correspondence between the elements of the modeling techniques or "language" and the phenomena that the researcher is trying to model.

A second disadvantage is that this method has a fairly high learning curve, although it is probably no more demanding than becoming well versed in any of the other techniques discussed in this volume. Third, it may be hard to find formal courses in these techniques, as courses in neural network modeling are not taught in every school. And when they are taught, they usually adopt a cognitive and cognitive neuroscience perspective, and do not focus on aspects of social reasoning and behavior. We hope that this will change. This technique is most appropriate for those who are comfortable thinking dynamically and in computational terms. However, researchers who use the available programs (such as Emergent) can do a tremendous amount without any programming knowledge, although programming knowledge is helpful.

Conclusion

In closing, we would like to remind our readers that knowing, for example, that the anterior cingulate cortex is a region involved in detecting conflict and signaling that something is wrong and needs attention does not by itself answer the question of how the brain solves the problem of cognitive dissonance resolution. But at the same time, proposing a computational model that just represents beliefs connected to each other in a semantic network surely doesn't account for the role that neuroanatomical systems play in directing processing. It is our view that using these methods in combination will lead to new insights and yield tremendous advances, if only researchers take advantage of them.

References

Adolphs, R., & Damasio, A. R. (2001). The interaction of affect and cognition: A neurobiological perspective. In J. P. Forgas (Ed.), *Handbook of affect and social cognition* (pp. 27–49). Mahwah, NJ: Erlbaum.

Albarracín, D. (2002). Cognition in persuasion: An analysis of information processing in response to persuasive communications. In M. P. Zanna (Ed.), *Advances in experimental social psychology* (Vol. 34, pp. 61–130). San Diego, CA: Academic Press.

Amodio, D. M., Harmon-Jones, E., Devine, P. G., Curtin, J. J., Hartley, S. L., & Covert, A. E. (2004). Neural signals for the detection of unintentional race bias. *Psychological Science, 15*(2), 88–93.

Ashton, M. C., Lee, K., Perugini, M., Szarota, P., de Vries, R. E., Di Blas, L., et al. (2004). A six-factor structure of personality-descriptive adjectives: Solutions from psycholexical studies in seven languages. *Journal of Personality and Social Psychology, 86*(2), 356–366.

Baker, S. M., & Petty, R. E. (1994). Majority and minority influence: Source–position imbalance as a determinant of message scrutiny. *Journal of Personality and Social Psychology, 67*(1), 5–19.

Banfield, J. F., Wyland, C. L., Macrae, C. N., Münte, T. F., & Heatherton, T. F. (2004). The cognitive neuroscience of self-regulation. In R. F. Baumeister & K. D. Vohs (Eds.), *Handbook of self-regulation: Research, theory, and applications* (pp. 62–83). New York: Guilford Press.

Bechara, A., Tranel, D., Damasio, H., & Damasio, A. R. (1996). Failure to respond autonomically to anticipated future outcomes following damage to prefrontal cortex. *Cerebral Cortex, 6*(2), 215–225.

Botvinick, M. M., Braver, T. S., Barch, D. M., Carter, C. S., & Cohen, J. D. (2001). Conflict monitoring and cognitive control. *Psychological Review, 108*(3), 624–652.

Botvinick, M. M., & Plaut, D. C. (2006). Short-term memory for serial order: A recurrent neural network model. *Psychological Review, 113*(2), 201–233.

Bugental, D. B. (2000). Acquisition of the algorithms of social life: A domain-based approach. *Psychological Bulletin, 126*, 187–219.

Cacioppo, J. T., Gardner, W. L., & Berntson, G. G. (1997). Beyond bipolar conceptualizations and measures: The case of attitudes and evaluative space. *Personality and Social Psychology Review, 1*(1), 3–25.

Cacioppo, J. T., Gardner, W. L., & Berntson, G. G. (1999). The affect system has parallel and integrative processing components: Form follows function. *Journal of Personality and Social Psychology, 76*(5), 839–855.

Clark, L. A., & Watson, D. (1999). Temperament: A new paradigm for trait psychology. In L. A. Pervin & O. P. John (Eds.), *Handbook of personality: Theory and research* (2nd ed., pp. 399–423). New York: Guilford Press.

Cunningham, W. A., Raye, C. L., & Johnson, M. K. (2004). Implicit and explicit evaluation: FMRI correlates of valence, emotional intensity, and control in the processing of attitudes. *Journal of Cognitive Neuroscience, 16*(10), 1717–1729.

Cunningham, W. A., & Zelazo, P. D. (2007). Attitudes and evaluations: A social cognitive neuroscience perspective. *Trends in Cognitive Sciences, 11*(3), 97–104.

Davidson, R. J. (2003). Affective neuroscience: A case for interdisciplinary research. In F. Kessel, P. L. Rosenfield, & N. B. Anderson (Eds.), *Expanding the boundaries of health and social science: Case studies in interdisciplinary innovation* (pp. 99–121). New York: Oxford University Press.

Davidson, R. J., Jackson, D. C., & Kalin, N. H. (2000). Emotion, plasticity, context, and regulation: Perspectives from affective neuroscience. *Psychological Bulletin, 126*(6), 890–909.

Depue, R. A., & Collins, P. F. (1999). Neurobiology of the structure of personality: Dopamine, facilitation of incentive motivation, and extraversion. *Behavioral and Brain Sciences, 22*(3), 491–569.

Digman, J. M. (1997). Higher-order factors of the Big Five. *Journal of Personality and Social Psychology, 73*, 1246–1256.

Eisenberger, N. I., Lieberman, M. D., & Williams, K. D. (2003). Does rejection hurt?: An fMRI study of social exclusion. *Science, 302*, 290–292.

Eiser, J. R., Fazio, R. H., Stafford, T., & Prescott, T. J. (2003). Connectionist simulation of attitude learning: Asymmetries in the acquisition of positive and negative evaluations. *Personality and Social Psychology Bulletin, 29*(10), 1221–1235.

Eysenck, H. J. (1983). Psychophysiology and personality: Extraversion, neuroticism and psychoticism. In A. Gale & J. A. Edwards (Eds.), *Psychological correlates of human behavior: Vol. 3. Individual differences and psychopathology* (pp. 13–30). San Diego, CA: Academic Press.

Eysenck, H. J. (1994). Personality: Biological foundations. In P. A. Vernon (Ed.), *The neuropsychology of individual differences* (pp. 151–207). San Diego, CA: Academic Press.

Fiske, A. P. (1992). The four elementary forms of sociality: Framework for a unified theory of social relations. *Psychological Review, 99,* 689–723.

Funder, D. C. (2001). Personality. *Annual Review of Psychology, 52,* 197–221.

Goldberg, L. R. (1981). Language and individual differences: The search for universals in personality lexicons. In L. Wheeler (Ed.), *Review of personality and social psychology* (Vol. 2, pp. 141–165). Beverly Hills, CA: Sage.

Gray, J. A. (1987). The neuropsychology of emotion and personality. In S. M. Stahl, S. D. Iversen, & E. C. Goodman (Eds.), *Cognitive neurochemistry* (pp. 171–190). New York: Oxford University Press.

Gray, J. A. (1991). The neuropsychology of temperament. In J. Strelau & A. Angleitner (Eds.), *Explorations in temperament: International perspectives on theory and measurement* (pp. 105–128). New York: Plenum Press.

Gray, J. A., & McNaughton, N. (2000). *The neuropsychology of anxiety: An enquiry into the functions of the septo-hippocampal system* (2nd ed.). New York: Oxford University Press.

Greenwald, A. G. (1989). Why attitudes are important: Defining attitude and attitude theory 20 years later. In A. R. Pratkanis, S. J. Breckler, & A. G. Greenwald (Eds.), *Attitude structure and function* (pp. 429–440). Hillsdale, NJ: Erlbaum.

Harmon-Jones, E. (2004). Contributions from research on anger and cognitive dissonance to understanding the motivational functions of asymmetrical frontal brain activity. *Biological Psychology, 67*(1–2), 51–76.

Harmon-Jones, E., & Sigelman, J. (2001). State anger and prefrontal brain activity: Evidence that insult-related relative left-prefrontal activation is associated with experienced anger and aggression. *Journal of Personality and Social Psychology, 80*(5), 797–803.

John, O. P., & Srivastava, S. (1999). The Big Five trait taxonomy: History, measurement, and theoretical perspectives. In L. A. Pervin & O. P. John (Eds.), *Handbook of personality: Theory and research* (2nd ed., pp. 102–138). New York: Guilford Press.

Kenrick, D. T., & Trost, M. R. (1997). Evolutionary approaches to relationships. In S. Duck (Ed.), *Handbook of personal relationships: Theory, research, and interventions* (pp. 151–177). Chichester, UK: Wiley.

Lee, K., & Ashton, M. C. (2004). Psychometric properties of the HEXACO Personality Inventory. *Multivariate Behavioral Research, 39,* 329–358.

Majani, E., Erlarson, R., & Abu-Mostafa, Y. (1989). The induction of mul-
tiscale temporal structure. In D. S. Touretzky (Ed.), *Advances in neural
information processing systems* (pp. 634–642). San Mateo, CA: Morgan
Kaufmann.

McCrae, R. R., & Costa, P. T., Jr. (1999). A five-factor theory of personality. In
L. A. Pervin & O. P. John (Eds.), *Handbook of personality: Theory and
research* (2nd ed., pp. 139–153). New York: Guilford Press.

Miller, L. C., & Read, S. J. (1987). Why am I telling you this?: Self-disclosure
in a goal-based model of personality. In V. J. Derlega & J. H. Berg (Eds.),
Self-disclosure: Theory, research, and therapy (pp. 35–58). New York: Plenum Press.

Miller, L. C., & Read, S. J. (1991). On the coherence of mental models of persons
and relationships: A knowledge structure approach. In G. J. O. Fletcher &
F. D. Fincham (Eds.), *Cognition in close relationships* (pp. 69–99). Hillsdale, NJ: Erlbaum.

Mischel, W., & Shoda, Y. (1995). A cognitive–affective system theory of personality: Reconceptualizing situations, dispositions, dynamics, and invariance
in personality structure. *Psychological Review, 102*(2), 246–268.

Mischel, W., & Shoda, Y. (1998). Reconciling processing dynamics and personality dispositions. *Annual Review of Psychology, 49,* 229–258.

Monroe, B. M., & Read, S. J. (2008). A general connectionist model of attitudes
and attitude change: The ACS (attitudes as constraint satisfaction) model.
Psychological Review, 115, 733–739.

Ochsner, K. N., Ray, R. D., Cooper, J. C., Robertson, E. R., Chopra, S., Gabri-
eli, J. D., et al. (2004). For better or for worse: Neural systems supporting
the cognitive down- and up-regulation of negative emotion. *NeuroImage,
23*(2), 483–499.

O'Doherty, J., Kringelbach, M. L., Rolls, E. T., Hornak, J., & Andrews, C.
(2001). Abstract reward and punishment representations in the human
orbitofrontal cortex. *Nature Neuroscience, 4*(1), 95–102.

O'Reilly, R. C. (1996). Biologically plausible error-driven learning using local
activation differences: The generalized recirculation algorithm. *Neural
Computation, 8*(5), 895–938.

O'Reilly, R. C., & Munakata, Y. (2000). *Computational explorations in cognitive neuroscience: Understanding the mind by simulating the brain.* Cambridge, MA: MIT Press.

O'Reilly, R. C., & Munakata, Y. (2003). Psychological function in computational models of neural networks. In I. B. Weiner (Series Ed.) & M. Gal-
lagher & R. J. Nelson (Vol. Eds.), *Handbook of psychology: Vol. 3. Biological psychology* (pp. 637–654). New York: Wiley.

Panksepp, J. (1998). *Affective neuroscience: The foundations of human and
animal emotions.* New York: Oxford University Press.

Peabody, D., & De Raad, B. (2002). The substantive nature of psycholexical
personality factors: A comparison across languages. *Journal of Personality
and Social Psychology, 83,* 983–997.

Pelphrey, K. A., Morris, J. P., & McCarthy, G. (2004). Grasping the intentions
of others: The perceived intentionality of an action influences activity in

the superior temporal sulcus during social perception. *Journal of Cognitive Neuroscience, 16*(10), 1706–1716.

Phelps, E. A., O'Connor, K. J., Cunningham, W. A., Funayama, E. S., Gatenby, J. C., Gore, J. C., et al. (2000). Performance on indirect measures of race evaluation predicts amygdala activation. *Journal of Cognitive Neuroscience, 12*(5), 729–738.

Pratkanis, A. R., Breckler, S. J., & Greenwald, A. G. (Eds.). (1989). *Attitude structure and function.* Hillsdale, NJ: Erlbaum.

Read, S. J., & Miller, L. C. (1989). The importance of goals in personality: Toward a coherent model of persons. In R. S. Wyer, Jr. & T. K. Srull (Eds.), *Social intelligence and cognitive assessments of personality* (pp. 163–174). Hillsdale, NJ: Erlbaum.

Read, S. J., Vanman, E. J., & Miller, L. C. (1997). Connectionism, parallel constraint satisfaction processes, and gestalt principles: (Re)introducing cognitive dynamics to social psychology. *Personality and Social Psychology Review, 1*(1), 26–53.

Rothbart, M. K., & Bates, J. E. (1998). Temperament. In W. Damon (Series Ed.) & N. Eisenberg (Vol. Ed.), *Handbook of child psychology: Vol. 3. Social, emotional, and personality development* (5th ed., pp. 105–176). New York: Wiley.

Saucier, G., & Ostendorf, F. (1999). Hierarchical subcomponents of the Big Five personality factors: A cross-language replication. *Journal of Personality and Social Psychology, 76,* 613–627.

Saucier, G., & Simonds, J. (2006). The structure of personality and temperament. In D. K. Mroczek & T. D. Little (Eds.), *Handbook of personality development* (pp. 109–128). Mahwah, NJ: Erlbaum.

Schwarz, N. (2007). Attitude construction: Evaluation in context. *Social Cognition, 25*(5), 638–656.

Spoont, M. R. (1992). Modulatory role of serotonin in neural information processing: Implications for human psychopathology. *Psychological Bulletin, 112*(2), 330–350.

Tellegen, A., & Waller, N. G. (in press). Exploring personality through test construction: Development of the Multidimensional Personality Questionnaire. In G. J. Boyle, G. Matthews, & D. H. Saklofske (Eds.), *Handbook of personality theory and testing* (Vol. II). London: Sage.

Van Overwalle, F. (2007). *Social connectionism: A reader and handbook for simulations.* New York: Psychology Press.

Van Overwalle, F., & Siebler, F. (2005). A connectionist model of attitude formation and change. *Personality and Social Psychology Review, 9*(3), 231–274.

Walter, H., Adenzato, M., Ciaramidaro, A., Enrici, I., Pia, L., & Bara, B. G. (2004). Understanding intentions in social interaction: The role of the anterior paracingulate cortex. *Journal of Cognitive Neuroscience, 16*(10), 1854–1863.

Widrow, B., & Hoff, M. E. (1960). Adaptive switching circuits. *Institute of Radio Engineers, Western Electronic Show and Convention, Convention Record, Part 4,* 96–104.

Wiggins, J. S., & Trapnell, P. D. (1996). A dyadic-interactional perspective on the five-factor model. In J. S. Wiggins (Ed.), *The five-factor model of personality: Theoretical perspectives* (pp. 88–162). New York: Guilford Press.

Wood, W., & Neal, D. T. (2007). A new look at habits and the habit-goal interface. *Psychological Review, 114*(4), 843–863.

Zebrowitz, L. A., Fellous, J., Mignault, A., & Andreoletti, C. (2003). Trait impressions as overgeneralized responses to adaptively significant facial qualities: Evidence from connectionist modeling. *Personality and Social Psychology Review, 7*(3), 194–215.

Zuckerman, M. (2002). Zuckerman–Kuhlman Personality Questionnaire (ZKPQ): An alternative five-factorial model. In B. de Raad & M. Perugini (Eds.), *Big Five assessment* (pp. 376–392). Seattle, WA: Hogrefe & Huber.

13

Molecular Biology and Genomic Imaging in Social and Personality Psychology

Turhan Canli

Efforts to understand the biological basis of individual differences have been catalyzed in the past 15 years by advances in molecular biology and in neuroimaging. Molecular biologists have uncovered the basic nucleotide sequence of the human genome's DNA, have begun to identify common variations within this sequence, and have identified common gene variations that are associated with individual differences in personality traits. They have also begun to identify mechanisms for gene–environment interactions involving the so-called "epigenome," which consists of molecules that are associated with the genome, but not part of the DNA itself. In parallel, neuroscientists have begun using noninvasive means to measure brain activation of healthy individuals, making significant progress toward revealing the neural circuitry underlying complex behaviors. In the past few years, these two lines of research have become interwoven: Interdisciplinary teams of researchers have conducted brain imaging studies on individuals who have been genotyped. This line of research has been called "imaging genetics" by some (Hariri, Drabant,

& Weinberger, 2006). I prefer the term "genomic imaging" (Canli, 2006; Congdon & Canli, in press), because of the increasing use of technologies that move from the analysis of individual genes to analysis of the whole genome, which will undoubtedly find applications in neuroimaging. In this chapter, I illustrate the ways in which molecular biology and genomic imaging are highly relevant to social and personality psychology, point out experimental considerations, and give some practical advice on how to integrate these approaches into one's research.

Relevance to Social and Personality Psychology

Why should social and personality psychologists care about the methods used in molecular biology and in genomic imaging? I argue that these methods offer powerful tools for understanding the role of the environment and its interaction with the individual's (epi)genome, as well as for learning how these interactions shape individual differences in behavior. Moreover, these methods offer tools for understanding how individual differences in behavior may affect an individual's biology, with significant importance for health psychology. Broadly speaking, research on any topic within social and personality psychology that involves individual differences (e.g., aggression, other traits, or attachment), or in which the environment plays a critical role (e.g., culture, early childhood experience, or aging), could include methods from molecular biology or genomic imaging.

Another important point is that social and personality psychologists who are well versed in contemporary molecular biology can be powerful advocates of their discipline in their interactions with molecular biologists. Biologists may make important discoveries at the molecular level, but have no exposure to psychology that would enable them to imagine how this discovery may be relevant to human behavior. Although connections between vastly different levels of analysis must be drawn with care, integration of research across levels of analysis may lead to important advances in both fields.

Finally, social and personality psychologists can look to biological measures for validation of their theoretical constructs. For example, several brain imaging studies have found highly significant correlations between self-reported personality traits and individual differences in neural activation, suggesting that self-report measures can map onto reliable (biologically based) individual differences. Thus biological approaches give social and personality psychologists novel tools for assessing the validity of multiple conceptualizations of a given construct.

Genetics and the Personality Trait of Neuroticism

To illustrate the relevance of molecular biology and genomic imaging to social psychology, I present a brief illustration of research on the personality trait of neuroticism. (I have presented a more comprehensive neurogenetic model of neuroticism elsewhere; see Canli, 2008). Neuroticism is a personality trait associated with heightened negative affect that figures prominently in a number of influential models of personality, such as Eysenck's model (Eysenck, 1990) or the "Big Five" taxonomy (John & Srivastava, 1999).

Like all personality traits, neuroticism has a high degree of heritability: Twin and adoption studies using a quantitative genetic approach estimate that about 40–60% of the variance for such traits as neuroticism is accounted for by genetic factors (Carey, 2003). Lesch and colleagues (1996) reported a significant association between self-reported neuroticism and a common variation (polymorphism) within the gene that encodes the serotonin transporter. This transporter regulates the reuptake of serotonin after its release into the synaptic cleft between two neurons. The polymorphism is located within the regulatory region of the gene, which determines how much serotonin transporter is produced, and it has a short (s) and a long (l) variant. Because each individual carries two copies of the gene (one from each parent), the possible combinations are s/s, s/l, and l/l. Lesch and colleagues discovered that those with either the s/s or s/l variant of this gene reported significantly higher levels of neuroticism than those with the l/l variant.

The effect size of the influence of this polymorphism is small, however. Lesch and colleagues (1996) found that the presence of the s variant accounted for only 7–9% of the genetic variance in measured neuroticism, suggesting that at least another 10–13 genes with similar effect size (or many more with smaller effect size) influence this trait.

Genomic Imaging

Following the report of the association between self-reported neuroticism and the serotonin transporter polymorphism, later studies began to probe the neural correlates of this association. Fallgatter, Jatzke, Bartsch, Hamelbeck, and Lesch (1999) measured event-related potentials (ERPs) during performance of a cognitive response control task (the "go/no-go" task) and found that this polymorphism was associated with individual differences in task-related activation of the prefrontal cortex and limbic system. A later study by the same group found that presence of the s variant was associated with higher activity of the anterior cingulate cortex, a brain region at the intersection of cognition and emotion, in a go/no-go task (Fallgatter, Bartsch, & Herrmann, 2002).

The field of genomic imaging was catalyzed by a seminal report by Hariri and colleagues (2002), who used functional magnetic resonance imaging (fMRI) to measure brain responses to emotional stimuli in individuals who were genotyped for the serotonin transporter polymorphism. Participants were either carriers of the s variant (S group) or noncarriers (i.e., they had two copies of the l variant; L group). While being scanned, these individuals made matching decisions on images of angry or fearful facial expressions, or of vertical and horizontal oval shapes. These investigators found that the S and L groups differed significantly in activation of the amygdala, a brain region involved in emotional processing. Relative to the neutral condition, there was significantly greater amygdala activation to emotional stimuli in the S group, but not the L group. These findings were interpreted as showing that the association between trait negative affect (i.e., neuroticism) and the s variant was due, at least in part, to enhanced amygdala reactivity to negative stimuli. Since the publication of this study, several other imaging studies have replicated this observation with a range of task paradigms and different participant populations, as confirmed in a recent meta-analysis (Munafo, Brown, & Hariri, 2008).

Design Issues in fMRI: Selection of the Baseline Condition

As reviewed by Whalen (Chapter 14, this volume), fMRI data analysis requires calculating the relative difference in activation between at least two conditions: the experimental and the control condition. In the case of the Hariri and colleagues (2002) study discussed above (as well as almost all replication studies), the experimental condition involved presentation of emotional stimuli, and the control condition involved presentation of emotionally neutral stimuli. The conclusion that the association between neuroticism and the s variant can be explained in terms of enhanced amygdala reactivity to negative stimuli rests on the assumption that the relative activation difference between the two conditions is driven by greater activation during presentation of negative stimuli, and that there is no activation of interest during the control condition. I have illustrated this assumption in Figure 13.1 (top).

Although this interpretation of the data is intuitively appealing, the relative activation difference can also be explained in a different way (illustrated in Figure 13.1, bottom): It is possible that there is no significant activation increase during presentation of negative stimuli, but

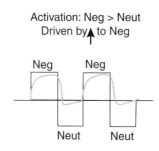

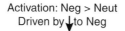

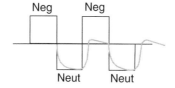

FIGURE 13.1. Hemodynamic response to negative and neutral stimuli. The square wave illustrates the two task conditions; the curving line illustrates the hemodynamic response. Both panels illustrate greater activation in the negative than in the neutral condition. The top panel indicates significant activation during the negative (but not neutral) condition. The bottom panel indicates significant activation during the neutral (but not negative) condition.

instead a significant activation *decrease* during presentation of *neutral* stimuli. In other words, the reported greater amygdala activation in the S group during the negative as opposed to the neutral condition (Neg > Neut) may be due to activation (Figure 13.1, curving line, representing the hemodynamic response curve) that either *increases* during the negative condition (Figure 13.1, top) or *decreases* during the neutral condition (Figure 13.1, bottom). Because the published studies directly contrasted the emotional and neutral conditions with each other, these two interpretations could not be dissociated.

The decreased activation during neutral stimulus processing may be less intuitive, but it has biological credibility in the context of theories about the brain's default state of activity. Raichle and colleagues (2001) analyzed data from a number of imaging studies and concluded that some brain regions (the amygdala included) appear to be characterized by elevated levels of activity when idle or "at rest" (i.e., a participant is not engaged in any particular cognitive task), from which they then show a decrease in activation when a participant is occupied with some (emotionally neutral) cognitive task. In the context of the sero-tonin transporter gene's effect on neural activation, this would suggest the intriguing possibility that individuals who carry the s variant may be characterized by an elevated level of amygdala activation when at rest (i.e., not instructed to engage in any particular cognitive process), from which they show a deactivation when processing neutral stimuli.

To address this possibility, my colleagues and I therefore designed an imaging study using two baseline conditions to dissociate the respective contributions of the negative and neutral task conditions (Canli et al., 2005). We used an emotional word Stroop task, in which participants viewed neutral, negative, and positive words printed in different colors, and pressed a response button corresponding to the color of the printed word (this paradigm is commonly used to study implicit emotional pro-cessing). Importantly, we also included a fixation/rest condition, during which participants passively viewed a fixation cross placed in the middle of the screen, with no particular instruction to do anything. Since all stimuli were presented in blocks of 24 sec, this meant that during the fixation/rest condition, participants' mind were free to wander in any way they wanted ("at rest" does not mean that the brain is in a state of inactivity; rather, it suggests that the brain is resting from following any particular task instructions). These different conditions allowed us to compare brain activation to negative versus neutral stimuli, but also to examine activation to negative and to neutral stimuli independently of each other, by comparing each condition to the fixation/rest condition. We replicated the finding that the S group showed significantly greater amygdala activation to negative, compared to neutral, stimuli than the L group did (Figure 13.2, left panel). However, by comparing each of these conditions separately to the second fixation/rest condition, we then showed that this difference was driven by a decrease in activation during the neutral condition (Figure 13.2, middle panel), and not by an increase in activation during the negative condition (Figure 13.2, right panel).

Our report prompted Heinz and colleagues to reanalyze data from their previously published study (Heinz et al., 2005), in which they had reported greater amygdala activation in the S group than in the L group in response to negatively (but not positively) valenced images. In their reanalysis (Heinz et al., 2007), they now contrasted amygdala activation during the neutral picture condition with a rest condition, and replicated our result of a relatively decreased activation during the neutral condi-tion in the S group.

Although we now had independent confirmation of decreased amygdala activation in the S group during the neutral condition, com-pared to a resting condition, there is no agreement about the interpreta-

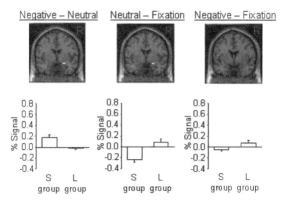

FIGURE 13.2. Amygdala activation to negative, neutral, and fixation stimuli. Bar graphs show percentage of signal change (± SEM) across a significant cluster in the amygdala. From Canli et al. (2005). Copyright 2005 by the National Academy of Sciences. Reprinted by permission.

tion of these results. Heinz and colleagues (2007) suggest that s variant carriers show elevated activation in response to an undefined and potentially threatening environment, as encountered during the rest condition in the scanner. This interpretation suggests that elevated amygdala activation in s variant carriers represents a response to the environment that affects the state of the individual. In contrast, we suggest that elevated amygdala activation in s variant carriers represents a chronic, trait-like condition, not a response to the environment (Canli & Lesch, 2007). Thus elevated amygdala activation in s variant carriers represents a trait of these individuals. In order to support our hypothesis further, we conducted a so-called "perfusion scan," which measures absolute blood flow. When we placed participants in the scanner with no task instructions (i.e., in a "resting" condition), we found that absolute levels of amygdala blood flow were significantly higher in the S group than in the L group (Canli et al., 2006). This observation was also independently replicated (Rao et al., 2007). Yet the interpretational ambiguity remains: Is this elevated activation in s variant carriers more like a state in response to the scanner environment, or more like a trait of the individual? Future work outside the scanner will have to address this question.

Given that the debate involves the interpretation of the data, rather than replicability, why does it matter whether observed activation differences reflect state-like short-term responses to the environment or trait-like chronic activation? It matters because each may be associated with different health consequences and molecular mechanisms, as is the case for acute versus chronic stress (Calcagni & Elenkov, 2006; McEwen,

2007). This is important because the presence of the s variant is associated with vulnerability for depression (in the presence of life stress), and understanding whether amygdala activation represents acute or chronic processes could therefore lead to different approaches in the development of future interventions and treatments.

Designing Analyses to Include Environmental Factors

Of particular interest to social and personality psychologists may be methods that integrate genetic and environmental variables. Quantitative genetics had long established that the environment, particularly the unshared environment that defines an individual's unique life history, plays about as much of a role as genes do (Carey, 2003). With respect to the serotonin transporter gene polymorphism, Caspi and colleagues (2003) demonstrated that presence of the s variant, in conjunction with a history of stressful life events, significantly increased individuals' vulnerability to depression. Carriers of the s variant were up to twice as likely to become depressed after stressful events such as bereavement, romantic disasters, illness, or job loss, and childhood maltreatment significantly increased this probability. These associations are further supported by replication studies (Kaufman et al., 2004; Kendler, Kuhn, Vittum, Prescott, & Riley, 2005), although partial replications suggest further moderation by gender (Eley et al., 2004; Grabe et al., 2005) and social support (Kaufman et al., 2004). Two studies (Gillespie, Whitfield, Williams, Heath, & Martin, 2005; Surtees et al., 2005) failed to replicate this gene × environment (G × E) effect altogether, but also used older subject populations than the other studies, suggesting that age may also be an important variable.

To investigate G × E interactions at the brain systems level and their impact on psychological processes relevant to depression vulnerability, we conducted an imaging study that also included self-report measures of life stress history and levels of rumination (Canli et al., 2006). Life stress history was based on a self-report questionnaire developed from items in the Life History Calendar (Caspi, Moffitt, Thornton, & Freedman, 1996), and contained 28 items related to work, financial and legal problems, death and serious illness, family and relationships, and other stressful life events. Participants checked a box indicating whether (and, if so, when, how often, or how long) they had ever experienced a particular event. For our analyses, "life stress" was quantified as the number of categories endorsed by each participant.

To evaluate the interaction of genotype and life stress on neural activation, we conducted a multiple-regression analysis within a standard fMRI analysis program (SPM2), into which we entered four variables: genotype (dummy-coded to indicated the presence or absence of the s variant); number of experienced life stress categories; the interaction term of genotype and life stress; and age. We ran the analysis to identify voxels in the brain that showed a significant interaction, while partialing out any main effects due to genotype, life stress, or age.

Both fMRI and perfusion data showed that the amygdala (and also the hippocampus, a region shown to play a role in depression and stress) (Campbell, Marriott, Nahmias, & MacQueen, 2004; Frodl et al., 2004; Hastings, Parsey, Oquendo, Arango, & Mann, 2004; McEwen & Sapolsky, 1995; Rusch, Abercrombie, Oakes, Schaefer, & Davidson, 2001; Sheline, Gado, & Kraemer, 2003) showed a G × E effect: Life stress was positively correlated with higher resting activation in the S group, but negatively correlated in the L group (Figure 13.3). Life events also differentially affected self-reported rumination, as a function of serotonin transporter genotype: Individuals in the S group exhibited *increased* rumination associated with life stress, whereas individuals in the L group exhibited *decreased* rumination (Figure 13.4).

For social and personality psychologists, these findings may inspire work to investigate the psychological mechanisms that produce these interaction effects. For example, could the association between life stress and decreased rumination in the L group reflect some kind of a training effect for coping skills? If so, why would coping skills become strengthened with life stress in the L group, but weakened in the S group? Do these groups differ in the kinds of life stress experiences they accrue, and to what extent do the S and L groups differ in the extent to which they

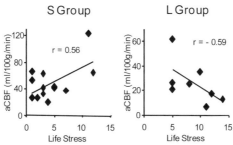

FIGURE 13.3. Absolute cerebral blood flow (aCBF) in amygdala. Scatterplots from a cluster within the amygdala show a significant interaction of life stress and aCBF. From Canli et al. (2006). Copyright 2006 by the National Academy of Sciences. Reprinted by permission.

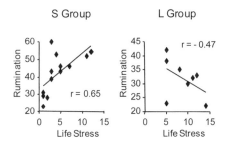

FIGURE 13.4. G × E effect on self-reported rumination. Left and right columns show scatterplots of self-reported rumination as a function of life stress. From Canli et al. (2006). Copyright 2006 by the National Academy of Sciences. Reprinted by permission.

seek or avoid life stress experiences? If coping skills are a critical mechanism, do individuals who carry the s variant have poor coping skills that can be improved with training? Clearly, understanding the observed G × E interactions will require significant contributions from social and personality psychologists.

Understanding Environmental Influences through Epigenetics

Social life experience changes gene expression. This profound insight is based on the work of Weaver and colleagues (2004), who studied how maternal behavior changes the genetic structure of rat pups. They started with the well-known observation that rats that experience poor maternal care as pups (receiving little licking and grooming) grow up to show strong stress responses. Focusing on the gene that codes for the glucocorticoid receptor in the hippocampus (both the receptor and the hippocampus are related to the stress response), they found that poor maternal care altered the physical shape of the receptor gene. The process did not involve changes in the DNA itself, but rather in the molecules that regulate DNA gene expression (the epigenome). Specifically, they discovered that poor maternal care altered DNA methylation, in which a methyl group is attached to the cytosine base of the DNA, to act as a docking site for molecules that can alter its physical shape in a way that changes the gene expression. Using a cross-fostering paradigm in which pups were born to mothers that exercised either good or poor maternal care and then were switched to the other kind, they showed that differences in DNA methylation were not inherited, but rather reflected rearing experience. DNA methylation acted as an epigenetic switch that altered the production of the glucocorticoid receptor, which may explain why maternal care affects stress reactivity. Importantly, they also showed that this form of "epigenetic programming" by early life experience was reversible in principle.

For social and personality psychologists, several exciting and important questions are inspired by this line of research. Do epigenetic processes affect human gene expression? Is there a critical period for these processes, or can they operate at any stage in life? Are they reversible through social interactions or other psychological interventions? Are some interventions more effective than others? What kinds of behaviors other than stress responses may be modulated in this way? Finding the answers to these questions may well define a major research agenda for future generations of social and personality psychologists.

Other Methodological and Practical Issues

A Priori Hypothesis Testing versus Data Mining

A key decision early in designing an experiment is whether the study is designed to test an a priori hypothesis or not. This decision is likely to affect the sample size, and can also affect recruitment procedures and analysis methods. For example, if I design a study specifically to address a hypothesized difference between the S and L groups, I may only need to conduct a small set of targeted statistical comparisons. An imaging study contrasting two groups may only require about 12 individuals in each group. In contrast, if I don't have any a priori hypotheses, I may have to conduct a very large number of analyses and to control for multiple comparisons, reducing my statistical power or having to increase my sample size (some published imaging studies have reported samples of well over 100 participants). Also, if my study is designed a priori to compare two genotype groups, I may choose to preselect participants on the basis of their genotype to ensure that both cells have the same sample size. With preselection, I also have the option to control or match for other variables that I think may affect results across both groups. The drawback is that preselection turns the recruitment into a two-step process in which some individuals will be rejected from inclusion in the study because their genotype is oversampled.

Having an a priori hypothesis makes for a clean, crisp study with clear objectives. On the other hand, it is also somewhat limiting, in that only one gene (or a very small number of genes) is studied. Perhaps the dependent variable of interest is not as much affected by one's favorite gene as by another. Given that once the DNA is collected, it can be analyzed to yield information about potentially millions of other gene variations (e.g., if one uses gene chip technology), ignoring this additional information would be wasteful. As one becomes interested in larger numbers of gene polymorphisms, or interactions among genes or between genes and other variables, the sample size inevitably needs to increase. This becomes particularly salient in neuroimaging studies, where the cost of one participant runs in the hundreds of dollars. Similarly, genetic analyses of hundreds of thousands (soon millions) of polymorphisms also cost several hundred dollars per participant.

Ethnic Representation versus Stratification

In general, federal research funding guidelines require that the recruited participants represent a broad range of ethnic groups. Yet genetic studies are vulnerable to "ethnic stratification." That is, different ethnicities may differ not only genetically, but also in many other respects that may reflect cultural or societal differences; thus observed differences believed to reflect genetic variation may reflect nongenetic factors if the sample consists of different ethnicities, and particularly if the representation of these ethnicities differs across groups within the study. Furthermore, genetic variation may differ dramatically among ethnicities; for example, the allele frequencies of the serotonin transporter l variant among African Americans, European Americans, and Japanese are 70%, 59%, and only 17%, respectively (Gelernter, Kranzler, & Cubells, 1997). Thus, without adequate controls during recruitment for the L group, a study is likely to oversample some ethnicities and undersample others. To avoid these stratification confounds, it is therefore common in many genetic studies to recruit ethnically homogeneous populations. In our genomic imaging work, we use diverse ethnic samples to maximize generalizability, but statistically test for significant group differences with respect to subject demographics and performance variables. When participants are preselected on the basis of genotype, variant frequency and demographic differences can be minimized.

DNA Collection, Storage, and Analysis

A defining feature of progress in molecular biology is its breakneck pace. Methods constantly evolve, and publications keep identifying new candidate genes on a monthly, if not weekly, basis. I therefore recommend designing the research protocol (including consent forms) in a manner that ensures a high degree of flexibility, so that future analyses of collected DNA are possible. These analyses may look for genes that are currently unknown, or may use technologies that currently do not exist. These analyses may not even focus on DNA per se, but rather on the molecules associated with its expression and regulation that make up the epigenome. When research is set up with this degree of flexibility in mind, it is possible to reanalyze old data in light of new genetic information.

To ensure the greatest amount of flexibility in future analyses, I recommend obtaining DNA through blood draw. This will generate a practically limitless amount of DNA for future analyses, which can be stored with no loss of DNA quality. For ease of administration, cheek swabs or mouth wash solutions are similarly effective. However, researchers should be aware that cheek swabs (I have no personal experience with wash solutions) do not yield nearly as much DNA as blood does, and that the quality of the DNA deteriorates after a few years to the point of being useless. This is fine if investigators want to collect DNA conveniently from large numbers of people (such as subject pool participants), are only interested in a few candidate genes, and do not plan to analyze a given sample more than 2 years into the future.

Obviously, this type of research needs to be done in a manner consistent with the local institutional review board's guidelines regarding the communication of genetic information to the participants, and with other ethical considerations (such as potential risks or unanticipated discoveries). In general, however, our studies do not seek to identify disease-related genes (e.g., it is unlikely that genes related to social behavior will be comparable to cancer-linked genes), and the effect sizes for any single gene of interest are too small to be of any meaningful predictive value for an individual participant.

Collaborations

For a social or personality psychologist, collaboration with a molecular biologist is the fastest, cheapest way to get started. (Our foray into this field was greatly facilitated by collaborating with Klaus Peter Lesch.) Even among researchers who are experienced in combining methods from psychology and molecular biology, collaborations may become more common. One example comes from genomic imaging: Whereas a one-sample fMRI study may only require a sample of 12 subjects, genomic imaging studies now typically require several dozen participants, and current grant proposals may request funding for hundreds or even thousands of participants. With ever-tightening federal research budgets, it is becoming more difficult for individual labs to obtain this level of funding—moving genomic imaging more into the realm of "Big Science," with the formation of consortia or multi-institutional collaborations.

Another aspect of these collaborations is the need for replication and verification in studies using different labs or methods. A recent paper in *Science* reported on a novel gene variation related to individual differences in memory (Papassotiropoulos et al., 2006). This study was a tour de force in which a novel gene variation was discovered and related to memory performance in one sample of Swiss participants, then replicated in a U.S. sample, and replicated again in a second Swiss sample. As reported in the same paper, this gene was then functionally studied in the hippocampus of the human brain with fMRI and causally linked to memory performance in transgenic mice. This convergence of research disciplines, methodologies, and levels of analysis sets a high bar for future work, and is all but impossible to conduct in single-principal-investigator laboratory settings. In recognition of this fact, the National Institutes of Health now allow for grant applications to list multiple individuals as principal investigators (as opposed to the older "co-P.I." designation).

Training and Education

Even social and personality psychologists who only seek to collaborate with molecular biologists will benefit from additional training or education in contemporary biology. As I have stated earlier, this field is so fast-moving that one's knowledge of biology at the high school or even college level is hopelessly limited and outdated. It will be difficult to engage in a dialogue with a colleague in another field if one has no common language to communicate.

I had no training in molecular biology when I started my first faculty appointment. Through a colleague, I learned of a 2-week summer workshop at Smith College in Massachusetts, called the New England Biolabs Molecular Biology Summer Workshop (*www.science.smith.edu/neb*). The designers of this workshop make no assumptions about participants' prior knowledge in molecular biology. Students spend 10–12 hours a day for 2 weeks in lectures and in the lab, and gain hands-on experience from Day 1. The workshop has been taught for 23 years; it is offered three times each summer; and its contents are continually updated to include the latest techniques. It is so efficiently designed and run that after 2 weeks, students will have knowledge and hands-on experience equivalent to at least 1 year of graduate-level molecular biology. It is obviously very intense, but also a lot of fun—embracing a "work hard, play hard" attitude, with excellent room and board and great camaraderie. Completing this course will suffice to make participants feel comfortable reading and conversing in the literature of molecular biology, or it may be the beginning of starting a molecular biology branch within their existing labs (as it has been in my case). Researchers who are too busy to attend this workshop should consider sending their students.

In addition to the Smith College workshop, Cold Spring Harbor Laboratory offers a large number of workshops and courses throughout the year (*meetings.cshl.edu*). The offerings vary from year to year, but always feature leading scientists as organizers and speakers. In a similar vein, the summer courses offered by Woods Hole Marine Biology Laboratory (*www.mbl.edu/education/courses/summer*) also have a fantastic reputation. I am sure that this is not an exhaustive list, but it should be a useful starting point for researching training and educational opportunities.

Concluding Comments

I hope that this chapter will inspire some readers to consider integrating molecular biology or genomic imaging into their research. Principal investigators with already established laboratories and research themes may consider how to spend their next sabbatical, if only by catching up with some reading of review articles or introductory textbooks. Advanced graduate students may be inspired to consider postdoctoral training in some of the techniques I have described. Beginning graduate students or undergraduates may feel encouraged to take an introductory class in molecular biology. The methods, though pioneered by molecular biologists, surely will have endless applications in psychology.

Acknowledgment

The work discussed here was supported by the National Science Foundation (Grant No. BCS-0224221).

References

Calcagni, E., & Elenkov, I. (2006). Stress system activity, innate and T helper cytokines, and susceptibility to immune-related diseases. *Annals of the New York Academy of Sciences, 1069,* 62–76.

Campbell, S., Marriott, M., Nahmias, C., & MacQueen, G. M. (2004). Lower hippocampal volume in patients suffering from depression: A meta-analysis. *American Journal of Psychiatry, 161*(4), 598–607.

Canli, T. (2006). Genomic imaging of extraversion. In T. Canli (Ed.), *Biology of personality and individual differences* (pp. 93–115). New York: Guilford Press.

Canli, T. (2008). Toward a neurogenetic theory of neuroticism. *Annals of the New York Academy of Sciences, 1129,* 153–174.

Canli, T., & Lesch, K. P. (2007). Long story short: The serotonin transporter in emotion regulation and social cognition. *Nature Neuroscience, 10*(9), 1103–1109.

Canli, T., Omura, K., Haas, B. W., Fallgatter, A. J., Constable, R. T., & Lesch, K. P. (2005). Beyond affect: A role for genetic variation of the serotonin transporter in neural activation during a cognitive attention task. *Proceedings of the National Academy of Sciences USA, 102,* 12224–12229.

Canli, T., Qiu, M., Omura, K., Congdon, E., Haas, B. W., Amin, Z., et al. (2006). Neural correlates of epigenesis. *Proceedings of the National Academy of Sciences USA, 103,* 16033–16038.

Carey, G. (2003). *Human genetics for the social sciences* (Vol. 4). Thousand Oaks, CA: Sage.

Caspi, A., Moffitt, T. E., Thornton, A., & Freedman, D. (1996). The life history calendar: A research and clinical assessment method for collecting retrospective event-history data. *International Journal of Methods in Psychiatry Research, 6*(2), 101–114.

Caspi, A., Sugden, K., Moffitt, T. E., Taylor, A., Craig, I. W., Harrington, H., et al. (2003). Influence of life stress on depression: Moderation by a polymorphism in the 5-HTT gene. *Science, 301,* 386–389.

Congdon, E., & Canli, T. (2008). Genomic imaging of personality: Towards a molecular neurobiology of impulsivity. In G. Boyle, G. Matthews, & D. Saklowsky (Eds.), *The Sage handbook of personality, theory and assessment: Personality measurement and testing* (Vol. 2, pp. 334–351). Thousand Oaks, CA: Sage.

Eley, T. C., Sugden, K., Corsico, A., Gregory, A. M., Sham, P., McGuffin, P., et al. (2004). Gene–environment interaction analysis of serotonin system markers with adolescent depression. *Molecular Psychiatry, 9*(10), 908–915.

Eysenck, H. J. (1990). Biological dimensions of personality. In L. A. Pervin (Ed.), *Handbook of personality: Theory and research* (pp. 244–276). New York: Guilford Press.

Fallgatter, A. J., Bartsch, A. J., & Herrmann, M. J. (2002). Electrophysiological measurements of anterior cingulate function. *Journal of Neural Transmission, 109*(5–6), 977–988.

Fallgatter, A. J., Jatzke, S., Bartsch, A. J., Hamelbeck, B., & Lesch, K. P. (1999). Serotonin transporter promoter polymorphism influences topography of inhibitory motor control. *International Journal of Neuropsychopharmcology, 2*(2), 115–120.

Frodl, T., Meisenzahl, E. M., Zill, P., Baghai, T., Rujescu, D., Leinsinger, G., et al. (2004). Reduced hippocampal volumes associated with the long variant of the serotonin transporter polymorphism in major depression. *Archives of General Psychiatry, 61*(2), 177–183.

Gelernter, J., Kranzler, H., & Cubells, J. F. (1997). Serotonin transporter protein (SLC6A4) allele and haplotype frequencies and linkage disequilibria in African- and European-American and Japanese populations and in alcohol-dependent subjects. *Human Genetics, 101*(2), 243–246.

Gillespie, N. A., Whitfield, J. B., Williams, B., Heath, A. C., & Martin, N. G.

(2005). The relationship between stressful life events, the serotonin transporter (5-HTTLPR) genotype and major depression. *Psychological Medicine, 35*(1), 101–111.

Grabe, H. J., Lange, M., Wolff, B., Volzke, H., Lucht, M., Freyberger, H. J., et al. (2005). Mental and physical distress is modulated by a polymorphism in the 5-HT transporter gene interacting with social stressors and chronic disease burden. *Molecular Psychiatry, 10*(2), 220–224.

Hariri, A. R., Drabant, E. M., & Weinberger, D. R. (2006). Imaging genetics: Perspectives from studies of genetically driven variation in serotonin function and corticolimbic affective processing. *Biological Psychiatry, 59*(10), 888–897.

Hariri, A. R., Mattay, V. S., Tessitore, A., Kolachana, B., Fera, F., Goldman, D., et al. (2002). Serotonin transporter genetic variation and the response of the human amygdala. *Science, 297*, 400–403.

Hastings, R. S., Parsey, R. V., Oquendo, M. A., Arango, V., & Mann, J. J. (2004). Volumetric analysis of the prefrontal cortex, amygdala, and hippocampus in major depression. *Neuropsychopharmacology, 29*(5), 952–959.

Heinz, A., Braus, D. F., Smolka, M. N., Wrase, J., Puls, I., Hermann, D., et al. (2005). Amygdala–prefrontal coupling depends on a genetic variation of the serotonin transporter. *Nature Neuroscience, 8*(1), 20–21.

Heinz, A., Smolka, M. N., Braus, D. F., Wrase, J., Beck, A., Flor, H., et al. (2007). Serotonin transporter genotype (5-HTTLPR): Effects of neutral and undefined conditions on amygdala activation. *Biological Psychiatry, 61*(8), 1011–1014.

John, O. P., & Srivastava, S. (1999). The Big Five trait taxonomy: History, measurement, and theoretical perspectives. In L. A. Pervin & O. P. John (Eds.), *Handbook of personality: Theory and research* (2nd ed., pp. 102–138). New York: Guilford Press.

Kaufman, J., Yang, B. Z., Douglas-Palumberi, H., Houshyar, S., Lipschitz, D., Krystal, J. H., et al. (2004). Social supports and serotonin transporter gene moderate depression in maltreated children. *Proceedings of the National Academy of Sciences USA, 101*, 17316–17321.

Kendler, K. S., Kuhn, J. W., Vittum, J., Prescott, C. A., & Riley, B. (2005). The interaction of stressful life events and a serotonin transporter polymorphism in the prediction of episodes of major depression: A replication. *Archives of General Psychiatry, 62*(5), 529–535.

Lesch, K. P., Bengel, D., Heils, A., Sabol, S. Z., Greenberg, B. D., Petri, S., et al. (1996). Association of anxiety-related traits with a polymorphism in the serotonin transporter gene regulatory region. *Science, 274*, 1527–1531.

McEwen, B. S. (2007). Physiology and neurobiology of stress and adaptation: Central role of the brain. *Physiological Review, 87*(3), 873–904.

McEwen, B. S., & Sapolsky, R. M. (1995). Stress and cognitive function. *Current Opinion in Neurobiology, 5*(2), 205–216.

Munafo, M. R., Brown, S. M., & Hariri, A. R. (2008). Serotonin transporter (5-HTTLPR) genotype and amygdala activation: A meta-analysis. *Biological Psychiatry, 63*(9), 852–857.

Papassotiropoulos, A., Stephan, D. A., Huentelman, M. J., Hoerndli, F. J., Craig, D. W., Pearson, J. V., et al. (2006). Common Kibra alleles are associated with human memory performance. *Science, 314,* 475–478.

Raichle, M. E., MacLeod, A. M., Snyder, A. Z., Powers, W. J., Gusnard, D. A., & Shulman, G. L. (2001). A default mode of brain function. *Proceedings of the National Academy of Sciences USA, 98*(2), 676–682.

Rao, H., Gillihan, S. J., Wang, J., Korczykowski, M., Sankoorikal, G. M., Kaercher, K. A., et al. (2007). Genetic variation in serotonin transporter alters resting brain function in healthy individuals. *Biological Psychiatry, 62*(6), 600–606.

Rusch, B. D., Abercrombie, H. C., Oakes, T. R., Schaefer, S. M., & Davidson, R. J. (2001). Hippocampal morphometry in depressed patients and control subjects: Relations to anxiety symptoms. *Biological Psychiatry, 50*(12), 960–964.

Sheline, Y. I., Gado, M. H., & Kraemer, H. C. (2003). Untreated depression and hippocampal volume loss. *American Journal of Psychiatry, 160*(8), 1516–1518.

Surtees, P. G., Wainwright, N. W., Willis-Owen, S. A., Luben, R., Day, N. E., & Flint, J. (2005). Social adversity, the serotonin transporter (5-HTTLPR) polymorphism and major depressive disorder. *Biological Psychiatry, 59,* 224–229.

Weaver, I. C., Cervoni, N., Champagne, F. A., D'Alessio, A. C., Sharma, S., Seckl, J. R., et al. (2004). Epigenetic programming by maternal behavior. *Nature Neuroscience, 7*(8), 847–854.

14

Functional Magnetic Resonance Imaging in the Affective and Social Neurosciences

Tom Johnstone
M. Justin Kim
Paul J. Whalen

O ver the last 10 years, there has been an unprecedented expansion in brain imaging research. With the availability of magnetic resonance imaging (MRI) scanners steadily growing, and with the refinement of functional MRI (fMRI) techniques, the pool of brain imaging researchers has expanded beyond neuroscience and medical imaging departments into psychology departments throughout the world. Early adopters of fMRI in psychology departments were visual psychophysicists interested in mapping the visual processing areas of the brain. Researchers of perception, language, and cognition soon followed, often building upon the theoretical framework provided by animal researchers and neuropsychologists. In addition, affective and social neuroimagers have begun to offer data to make their case that functional brain imaging can add valuable insights to the existing experimental descriptions of human behavior already put forward by affective and social psychologists. Ideally, these insights will enable us to ask new questions to enrich these fields further. The purpose of this chapter, then, is to identify ways in which functional brain imaging may be usefully employed in the social and affective sciences, and to highlight both the advantages and the potential pitfalls of functional brain imaging as a technique for studying the human brain within a social and affective context.

What Does fMRI Measure?

It is generally understood that fMRI is not a measure of neural activity. It is a measure of the ratio of deoxygenated to oxygenated blood, commonly referred to as "blood-oxygenation-level-dependent" (BOLD) contrast. Through some good fortune, oxygenated blood and deoxygenated blood have slightly different magnetic properties; this difference makes it possible to detect the ratio by combining a large electromagnet and radio waves (for details of the physics of BOLD measurements, see Moonen, Bandettini, & Aguirre, 1999). What is clear is that fMRI is based on the experimentally verified assumption that changes in oxygenation in a given region are useful proxies for changes in neuronal activation in that region.

Still not entirely understood is what exactly this oxygenated-to-deoxygenated ratio reflects in terms of neural activity. Is it the activity of neurons within this very region communicating with other brain regions? Is it the activity of other regions communicating with this observed region? Or could it be the activity of neurons within this region communicating with other neurons within this same region? One line of research indicates that the BOLD signal scales roughly linearly with the local summed activity of dendrites, known as the "local field potential" (Goense & Logothetis, 2008; Logothetis, Pauls, Augath, Trinath, & Oeltermann, 2001; Logothetis & Wandell, 2004). These data suggest that BOLD contrast may represent an indirect and approximate measure of dentritic activity averaged over a certain neural region. This would mean that BOLD contrast is not a measure of neuron spiking, but instead that it reflects signals coming into a particular neural region, as well as signals being passed between neurons within the region (though not outgoing signals to other parts of the brain). As research concerning the nature of the BOLD signal continues, the best we can do as we interpret observed BOLD activations is to understand that these different possibilities exist.

Some Advantages of fMRI

The major advantage of fMRI over other techniques of measuring brain activity is its combined spatial and temporal resolution. fMRI can measure BOLD contrast with a spatial resolution of a few millimeters and with a temporal resolution of a few seconds. This compares favorably with electroencephalography (EEG), which can only measure the effects of brain activity at the scalp surface with a resolution of a few centimeters, and with positron emission tomography (PET), which has a temporal resolution of minutes. Thus fMRI is ideally suited to measurement of various brain processes. For example, fairly extensive areas of primary and secondary auditory cortex show sustained activity in response to common sounds, including speech. Large visual processing areas in the occipital cortex and adjacent parts of the parietal and temporal lobes show sustained activity to different types of visual stimuli. Where the temporal and spatial resolution of fMRI comes in handy is in more fine-grained distinctions between subregions that specialize in one particular type of visual or auditory processing. For example, Epstein and Kanwisher (1998) and O'Craven and Kanwisher (2000) have found that distinct parts of the inferior occipital and temporal lobes are involved in processing information about faces and people, as opposed to places. Similar regions in auditory cortex have been identified that respond selectively to human speech sounds (Belin, Zatorre, & Ahad, 2002; Belin, Zatorre, Lafaille, Ahad, & Pike, 2000).

Sustained neural activity in delineated areas of prefrontal cortex and parietal cortex has also been measured during working memory tasks involving maintenance of items in memory. These sorts of processes should thus be amenable to examination with fMRI, as has in fact been demonstrated in many neuroimaging studies (Buckner & Koutstaal, 1998; Cohen et al., 1997; D'Esposito et al., 1995; Feredoes & Postle, 2007; McCarthy et al., 1994). Furthermore, the temporal resolution of fMRI has permitted the separate examination of encoding, maintenance, and retrieval stages in a working memory task. In such a way, fMRI potentially provides researchers in social psychology with a means to examine the neural processes that support the various stages of social behavior.

Some Limitations of fMRI

Many neural processes fall outside of this spatial and temporal resolution, however. For example, many neural processes involved in perception and cognition last just a few milliseconds, and so will not be captured by fMRI unless the experiment is designed in such a way as to allow the accumulation of several such processes. Batty and Taylor (2003) used EEG to measure event-related potentials (ERPs) to emotional facial expressions. They demonstrated effects of emotion (vs. nonemotion) as early as 90 msec after stimulus onset, and differences between emotion expressions after just 140 msec. Importantly, later ERPs showed a different pattern across emotion expressions, presumably due to the engagement of later-stage processing of a different type. The same experiment performed with fMRI would not be able to identify these different stages of processing; rather, the measured response to a given expression would be the cumulative result of all processing stages. For the measurement of fast neural responses, EEG/ERPs or magnetoencephalography would thus be a more appropriate choice—although these techniques do not offer the three-dimensional spatial resolution of fMRI, since they are based on measurements from the scalp surface, and thus reflect the distal aggregate electromagnetic effects of underlying neural activity.

A further consideration with fMRI is that BOLD contrast is a relative and arbitrarily scaled measurement, as explained above. Although BOLD varies with dentritic activity, we have no way of quantifying exactly how much activity is occurring, or even how much more activity (as a difference or a ratio) occurs in one experimental condition than in another. This has a number of implications for emotion and social psychology research, particularly for studies involving individual differences or special populations. Perhaps the most important is that although all measured changes in fMRI signal obviously occur with respect to some underlying baseline neural activity, fMRI cannot tell us anything about the level of baseline activity (e.g., Stark & Squire, 2001). Furthermore, fMRI researchers must make the assumption that the amount of BOLD signal change in response to an experimental manipulation is unrelated, or at most linearly related, to the (unmeasurable) level of baseline neural activity. This assumption is questionable on basic neurophysiological grounds (Hyder, Rothman, & Shulman, 2002; Vazquez et al., 2006), as well as on psychological grounds. Consider, for example, a researcher who wishes to study the neural mechanisms underlying anxiety disorders by comparing brain activation in a clinical group with that in a group of low-anxiety individuals. It is reasonable to expect that upon entering the scanner, anxious individuals will have elevated activity in the brain regions involved in anxiety. To what extent, then, might the researcher expect their fMRI BOLD responses to increase further with the experimental manipulations? Might there be a ceiling effect in the anxious participants' fMRI BOLD responses, due to their elevated baseline activity? Is it valid to compare fMRI BOLD signal changes between a group with low resting baseline and one with higher resting baseline? Without the means of measuring the baseline level of neural activity, the researcher has no way of answering these questions (see Whalen et al., 2008).

fMRI measurements also drift slowly over time, in such a way that fMRI cannot typically be used to measure any change to neural activity that occurs over a time period of more than a few minutes (though some newer fMRI techniques, such as arterial spin labeling [ASL], promise to address this limitation; Wang et al., 2003). So if a researcher's interest is in long-term changes in neural activity, or characterizing resting neural activity as a function of social context or individual differences in mood, then fMRI is probably not a good measurement choice. A further consequence of the relative nature of fMRI BOLD contrast is that comparisons of brain activation between different brain regions are difficult. This is because the magnitude of BOLD response in different neural regions to a given experimental manipulation will depend not only on changes in neural activity, but also on characteristics of the underlying brain anatomy and physiology. Even if we were able to measure those aspects of anatomy and physiology, their relationship with the BOLD response is not yet well enough understood to enable accurate comparisons of BOLD between different brain regions. As a consequence, any claim based on fMRI that, for example, auditory cortex was more or less active than visual cortex in response to a social stimulus would be methodologically questionable. In certain cases, then, PET would be a more appropriate brain imaging choice, since it can be used for absolute baseline and change measurements of cerebral metabolism—though its more invasive nature (involving radioactive tracers) precludes its use in many studies. Alternatively, ASL and other more absolutely quantifiable fMRI techniques are under development and are likely to be applicable to such research designs in the near future (Detre & Wang, 2002; see also this chapter's "Future Directions . . . " section).

Experimental Design Considerations

In order to get the most from an fMRI experiment, great consideration must be given to the ordering, duration, and timing of experimental conditions and stimuli. All of the same basic rules for psychology experiments also apply to brain imaging experiments. Conditions need to be properly counterbalanced or randomized to control for habituation, fatigue, or other order confounds. A suitable number of repetitions of each experimental condition is needed to produce reliable data. The exact number will depend not only on the inherent reliability of fMRI, but also on the reliability of the behavior under observation. In addition to more general rules for experimental design, fMRI poses some further constraints, which we now discuss.

Block Designs versus and Event-Related Designs

A brief burst of neural activity corresponding to presentation of a short discrete stimulus or event will produce a more gradual BOLD response lasting about 15 sec. Due to noisiness of the BOLD signal, multiple repetitions of each condition are required in order to achieve sufficient reliability and statistical power. Block designs and event-related designs achieve this through slightly different means.

In a block design, multiple stimulus repetitions from a given experimental condition are strung together in a condition block, which alternates with one or more other condition blocks or control blocks. The advantage of such an approach is that the BOLD signal from multiple repetitions of closely spaced stimuli scales additively with the number of repetitions (Boynton, Engel, Glover, & Heeger, 1996); the more repetitions, the bigger and more reliable the signal. Because successive trials within a condition block are all the same condition, there is no fMRI-imposed lower limit to the intertrial interval (ITI), meaning that more repetitions can be fitted within a block of a given duration than would be the case with stimuli of different conditions. Block designs thus remain the most statistically powerful designs for fMRI experiments, all other considerations being equal (Bandettini & Cox, 2000). When a researcher is adopting a block design, three decisions need to be made:

- How long should each block be?
- How many blocks of each condition are needed?
- Should a resting baseline be included?

Based on knowledge of the noise characteristics of fMRI BOLD contrast, the answer to the first question is in the range of 20–40 sec (Skudlarski, Constable, & Gore, 1999; Smith, Jenkinson, Beckmann, Miller, & Woolrich, 2007). With blocks shorter than 20 sec, the statistical power advantage of a block design starts to disappear, particularly if psychological/behavioral constraints require a reasonably long ITI. With blocks longer than 40 sec, the random, slow fluctuations in fMRI BOLD signal start to compromise the reliability of the mean activation measured over the duration of a block. Of course, the psychological phenomena under question will add their own constraints, so this ideal range of block durations should be seen as a guideline only.

Because each block of a block design typically includes multiple repetitions of the same stimulus condition, it is not necessary to include many blocks. Many block design experiments are successful with between two and four blocks per condition. Once again, more blocks may be required for behavioral reasons (i.e., to achieve a reliable behavioral effect).

Finally, we strongly recommend including a resting baseline condition. Such a condition usually consists of having subjects look at a fixation cross on an otherwise blank screen. The amount of time spent in this condition is best when it matches the amount of time subjects are engaged in other experimental conditions of interest. The importance of including a resting baseline has been highlighted in some recent research showing that contrasts between an experimental condition and a resting baseline can be more reliable than contrasts between two experimental conditions. The idea is that a well-controlled resting baseline will be less variable than responses to many experimental stimuli. For example, Johnstone and colleagues (2005) reported that BOLD contrast in the amygdala showed greater test–retest reliability when calculated between responses to viewed fear faces and a passive fixation baseline than between responses to fear faces and responses to neutral faces. Obviously such condition–baseline contrasts do not have the task specificity of condition–condition contrasts, so inclusion of at least two active conditions is usually a good idea. In this way the condition–baseline contrast can be used for maximum sensitivity and reliability, whereas the condition–condition contrast can be used to answer questions about specific stimulus types or conditions. Inclusion of a resting baseline also makes basic fMRI quality control easier, since it is easy to check in primary sensory cortices for basic stimulus–baseline activation. For example, in a paradigm that uses visual stimuli, lack of stimulus–baseline activation in visual cortex would alert the experimenter to basic signal problems with the scanner, as well as to participants who were not paying attention, had their eyes closed, or fell asleep (not an uncommon problem in fMRI experiments, particularly with sleep-deprived undergraduate participants).

Although block designs are more statistically efficient (offering approximately 50% better signal-to-noise ratio than event-related designs; Bandettini & Cox, 2000), event-related designs are more suitable and often necessary in many experimental situations. In an event-related design, presentations of trials from different experimental conditions are interspersed in a random order, rather than being blocked together by condition (Buckner, 1998). This type of design avoids potential problems of habituation to specific stimulus types that might occur in a block design. In the affective and social sciences, event-related designs also avoid the problem of cumulative effects of emotional or social stimuli on a participant's mood. Moreover, event-related designs are necessary when it is important that the participants not know in advance what type of stimulus will be presented. Finally, event-related designs allow subsequent analysis on a trial-by-trial basis, using behavioral measures such as judgment times, subjective reports, or physiological responses to correlate with measured BOLD responses.

The minimum number of events, or trials per condition, needed in an event-related design must above all else be determined by considering how many such trials would be required to achieve a reliable behavioral effect in a nonimaging study. In addition, the low signal and high noise of fMRI mean that experimenters would do well to include as many trials as possible within a scan session. For example, Huettel and McCarthy (2001) have shown that even in a fairly simple cognitive task, 50 repetitions of a given condition only resulted in 50% of activated voxels being detected—though with a greater number of participants this number can fall to as low as 20 (Thirion et al., 2007), or perhaps even lower for paradigms or stimuli that are particularly potent, such as pain (e.g., Salomons, Johnstone, Backonja, & Davidson, 2004). The statistics underlying the analysis of slowly varying hemodynamic signals impose further constraints on the timing of trials in an event-related fMRI design. Because the BOLD response is relatively slow, if trials are spaced too close together, then the BOLD responses from successive trials will overlap. This is a strength of block designs, because overlapping BOLD responses add together, leading to a bigger aggregate response. In an event-related design, however, it can prevent the BOLD responses from different trials, and different trial types, from being separately quantifiable. The easiest and most obvious solution to this is to space successive trials at least as far apart as the expected duration of the BOLD response to a single stimulus (e.g., 12 sec apart for brief stimuli, but longer for stimuli lasting more than about 1 sec; Bandettini & Cox, 2000).

Some simple math shows that this will not always lead to an ideal experimental design. Take, for example, an experiment in which we want to examine the differential brain responses to 1-sec presentations of happy, fearful, or neutral facial expressions, each of which shows eyes directed straight ahead or averted. Thus the experiment consists of six conditions. Let's say that from previous behavioral pilot testing, we know that we need 30 repetitions of each condition to achieve suitable statistical power to detect an expression × eye gaze interaction in a 3 (expression) × 2 (eye gaze) within-subjects analysis of variance. Allowing 12 sec per trial, this would amount to $12 \times 6 \times 30$ sec, or 36 min for the experiment. Although this experiment length might be reasonable for some participant samples, it may be too long for adolescent or older participants, for participants with social anxiety, or for other specific participant groups. In order to get the most "bang for the buck," many researchers will also want to run two or more tasks in the one scanning session. Thus finding a way to reduce the time for a single task is invaluable.

The accepted way to do this for event-related designs is to use variable-length ITIs (i.e., "jitter"). By doing so, we can use the fact that overlapping BOLD responses add together in an approximately linear fashion, and so can be linearly separated if we use variable ITIs with known timing. Although the math underlying this technique is beyond the scope of this chapter (Birn, Cox, & Bandettini, 2002; Dale, 1999; Liu, Frank, Wong, & Buxton, 2001; Smith et al., 2007), the upshot is that trials can be spaced apart by an average ITI much shorter than would otherwise be necessary. In fact, to detect the difference in activation between two conditions, the shorter the mean ITI the better, down to a limit imposed by nonlinear saturation effects when successive trials are very close to one another. Mean ITIs of as low as 2–3 sec can lead to maximum statistical power with some designs (Friston, Zarahn, Josephs, Henson, & Dale, 1999); however, it is important to note than such short ITIs allow for the measurement of the difference in activation between conditions, but limit the ability to detect brain activation common to all conditions. To detect both differential and common activation, a somewhat longer ITI is preferable. Using our example of the face expressions experiment, we could use ITIs randomly varying between 2 and 10 sec, with an average ITI of 6 sec, which would result in an experiment length of $6 \times 6 \times 30$ sec, or 18 min—less than half the duration required for a slow event-related design—while retaining similar statistical power.

Three things are worth noting with respect to experimental design and timing. The first is that even if overall experimental time is not a major consideration, using variable ITIs makes it possible to increase statistical power. In our example, if time were not an issue, we could use variable ITIs to double the number of trials per condition (relative to a well-spaced design) without lengthening the experimental duration, and thus increase the reliability of our data. More sophisticated methods for choosing optimal experimental timing can yield even greater statistical power (Birn et al., 2002; Buracas & Boynton, 2002; Murphy, Bodurka, & Bandettini, 2007; Murphy & Garavan, 2005; Hagberg, Zito, Patria, & Sanes, 2001; Wager & Nichols, 2003). The second point is one that we repeatedly return to: The timing of an event-related design must make sense in a behavioral context. If it doesn't make sense to space trials closely or use variable ITIs in a behavioral experiment, then it almost certainly doesn't in an fMRI experiment either. The final point is that the ordering and timing of trials are critical if the results are to be statistically analyzable. Table 14.1 presents a summary of factors to consider in designing different types of fMRI experiments.

TABLE 14.1. Considerations for Different Types of fMRI Designs

Design type	Comments
Block designs	Have the strongest statistical power, compared to other types.
	Length of each block: 20–40 sec. Number of blocks per condition: Minimum 2–4 blocks. Resting baseline condition is highly recommended.
	Collection of behavioral and other measures is possible for correlation/regression analysis across participants.
Event-related designs	Number of events per condition depends on behavioral effect, but typically minimum of 20.
	Minimum ITI for evenly spaced events: 12 sec. Minimum ITI for jittered events: As low as 2–3 sec.
	Using jittered ITIs and randomized event order can increase statistical power, improve ecological validity, and reduce habituation/anticipation.
	Collection of behavioral and other measures is possible for correlation/regression analysis within and across participants.
Mixed designs	Useful when separating sustained from transient brain activity.
	Each event is presented using jittered ITIs within blocks; thus considerations for both block and event-related designs should be taken into account.
	Collection of behavioral and other measures is possible for correlation/regression analysis within and across participants.

Mixed Block and Event-Related Designs

More recently, researchers have recognized the need to take into account two distinct types of neural processes that occur in the brain during fMRI tasks. One type of brain activity is sustained throughout the trials of a task, regardless of individual trials; the other type of brain activity is specifically evoked by each trial of a task. Imagine that someone is taking a test such as the Graduate Record Examination. Once the clock starts ticking and the person begins reading the questions, certain neural circuits may enter a mode or a state that is optimized for written exams. However, in addition to this, other neural regions are reacting to each individual question on the test sheet. Naturally, brain regions turned on for the task itself rather than for each individual trial will show prolonged, sustained activations, while brain regions reacting to individual trials will exhibit short, transient activations. Reflecting the difference in the time course of brain activity, the former is often called "sustained activity," while the latter is dubbed "transient activity" (Visscher et al., 2003).

Since a simple block design or event-related design cannot separate these two types of brain activity, researchers have developed ways to combine block and event-related designs in fMRI. These "mixed designs" have been used for the purpose of dissociating sustained and transient trial-related activity in the brain (Donaldson, 2004; Donaldson, Petersen, Ollinger, & Buckner, 2001; Dosenbach et al., 2006; Visscher et al., 2003). In order to separate these two types of processes in fMRI data, trials are presented within task blocks interspersed with control blocks just as in a block design; within the task blocks, however, the onset of each trial is jittered, just as it would be in an event-related design. Having control blocks allows estimation of sustained brain activity separately from transient effects, and jittered trials enable dissociation of transient brain activity from sustained effects. Importantly, the interaction of sustained and transient manipulations can also be examined by measuring the difference in event-related responses between different blocks of sustained activity.

Mixed block and event-related designs are likely to be particularly suitable to social and affective neuroscience studies, in which the sustained social or emotional context has a direct impact on more transient socioaffective behaviors or responses. For example, Smith, Stephan, Rugg, and Dolan (2006) used a mixed design to examine the sustained effect of task requirements on retrieval of emotional information. Retrieval trials were presented as variable-ITI events embedded within blocks of one of two tasks—one requiring emotional information in order to make an accurate response, and one for which the emotional information was irrelevant. Smith and colleagues were able to demonstrate that connectivity among the hippocampus, amygdala, and orbitofrontal cortex during retrieval of emotional cues depend on whether the emotional cues were relevant or irrelevant to the task demands.

In another example, Bishop, Jenkins, and Lawrence (2007) used a mixed block and event-related design to examine how perceptual load (high vs. low, manipulated in blocks) would modulate activation of the amygdala to anxiety-relevant information (manipulated in an event-related manner with fearful vs. neutral facial expressions). They found that trait anxiety interacted with perceptual load in the engagement of prefrontal circuits thought to regulate amygdala output.

Studies of social interaction may also benefit from such mixed designs, enabling researchers to model sustained activation corresponding to attention to certain types of social stimuli (e.g., facial expressions of emotion, emotional speech) separately from transient activation corresponding to processing specific stimulus features (e.g., presence or absence of a given facial or vocal feature).

Combining fMRI with Other Online Measures: Behavior and Physiology

fMRI reveals activation at a spatial and temporal scale too coarse to enable us to say much about the fundamental neural processes involved. fMRI is also fundamentally correlational, telling us which brain regions coactivate with a particular behavior or response, but not which brain regions were responsible for producing the response. But fMRI data do not exist in isolation, and when combined with other complementary techniques can lead to valuable insights into the social–affective brain.

Take, for example, the question of the neural mechanisms that underlie social interaction problems in autism. Individuals with autism have a spectrum of symptoms, including severe disruption of social contact and interaction (Kanner, 1943). It has been observed that individuals with autism perform poorly on tasks involving the perception of emotional facial expressions (Celani, Battacchi, & Arcidiacono, 1999). Early brain imaging studies comparing individuals with autism to controls in facial expression tasks found a lack of activation in the fusiform gyrus, a brain region thought to be important for processing faces (Pierce, Muller, Ambrose, Allen, & Courchesne, 2001). The obvious conclusion was that autism involves loss of function of this brain region, with consequent poor performance in facial expression tasks, which would be expected to have a negative impact on social interaction skills more generally.

In a follow-up to these studies, however, Dalton and colleagues (2005) questioned whether the lack of fusiform activation was the cause of performance deficits, or whether it was itself caused by dysfunction in some other brain region, perhaps reflecting an attentional or affective deficit. To test this hypothesis, Dalton and colleagues measured the pattern of eye gaze fixations while individuals viewed pictures of different emotional facial expressions. In individuals with autism, not only fusiform gyrus but also amygdala activation was found to correlate with the amount of time individuals fixated on the eye region of the faces— one of the principal regions that conveys emotional information in the face (see Plate 14.1). The implication is that faces of strangers, which are particularly aversive stimuli to individuals with autism, provoke strong amygdala activation; this may underlie the tendency of those with autism to avoid focusing on the eye region, and thus may explain the prior autism findings of hypoactivation in the fusiform gyrus.

Individual Differences in Social and Affective Style, Personality, and Temperament

Many fMRI studies have two or more experimental conditions, and look for main effects of these conditions. This is especially true in the field of traditional visual and cognitive neuroscience, where individual differences are usually negligible, or considered as a confounding factor. However, in social and personality psychology studies, individual differences are often the main focus. For example, researchers conducting such a study may use a scale that measures empathy to collect a range of empathy scores across all subjects. These empathy scores can then be used to categorize subjects into subgroups (e.g., low empathizers and high empathizers), or entered as a covariate in a general linear model analysis. The same approach can be applied to fMRI data. Social neuroscientists interested in the neural correlates of empathy can collect empathy scores just as they would do in a behavioral experiment, and analyze them in conjunction with fMRI data collected during a task that evokes empathy. As with behavioral experiments, brain activity can be contrasted between groups (low vs. high empathizers), or empathy scores can be used as a regressor to identify brain regions within which activation correlates with the scores. Obviously, the word "empathy" in this example could be exchanged with any characteristic of social or affective style, personality, or temperament of interest. And since we would have a single value per subject, this analysis could be performed on fMRI data regardless of whether a block or an event-related design is used to collect them.

Another way of using fMRI to study individual differences is to parametrically model each response to a stimulus within each subject. To put it another way, when analyzing fMRI data, we could create a general linear model with subjective ratings for each and every stimulus entered as a regressor, convolved with an ideal hemodynamic response function. This would allow us to identify brain regions that show activation covarying with the magnitude of the subjective rating we have used. For example, let's assume that we have presented pictures of human faces during an fMRI experiment and collected attractiveness ratings for each face from all of the subjects. We could analyze the fMRI data by creating a general linear model as we would in a conventional subtraction analysis, but in this case we would also enter the (zero-meaned) attractiveness ratings as a regressor. As a result, we would have a statistical map for each individual showing brain regions in which activation linearly tracks the magnitude of attractiveness ratings for each subject. We could then use a further (second-level) analysis to identify brain regions that show such attractiveness activation across subjects. Here lies the major difference between this type of analysis and the former one: The former regression is performed during the second level (i.e., "group"-level) analysis only.

Functional and Effective Connectivity

Complex social behaviors involve the coordinated activity of multiple brain regions, so testing for fMRI activation in single brain regions is likely to be of limited use in social–affective neuroscience. Instead, we may be interested in investigating distributed networks of neural circuitry and determining how it is engaged or disengaged in different type of tasks. For example, we may want to know whether the activation we see in the amygdala during emotional face perception is functionally coupled to other regions of the brain, such as the orbitofrontal cortex, which is involved in learning and/or storage of hedonic information (Ghashghaei, Hilgetag, & Barbas, 2007; Iidaka et al., 2001; LoPresti et al., 2008).

Two different approaches to studying brain connectivity with fMRI are functional connectivity analysis and effective connectivity analysis. "Functional connectivity" is the temporal correlation between spatially remote neurophysiological events, whereas "effective connectivity" is defined as the influence one neuronal system exerts over another (Friston, 1994). By definition, output from functional connectivity analysis is purely correlational; even if two different brain regions show similar activation profiles across time, it does not necessarily mean that they are connected and directly influencing each other. In contrast, effective connectivity analysis attempts to infer directional influences of one region on another, at least to a certain degree.

Concretely, one simple way of applying functional connectivity analysis to our emotional face expression example would involve extracting time course data from the amygdala and performing a voxelwise cross-correlation analysis across the whole brain. More sophisticated techniques involve testing models of connectivity between multiple brain regions, using structural equation modeling (SEM; McIntosh & Gonzalez-Lim, 1994), dynamic causal modeling (Friston, Harrison, & Penny, 2003), or other related analytic techniques. Researchers have successfully confirmed that functional connectivity maps generated from voxels that were active during sensory or motor tasks corresponded to actual statistical maps of the auditory (Biswal, Yetkin, Haughton, & Hyde, 1996), visual (Lowe, Mock, & Sorenson, 1998), and motor

(Cordes et al., 2001; Lowe et al., 1998; Xiong, Parsons, Gao, & Fox, 1999) cortices, validating this approach. As with standard tests of brain activation, functional connectivity analyses can proceed voxelwise for the whole brain, though if we have predictions or hypotheses concerning a set of specific brain regions, it would be desirable to reduce the search volume to these a priori regions of interest (ROIs). Using an ROI-based functional connectivity analysis, Kim and colleagues (2004) found that the amygdala and the rostral anterior cingulate cortex were positively coupled during the processing of surprised facial expressions when combined with relevant contextual information. Thus this analysis proved useful in a task where the authors hypothesized that the amygdala would require assistance from the prefrontal cortex to use contextual information to understand the meaning of a given facial expression.

Effective connectivity analysis involves more advanced methods, such as psychophysiological interaction (PPI; Friston et al., 1997) analysis and SEM (McIntosh & Gonzalez-Loma, 1994). PPI analysis shows significant changes in the contribution of one brain region to another, as a function of experimental (psychological) context (Friston et al., 1997). Like functional connectivity analysis, PPI analysis can be performed across the whole brain without a priori regions of interest; however, once again, it is desirable to have a strong hypothesis and use PPI as a confirmatory rather than an exploratory analysis. This issue becomes especially important in SEM techniques. SEM takes into account the covariance matrix among multiple a priori regions of interest, and estimates the overall validity of the model as well as the strength and direction of the paths between the brain regions. Without a valid hypothesis for a brain network, SEM can lead to identifying a strongly significant but anatomically implausible model.

Increasing numbers of social and affective neuroscience researchers are taking advantage of these functional and effective connectivity analyses. As long as the researchers are aware of their caveats, these analyses have the potential to complement conventional statistical analysis by providing a more in-depth characterization of the neural mechanisms underlying a given social or affective process.

Considering Model Habituation or Familiarity Effects

As briefly mentioned earlier in this chapter, some brain regions tend to show a lesser degree of activation after repeated exposure to the same or similar stimuli. One prime example is the amygdala in response to fearful facial expressions. Amygdala activation to fearful facial expressions has been observed to show rapid habituation, regardless of explicit knowledge of perceiving the faces (e.g., use of masked or nonmasked facial stimuli) or study design (block or event-related; Breiter et al., 1996; Hare et al., 2008; Whalen et al., 1998). Moreover, the degree of amygdala habituation to fearful facial expressions has been found to be correlated with trait anxiety levels (Hare et al., 2008). Thus the rate of habituation itself could be a particularly interesting aspect of fMRI data.

The question arises of how we can quantify this habituation effect. Recall that a typical fMRI experiment consists of multiple repetitions of each event or block type, often distributed over multiple scan runs. Depending on how we define a habituation effect, there are two ways to calculate this: (1) early trials versus late trials within each run, or (2) early runs versus late runs. The former method is useful when we predict that the degree of brain activity will decline as a function of repetition or time within each run, whereas the latter method is more suitable if we think that habituation will occur throughout the entire experiment. We can certainly take advantage of both methods as well. For example, Somerville, Kim, Johnstone, Alexander, and Whalen (2004) calculated habituation effects of the amygdala in response to happy and neutral facial expressions within runs (e.g., block 1 > block 2 > block 3) and across runs (run 1 > run 2). Another possibility is to explicitly include a habituation factor in the general linear model by modifying each condition regressor by some function of time (e.g., an exponential decay; Tabert et al., 2007).

A remaining question, however, pertains to the underlying mechanism of this apparent habituation effect in the brain. The declination of brain activity over time may be solely due to habituation, but an alternative explanation would involve inputs from other brain areas that modulate brain activity in this region. In this case, we could achieve more complete understanding of our data by using the functional and effective connectivity methods described earlier to analyze the temporal profiles of these brain activations.

Future Directions in Social and Affective Brain Imaging

MRI of the human brain is a fairly recent development, and its application to social and affective neuroscience is even more recent. As such, the constant stream of new MRI techniques and analysis strategies announced at conferences and in journals can be quite daunting to the social neuroscientist. In this section, we highlight a few developments that may find their way into the social neuroscience toolbox in the near future.

Perfusion Imaging

Perfusion imaging, or ASL imaging, is a technique by which blood flow in arteries (which supply the brain with blood) is imaged—as opposed to blood flow in veins (which drain blood), as is the case with traditional BOLD imaging. ASL involves magnetically "tagging" the blood flowing into the brain by subjecting it to a brief radiofrequency burst. As the tagged blood perfuses into the small arteries in particular neural regions, it gives rise to an altered MRI signature. One advantage of ASL is that arterial blood flow changes that are associated with brain activation are more local than changes to venous draining blood flow changes, which may reflect downstream effects of large areas of neural tissue. ASL thus promises to provide better spatial resolution than BOLD imaging (Detre & Wang, 2002). In addition, ASL MRI can (at least in principle) be absolutely quantified, and thus ASL changes from different brain regions, different individuals, and different experimental sessions should be directly comparable. Even though absolute quantification of ASL images is not yet practical in most experimental contexts, ASL does have better temporal stability and test–retest reliability than BOLD (Leontiev & Buxton, 2007; Wang et al., 2003), thus making it attractive for the imaging of longer-term brain activation changes or studies involving repeated imaging sessions. The disadvantage of ASL is that it is less sensitive than BOLD, showing smaller signal change for a given experimental manipulation.

Diffusion Tensor Imaging

Diffusion tensor imaging (DTI) exploits the fact that water molecules diffuse at different rates through different types of brain tissue. In particular, water diffusion along the myelinated axons in white matter tracts (bundles of nerve fibers) is greater than across the tracts. DTI can thus be used to map the white matter tracts of the brain—the paths of nerve fibers that connect different neural regions (Le Bihan, 2003). DTI is a structural rather than a functional technique. In social and affective neuroscience, DTI is likely to be useful in interpreting data from functional and effective connectivity analyses—for example, by posing constraints on which neural regions are interconnected. Without DTI, knowledge of the neural connections between different brain regions must be based on studies with animals and on histological studies on postmortem human brains, neither of which is ideal for the study of healthy human brains. It may also be possible to use DTI to examine long-term changes to the neural connectivity between different brain regions associated with specific social–affective disorders (e.g., autism; Alexander et al., 2007; Barnea-Goraly et al., 2004), or in the study of the development of the human social brain.

Magnetic Resonance Spectroscopy

Most functional brain imaging studies address changes to the activity of different brain regions resulting from some experimental manipulation. Magnetic resonance spectroscopy (MRS) is a technique that can be used to measure concentrations of specific metabolites within the brain, including N-acetyl aspartate, lactate, creatine, and choline. MRS works by identifying magnetic resonance peaks at frequencies that correspond to known molecular resonances. Because the signal-to-noise ratio of MRI is low, MRS can currently only be applied to measure molecular concentrations of a small number of molecules in an a priori selected region of the brain. For the sensitive imaging of the concentrations of a different range of molecules across the whole brain, PET is a more suitable technology. Nonetheless, MRS may find uses in studies where individual differences in the concentration of a specific neurotransmitter in a given neural region are thought to underlie some affective behavior or disorder (see Pitman, Shin, & Rauch, 2001; Steingard et al., 2000; van Elst et al., 2001).

Summing Up: How Can fMRI Contribute to Social Neuroscience?

As we have seen in this chapter, fMRI can be applied in numerous ways to study the neural basis of human behavior. Standard BOLD imaging can measure increases in brain activation resulting from an experimental manipulation or corresponding to a specific behavior to within a few millimeters. Connectivity analyses can inform us about how different parts of the brain interact in social perception, expression and behavior. Many of the weaknesses of fMRI, such as its relative lack of temporal resolution, can be overcome with clever experimental design or through combination with other techniques (such as EEG).

As with all relatively new scientific approaches, a great deal of caution is required in designing, performing, and analyzing fMRI experiments. In particular, researchers need to be wary of using fMRI for fMRI's sake—that is, performing fMRI experiments merely because the scanner and funding to do so are available. Much of the research reported in the neuroimaging literature might be criticized on this point. An experiment that tells us which isolated brain regions are activated in a given task may give us no information at all about what processes are involved in that task, or how they are instantiated in the brain.

The problem of "inverse inference," or inferring process from brain activation, is also a potential pitfall. For inverse inference to be valid, we need to know enough about the detailed functioning of a given neural region to start with, yet this is rarely the case. For example, just because a particular brain region such as the anterior cingulate is involved in processing pain, this does not imply that activation of the same region during some other task must involve pain processing. Far more likely is that the anterior cingulate serves some other, more fundamental subprocess of pain processing that might equally be involved in processing any number of other types of stimuli.

The limitations of fMRI are all the more important to keep in mind for two reasons. One is the cost of fMRI studies. Researchers (and grant reviewers) need to ask whether the cost involved in brain imaging studies is justified by the added scientific value. Is an fMRI replication of a well-known social psychology experiment justified if the only conclusion that can be drawn is that "process X resides in the brain" (surely only an ardent dualist would need brain imaging proof of that), or that "process X activates regions A, B, and C of the brain" (telling us little or nothing about what regions A, B, and C do, except the trivial answer "process X")?

The second consideration is the weight that brain imaging findings seem to carry with the general public, and also parts of the research community. A recent study (McCabe & Castel, 2008) showed that experimental findings, when accompanied by brain imaging pictures, were given more credence than the same study without the fancy graphics. A related study (Weisberg, Keil, Goodstein, Rawson, & Gray, 2008) showed that non-neuroscience experts were more likely to accept a flawed explanation of human behavior when it was dressed up in pseudoscientific neuroscientific jargon than when the identical theory was presented in non-neuroscientific terms. Not only researchers, but also grant reviewers and journal editors and reviewers, need to keep this very much in mind, and ask themselves this question: "What does brain imaging really add to the study in question?"

Despite these limitations, there is much to be optimistic about. fMRI, when combined with well-thought-out, well-controlled, and theoretically motivated experimental designs and appropriate complementary measures, offers researchers an unprecedented tool for understanding the brain and all the behaviors it supports. The emerging fields of social and affective neuroscience promise to bring about a profound change in our understanding of our social and emotional lives.

References

Alexander, A. L., Lee, J. E., Lazar, M., Boudos, R., DuBray, M. B., Oakes, T. R., et al. (2007). Diffusion tensor imaging of the corpus callosum in autism. *NeuroImage, 34*(1), 61–73.

Bandettini, P. A., & Cox, R. W. (2000). Event-related fMRI contrast when using constant interstimulus interval: Theory and experiment. *Magnetic Resonance in Medicine, 43*(4), 540–548.

Barnea-Goraly, N., Kwon, H., Menon, V., Eliez, S., Lotspeich, L., & Reiss, A. L. (2004). White matter structure in autism: Preliminary evidence from diffusion tensor imaging. *Biological Psychiatry, 55*(3), 323–326.

Batty, M., & Taylor, M. J. (2003). Early processing of the six basic facial emotional expressions. *Brain Research: Cognitive Brain Research, 17*(3), 613–620.

Belin, P., Zatorre, R. J., & Ahad, P. (2002). Human temporal-lobe response to vocal sounds. *Brain Research: Cognitive Brain Research, 13*(1), 17–26.

Belin, P., Zatorre, R. J., Lafaille, P., Ahad, P., & Pike, B. (2000). Voice-selective areas in human auditory cortex. *Nature, 403*, 309–312.

Birn, R. M., Cox, R. W., & Bandettini, P. A. (2002). Detection versus estimation in event-related fMRI: Choosing the optimal stimulus timing. *NeuroImage, 15*(1), 252–264.

Bishop, S. J., Jenkins, R., & Lawrence, A. D. (2007). Neural processing of fearful faces: effects of anxiety are gated by perceptual capacity limitations. *Cerebral Cortex, 17*(7), 1595–1603.

Biswal, B. B., Yetkin, F. Z., Haughton, V. M., & Hyde, J. S. (1996). Functional connectivity in the auditory cortex studied with fMRI. *NeuroImage, 3*(Suppl.), 305.

Boynton, G. M., Engel, S. A., Glover, G. H., & Heeger, D. J. (1996). Linear systems analysis of functional magnetic resonance imaging in human V1. *Journal of Neuroscience, 16*(13), 4207–4221.

Breiter, H. C., Etcoff, N. L., Whalen, P. J., Kennedy, W. A., Rauch, S. L., Buckner, R. L., et al. (1996). Response and habituation of the human amygdala during visual processing of facial expression. *Neuron, 17*(5), 875–887.

Buckner, R. L. (1998). Event-related fMRI and the hemodynamic response. *Human Brain Mapping, 6*(5–6), 373–377.

Buckner, R. L., & Koutstaal, W. (1998). Functional neuroimaging studies of encoding, priming, and explicit memory retrieval. *Proceedings of the National Academy of Sciences USA, 95*(3), 891–898.

Buracas, G. T., & Boynton, G. M. (2002). Efficient design of event-related fMRI experiments using M-sequences. *NeuroImage, 16*(3, Pt. 1), 801–813.

Celani, G., Battacchi, M. W., & Arcidiacono, L. (1999). The understanding of the emotional meaning of facial expressions in people with autism. *Journal of Autism and Developmental Disorders, 29*(1), 57–66.

Cohen, J. D., Perlstein, W. M., Braver, T. S., Nystrom, L. E., Noll, D. C., Jonides, J., et al. (1997). Temporal dynamics of brain activation during a working memory task. *Nature, 386*, 604–608.

Cordes, D., Haughton, V. M., Arfanakis, K., Carew, J. D., Turski, P. A., Moritz,

C. H., et al. (2001). Frequencies contributing to functional connectivity in the cerebral cortex in "resting-state" data. *American Journal of Neuroradiology, 22*(7), 1326–1333.

Dale, A. M. (1999). Optimal experimental design for event-related fMRI. *Human Brain Mapping, 8*(2–3), 109–114.

Dalton, K. M., Nacewicz, B. M., Johnstone, T., Schaefer, H. S., Gernsbacher, M. A., Goldsmith, H. H., et al. (2005). Gaze fixation and the neural circuitry of face processing in autism. *Nature Neuroscience, 8*(4), 519–526.

D'Esposito, M., Detre, J. A., Alsop, D. C., Shin, R. K., Atlas, S., & Grossman, M. (1995). The neural basis of the central executive system of working memory. *Nature, 378*, 279–281.

Detre, J. A., & Wang, J. (2002). Technical aspects and utility of fMRI using BOLD and ASL. *Clinical Neurophysiology, 113*(5), 621–634.

Donaldson, D. I. (2004). Parsing brain activity with fMRI and mixed designs: What kind of a state is neuroimaging in? *Trends in Neurosciences, 27*(8), 442–444.

Donaldson, D. I., Petersen, S. E., Ollinger, J. M., & Buckner, R. L. (2001). Dissociating state and item components of recognition memory using fMRI. *NeuroImage, 13*(1), 129–142.

Dosenbach, N. U. F., Visscher, K. M., Palmer, E. D., Miezin, F. M., Wenger, K. K., Kang, H. C., et al. (2006). A core system for the implementation of task sets. *Neuron, 50*(5), 799–812.

Epstein, R., & Kanwisher, N. (1998). A cortical representation of the local visual environment. *Nature, 392*, 598–601.

Feredoes, E., & Postle, B. R. (2007). Localization of load sensitivity of working memory storage: Quantitatively and qualitatively discrepant results yielded by single-subject and group-averaged approaches to fMRI group analysis. *NeuroImage, 35*(2), 881–903.

Friston, K. J. (1994). Functional and effective connectivity in neuroimaging: A synthesis. *Human Brain Mapping, 2*, 56–78.

Friston, K. J., Buechel, C., Fink, G. R., Morris, J., Rolls, E., & Dolan, R. J. (1997). Psychophysiological and modulatory interactions in neuroimaging. *NeuroImage, 6*(3), 218–229.

Friston, K. J., Harrison, L., & Penny, W. (2003). Dynamic causal modelling. *NeuroImage, 19*(4), 1273–1302.

Friston, K. J., Zarahn, E., Josephs, O., Henson, R. N., & Dale, A. M. (1999). Stochastic designs in event-related fMRI. *NeuroImage, 10*(5), 607–619.

Ghashghaei, H. T., Hilgetag, C. C., & Barbas, H. (2007). Sequence of information processing for emotions based on the anatomic dialogue between prefrontal cortex and amygdala. *NeuroImage, 34*(3), 905–923.

Goense, J. B., & Logothetis, N. K. (2008). Neurophysiology of the BOLD fMRI signal in awake monkeys. *Current Biology, 18*, 631–640.

Hagberg, G. E., Zito, G., Patria, F., & Sanes, J. N. (2001). Improved detection of event-related functional MRI signals using probability functions. *NeuroImage, 14*(5), 1193–1205.

Hare, T. A., Tottenham, N., Galvan, A., Voss, H. U., Glover, G. H., & Casey, B. J. (2008). Biological substrates of emotional reactivity and regulation in adolescence during an emotional go/no-go task. *Biology Psychiatry, 63,* 927–934.

Huettel, S. A., McCarthy, G. (2001). The effects of single-trial averaging upon the spatial extent of fMRI activation. *NeuroReport, 12,* 2411–2416.

Hyder, F., Rothman, D. L., & Shulman, R. G. (2002). Total neuroenergetics support localized brain activity: Implications for the interpretation of fMRI. *Proceedings of the National Academy of Sciences USA, 99,* 10771–10776.

Iidaka, T., Omori, M., Murata, T., Kosaka, H., Yonekura, Y., Okada, T., et al. (2001). Neural interaction of the amygdala with the prefrontal and temporal cortices in the processing of facial expressions as revealed by fMRI. *Journal of Cognitive Neuroscience, 13*(8), 1035–1047.

Johnstone, T., Somerville, L. H., Alexander, A. L., Oakes, T. R., Davidson, R. J., Kalin, N. H., et al. (2005). Stability of amygdala BOLD response to fearful faces over multiple scan sessions. *NeuroImage, 25*(4), 1112–1123.

Kanner, L. (1943). Autistic disturbances of affective contact. *Nervous Child, 2,* 217–250.

Kim, H., Somerville, L. H., Johnstone, T., Polis, S., Alexander, A. L., Shin, L. M., et al. (2004). Contextual modulation of amygdala responsivity to surprised faces. *Journal of Cognitive Neuroscience, 16,* 1730–1745.

Le Bihan, D. (2003). Looking into the functional architecture of the brain with diffusion MRI. *Nature Reviews Neuroscience, 4*(6), 469–480.

Leontiev, O., & Buxton, R. B. (2007). Reproducibility of BOLD, perfusion, and CMRO2 measurements with calibrated-BOLD fMRI. *NeuroImage, 35*(1), 175–184.

Liu, T. T., Frank, L. R., Wong, E. C., & Buxton, R. B. (2001). Detection power, estimation efficiency, and predictability in event-related fMRI. *NeuroImage, 13*(4), 759–773.

Logothetis, N. K., Pauls, J., Augath, M., Trinath, T., & Oeltermann, A. (2001). Neurophysiological investigation of the basis of the fMRI signal. *Nature, 412,* 150–157.

Logothetis, N. K., & Wandell, B. A. (2004). Interpreting the BOLD Signal. *Annual Review of Physiology, 66*(1), 735–769.

LoPresti, M. L., Schon, K., Tricarico, M. D., Swisher, J. D., Celone, K. A., & Stern, C. E. (2008). Working memory for social cues recruits orbitofrontal cortex and amygdala: A functional magnetic resonance imaging study of delayed matching to sample for emotional expressions. *Journal of Neuroscience, 28*(14), 3718–3728.

Lowe, M. J., Mock, B. J., & Sorenson, J. A. (1998). Functional connectivity in single and multislice echoplanar imaging using resting-state fluctuations. *NeuroImage, 7*(2), 119–132.

McCabe, D. P., & Castel, A. D. (2008). Seeing is believing: The effect of brain images on judgments of scientific reasoning. *Cognition, 107*(1), 343–352.

McCarthy, G., Blamire, A. M., Puce, A., Nobre, A. C., Bloch, G., Hyder, F., et al. (1994). Functional magnetic resonance imaging of human prefrontal cortex activation during a spatial working memory task. *Proceedings of the National Academy of Sciences USA, 91*(18), 8690–8694.

McIntosh, A. R., & Gonzalez-Lim, F. (1994). Structural equation modeling and its application to network analysis in functional brain imaging. *Human Brain Mapping, 2*, 2–22.

Moonen, C. T. W., Bandettini, P. A., & Aguirre, G. K. (1999). *Functional MRI.* New York: Springer.

Murphy, K., Bodurka, J., & Bandettini, P. A. (2007). How long to scan?: The relationship between fMRI temporal signal to noise and necessary scan duration. *NeuroImage, 34*(2), 565–574.

Murphy, K., & Garavan, H. (2005). Deriving the optimal number of events for an event-related fMRI study based on the spatial extent of activation. *NeuroImage, 27*(4), 771–777.

O'Craven, K. M., & Kanwisher, N. (2000). Mental imagery of faces and places activates corresponding stimulus-specific brain regions. *Journal of Cognitive Neuroscience, 12*(6), 1013–1023.

Pierce, K., Muller, R. A., Ambrose, J., Allen, G., & Courchesne, E. (2001). Face processing occurs outside the fusiform "face area" in autism: Evidence from functional MRI. *Brain, 124*(Pt. 10), 2059–2073.

Pitman, R. K., Shin, L. M., & Rauch, S. L. (2001). Investigating the pathogenesis of posttraumatic stress disorder with neuroimaging. *Journal of Clinical Psychiatry, 62*(Suppl. 17), 47–54.

Salomons, T. V., Johnstone, T., Backonja, M. M., & Davidson, R. J. (2004). Perceived controllability modulates the neural response to pain. *Journal of Neuroscience, 24,* 7199–7203.

Skudlarski, P., Constable, R. T., & Gore, J. C. (1999). ROC analysis of statistical methods used in functional MRI: Individual subjects. *NeuroImage, 9*(3), 311–329.

Smith, A. P., Stephan, K. E., Rugg, M. D., & Dolan, R. J. (2006). Task and content modulate amygdala–hippocampal connectivity in emotional retrieval. *Neuron, 49*(4), 631–638.

Smith, S., Jenkinson, M., Beckmann, C., Miller, K., & Woolrich, M. (2007). Meaningful design and contrast estimability in fMRI. *NeuroImage, 34*(1), 127–136.

Somerville, L. H., Kim, H., Johnstone, T., Alexander, A. L., & Whalen, P. J. (2004). Human amygdala responses during presentation of happy and neutral faces: Correlations with state anxiety. *Biology Psychiatry, 55*(9), 897–903.

Stark, C. E. L., & Squire, L. R. (2001). When zero is not zero: The problem of ambiguous baseline conditions in fMRI. *Proceedings of the National Academy of Sciences USA, 98,* 12760–12766.

Steingard, R. J., Yurgelun-Todd, D. A., Hennen, J., Moore, J. E. C., Moore, C. M., Vakili, K., et al. (2000). Increased orbitofrontal cortex levels of choline in depressed adolescents as detected by *in vivo* proton magnetic resonance spectroscopy. *Biological Psychiatry, 48*(11), 1053–1061.

Tabert, M. H., Steffener, J., Albers, M. W., Kern, D. W., Michael, M., Tang, H., et al. (2007). Validation and optimization of statistical approaches for modeling odorant-induced fMRI signal changes in olfactory-related brain areas. *NeuroImage, 34*(4), 1375–1390.

Thirion, B., Pinel, P., Mériaux, S., Roche, A., Dehaene, S., & Poline, J.-P. (2007). Analysis of a large fMRI cohort: Statistical and methodological issues for group analyses. *NeuroImage, 35*(1), 105–120.

van Elst, L. T., Thiel, T., Hesslinger, B., Lieb, K., Bohus, M., Hennig, J., et al. (2001). Subtle prefrontal neuropathology in a pilot magnetic resonance spectroscopy study in patients with borderline personality disorder. *Journal of Neuropsychiatry and Clinical Neuroscience, 13*(4), 511–514.

Vazquez, A. L., Cohen, E. R., Gulani, V., Hernandez-Garcia, L., Zheng, Y., Lee, G. R., et al. (2006). Vascular dynamics and BOLD fMRI: CBF level effects and analysis considerations. *NeuroImage, 32*(4), 1642–1655.

Visscher, K. M., Miezin, F. M., Kelly, J. E., Buckner, R. L., Donaldson, D. I., McAvoy, M. P., et al. (2003). Mixed blocked/event-related designs separate transient and sustained activity in fMRI. *NeuroImage, 19*(4), 1694–1708.

Wager, T. D., & Nichols, T. E. (2003). Optimization of experimental design in fMRI: A general framework using a genetic algorithm. *NeuroImage, 18*(2), 293–309.

Wang, J., Aguirre, G. K., Kimberg, D. Y., Roc, A. C., Li, L., & Detre, J. A. (2003). Arterial spin labeling perfusion fMRI with very low task frequency. *Magnetic Resonance in Medicine, 49*(5), 796–802.

Weisberg, D. S., Keil, F. C., Goodstein, J., Rawson, E., & Gray, J. R. (2008). The seductive allure of neuroscience explanations. *Journal of Cognitive Neuroscience, 20*(3), 470–477.

Whalen, P. J., Johnstone, T., Somerville, L. H., Nitschke, J. B., Polis, S., Alexander, A. L., et al. (2008). A functional magnetic resonance imaging predictor of treatment response to venlafaxine in generalized anxiety disorder. *Biological Psychiatry, 63*(9), 858–863.

Whalen, P. J., Rauch, S. L., Etcoff, N. L., McInerney, S. C., Lee, M. B., & Jenike, M. A. (1998). Masked presentations of emotional facial expressions modulate amygdala activity without explicit knowledge. *Journal of Neuroscience, 18*(1), 411–418.

Xiong, J., Parsons, L. M., Gao, J. H., & Fox, P. T. (1999). Interregional connectivity to primary motor cortex revealed using MRI resting state images. *Human Brain Mapping, 8*(2–3), 151–156.

Index

Page numbers followed by *f* indicate figure, *t* indicate table